Praise for *Feed Your Pet Right*

"*Feed Your Pet Right* is . . . frank and fascinating, with abundant information that can be readily absorbed. It will make you an expert not only on the quality and contents of the canned foods and kibbles, but also on the doings of the manufacturers. You will realize how little you knew after you have read this splendid, highly scientific, star-quality book."

> —Elizabeth Marshall Thomas, author of
> *The Hidden Life of Dogs* and *The Social Lives of Dogs*

"One of the enduring topics of conversation among pet owners is what to feed our animals. Everybody has a strongly held opinion, but few have facts to back them. *Feed Your Pet Right* has those facts and gives them to you in a highly readable, fascinating, and entertaining way. You can find out what is really in commercial pet foods and how healthy they are, the truth about diets based on raw food, vegetarian only, and home-cooked foods and even look at the ethics of pet foods. This is a must read for every dog and cat owner."

> —Stanley Coren, author of *The Modern Dog,*
> *The Intelligence of Dogs,* and others

"This book is now the definitive work on what to feed pets. It is well researched and well written by two highly qualified, unbiased scientists who provide fascinating information putting many of the way-too-many pet food myths to rest. No longer will pet owners have to rely simply on what their breeder (or the person next door) says—instead they can just consult this book. I learned a lot from it and will use it as one of my bibles. Talk about food for thought! Two paws up!"

> —Nicholas H. Dodman, DVM and author of
> *The Well-Adjusted Dog* and *The Dog Who Loved Too Much*

"*Feed Your Pet Right* is mind-blowingly excellent!! It is brilliant in every way—comprehensive in scope and clearly impartial. The style of writing is accessible to any reader."

> —David Fraser, Emeritus Professor of Animal Science,
> University of Sydney

FEED
YOUR PET
RIGHT

The Authoritative Guide to
Feeding Your Dog and Cat

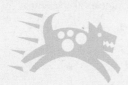

MARION NESTLE
and MALDEN C. NESHEIM

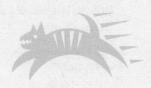

FREE PRESS
New York London Toronto Sydney

Free Press
A Division of Simon & Schuster, Inc.
1230 Avenue of the Americas
New York, NY 10020

First Free Press trade paperback edition May 2010

FREE PRESS and colophon are trademarks of Simon & Schuster, Inc.

For information about special discounts for bulk purchases, please contact Simon & Schuster Special Sales at 1-866-506-1949 or business@simonandschuster.com.

The Simon & Schuster Speakers Bureau can bring authors to your live event. For more information or to book an event contact the Simon & Schuster Speakers Bureau at 1-866-248-3049 or visit our website at www.simonspeakers.com.

Designed by Katy Riegel

Manufactured in the United States of America

10 9 8 7 6 5 4 3 2

Library of Congress Cataloging-in-Publication Data

Nestle, Marion.
    Feed your pet right : the authoritative guide to feeding your dog and cat / Marion Nestle and Malden C. Nesheim.
        p. cm.
    Includes bibliographical references and index. 1. Dogs—Food. 2. Cats—Food. 3. Dogs—Nutrition. 4. Cats—Nutrition. I. Nesheim, Malden C. II. Title.
SF427.4.N47 2010
636.7'084-dc22   2009031301

ISBN 978-1-4391-6642-0
ISBN 978-1-4391-6644-4 (ebook)

Contents

FEED
YOUR PET
RIGHT

1

Introduction

THIS BOOK IS about what dogs and cats eat—and should eat—to keep them at peak health for as long as they live. It is also about the food products available for feeding companion animals, the ingredients in those foods, the sources of those ingredients, the industry that makes the products, and what is and is not known about the best ways to feed these animals.* In this book, we provide dog and cat owners with the information they need to know about what their pets eat and why.

We are professors in the human nutrition departments at New York University (Marion Nestle) and Cornell University (Malden Nesheim). Both of us have had long careers in human nutrition and Malden Nesheim received much of his early training and experience in animal nutrition. But how we came to write a book about pet food and feeding is a story best told by Marion Nestle because *Feed Your Pet Right* evolved from *What to Eat,* a book she wrote in 2006 about food for people. *What to Eat* is not really a how-to book; it is a book about how to *think* about what to eat. Similarly, *Feed*

* This book discusses food for dogs and cats. It does not cover food for birds, fish, reptiles, or amphibians. Even though nearly 400 million of such creatures are kept as pets, their food accounts for less than 5 percent of the U.S. pet food market.

Your Pet Right is about how to decide for yourself what's best for your pet to eat and how to feel more confident about your choices.

MARION NESTLE EXPLAINS

For much of 2005 and 2006, I was spending every minute I could in supermarkets researching the topics I wrote about in *What to Eat*. That book, which started out as a guide to supermarkets, ended up as a reference work on the enormous range of issues—from basic nutrition to international politics—that confront anyone faced with food choices these days. As I wandered through supermarket aisles, I kept running across pet foods. In some stores, they occupied entire aisles, six shelves high. By the time I began paying attention to these products in a more serious way, I knew that food companies paid "slotting" fees (bribes, for all practical purposes) to many supermarkets for every inch of prime retail shelf space. It seemed obvious that pet foods must be a lively and profitable business for all concerned.

When I looked at the cans, pouches, and bags on those shelves, I was surprised by their labels. The Food and Drug Administration (FDA) has strict rules for what can and cannot go on the labels of foods for humans, but for historical reasons (which we explain later on) it regulates pet foods in an entirely different manner—as animal feed. The FDA requires the labels on feed for farm animals to list ingredients, but does not officially permit statements about benefits for special health conditions. Yet here were foods marketed for dogs and cats bearing claims that ingredients in the products could help reduce the risk of heart disease or diabetes, stimulate immune function, treat skin or joint disorders, or alleviate the infirmities of aging. The shelves were full of products advertised for dogs of different sizes and breeds, for puppies and kittens, for cats kept indoors, and for those fed vegetarian or all-meat diets.

But my initial look at the ingredient lists gave an entirely different impression: the products seemed much alike. Could it be possible that foods advertised for specific ages, breeds, lifestyles, and health conditions all contained virtually identical ingredients? If distinctions existed, they were not obvious at first glance. I also wondered about the health claims. Health claims on human foods are well known to confuse and mislead consumers but to strongly encourage sales. Indeed, manufac-turers of human foods deliberately add nutrients—vitamins, omega-3 fats, antioxidants—to products so companies can make health claims for those ingredients. Health claims usually have much more to do with marketing than health. I wondered if health claims on pet food labels had the same confusing effects on pet owners (or guardians, as some prefer).*

If for no other reason than to satisfy curiosity, I thought it would be a good idea to add a chapter to *What to Eat* about pet food choices. But by that time, the manuscript had expanded to more than six hundred pages and I was eager (desperate is more like it) to bring it to a close. Even though I suspected that pet owners were just as curious as I was, and just as interested in reliable information about what to feed their cats and dogs, I reluctantly abandoned the idea of including that chapter.

As soon as the book appeared, it was obvious that I had missed an opportunity. When giving talks about *What to Eat,* I began to hear about what I now think of as "the pet food gap." People asked, "Why can't you do the same for pet food? I don't have a clue what to feed my dog." "My cat will only eat this one brand and she hisses if I try anything else. How do I know if what I am feeding her is okay?" and "My veterinarian says one thing but books say another—and they say opposite things. Whose information should I trust?"

These questions were so similar to the ones that had started me work-ing on *What to Eat* that I was curious to pursue them further. I began by asking pet owners whether they felt they knew what to feed their cats or dogs. The answer: a resounding NO! Invariably, a deluge of questions followed, many of them highly specific. While some were easy to answer, some were not. The questions ended up guiding our research and this book deals with all of them. For example:

- Is commercial pet food any good? Can I trust it? (That's what this book is about.)
- Which is better—canned or dry dog food—or does it make any difference? (We deal with these questions in chapter 6.)

* We are well aware of concerns about the meaning of "owner" as applied to companion animals, and we struggled with how best to term the relationship. To us, ownership implies (or should imply) guardian-ship and stewardship. For simplicity, we use that term throughout this book.

- Why are pet food labels so hard to understand? What do they mean? (chapters 7 and 10)
- Are premium brands better? What does "all-natural" mean, and is it better? Should I give my pet organic foods? (chapter 12)
- Do I have to do anything special for my puppy or kitten? For my older pet? (chapter 13)
- Can I believe health claims on pet food labels? (chapter 14)
- How can I tell how much my pet should be eating? (chapter 15)
- Is it OK to give treats? What kind? What about tap water? (chapter 16)
- Should I give my pet vitamins or other nutritional supplements? (chapters 17 and 18)
- Is it OK to feed my pet a vegetarian diet? How about a vegan diet? What about grains? (chapter 19)
- Are raw-food diets OK? Are they really superior? (chapter 20)
- Is it okay to cook my own food for my pet? (chapter 21)
- Should I believe my veterinarian's advice about what foods to buy? (chapter 24)

From such questions, it was obvious that the matter of what to feed pets was just as important and just as confusing to owners as what to feed themselves and their families. Indeed, as I soon discovered, the question of what to feed pets can be far more important to people than what they feed themselves. If you have a pet, you are likely to adore your animal. You love pleasing your pet and food is an easy and satisfying way to express your love. You and other pet owners want to feed your animals properly, but the pet food marketplace is just as complicated, misleading, and confusing as the human food marketplace—and sometimes more so.

I thought it would be interesting and useful to answer such questions and to help clarify some of the choices involved in pet feeding and I convinced Malden Nesheim to join me in this project. The subsequent "we" represents both of us and reflects our joint perspective on the issues we cover in this book.

As we quickly learned, our particular perspective is unusual in this field. We approached this project out of genuine curiosity, with few preconceptions about what we might learn and without any specific goals in mind. Neither of us had any ties to the pet food industry, and we still do not. This book is the result of our attempt to bring as much objectivity as we could to examination of the pet food issues we discuss here.

WHO WE ARE

Neither of us lives with a pet at the moment. We travel too often and for too many days at a time to be able to give a dog or cat the attention and companionship it needs. But at various times in our lives, we owned, cared for, and sometimes bred dogs and cats, as well as our own or our children's hamsters, gerbils, guinea pigs, mice, parakeets, parrots, rabbits, rats, snakes, frogs, turtles, goldfish, aquarium fish, and on one occasion, a tarantula. At times in our family or professional life, one or both of us has raised or worked with mice, chickens, rabbits, pigs, cows, sheep, and horses. We like and get along well with animals, we love visiting our friends' and children's animals—together we boast of three grand-dogs and five grand-cats. We have enjoyed every minute of reading, writing, and thinking about these animals as we worked on this book. And now for more formal introductions:

Marion Nestle is a city girl. She was born in New York City, grew up in Los Angeles, but returned to Manhattan in 1988 and has been there ever since. She earned a doctorate in molecular biology and a master's in public health nutrition from the University of California at Berkeley, and has held jobs teaching and writing about human nutrition for more than thirty years at Brandeis University, the University of California School of Medicine in San Francisco, and, since 1988, at New York University. Her farm experience began in a childhood summer camp in Vermont where she took care of a dozen free-range Rhode Island Reds, but is otherwise limited to occasional farm visits. While working on this book, she was a member of the Pew Commission on Industrial Farm Animal Production, which released its final report in 2008. She is the author of three prize-winning books about human food issues: *Food Politics: How the Food Industry Influences Nutrition and Health* (2002, revised edition

2007), *Safe Food: The Politics of Food Safety* (2003, revised edition 2010), and *What to Eat* (2006). Her book on the pet food recalls of 2007, *Pet Food Politics: The Chihuahua in the Coal Mine,* was published in 2008.

Malden Nesheim started off in life as a farm boy. He was one of eight children growing up on an Illinois farm that kept cows, steers, sheep, pigs, horses, and chickens, and supported any number of working cats and dogs. He majored in agricultural science at the University of Illinois (Champaign-Urbana), and holds master's and doctoral degrees in animal nutrition. For many years, he was a professor of animal nutrition at Cornell University, followed by many more years as director of Cornell's Division of Nutritional Sciences, its vice president for budget and planning, and provost. He is a coauthor of *Nutrition of the Chicken* (1982), the definitive book on this subject, and *Poultry Production* (10th to 13th editions) as well as many articles in professional journals on various aspects of animal and human nutrition. He is a recipient of an award from the American Feed Manufacturers Association for research in animal nutrition, and is a past president of the American Institute of Nutrition. He is now professor emeritus, but continues to be active in the Division of Nutritional Sciences at Cornell.

As you can see from these biographies, both of us have long careers in academic research. We approached this project as we would any other such project: we or our assistants went to libraries, read books and journals, and consulted Internet websites. We subscribed to *Petfood Industry* and other trade journals. Beyond that, we tried to obtain as much firsthand experience as the pet food industry would allow. We visited stores selling pet foods, bought products, collected their labels, and donated the foods to our local SPCA shelters. When permitted, we went to meetings of pet food and ingredient suppliers, and of animal scientists giving presentations on their research. We talked to pet owners but also to the owners of pet food companies and stores, ingredient manufacturers, and animal scientists. We visited every manufacturing plant that would let us in and spoke with their owners and managers. We toured veterinary clinics and hospitals. We talked to veterinary students, representatives of veterinary colleges, and practicing veterinarians.

Much of the opinion we now hold on matters discussed in this book is based on these experiences. But, as we later explain, the industry that makes pet foods is unusually closed and secretive. We were refused many requests to visit and hardly any industry representatives agreed to talk to us on the record. We greatly appreciated the generosity of the companies that did open their doors to us and the many individuals who freely provided us with introductions, explanations, and information, and we acknowledge their contributions at the end of this book.

WHY PET FOODS COUNT

When we told friends and colleagues we were writing a book about foods for cats and dogs, we heard two kinds of reactions. Pet lovers told us: "Oh good. Get it done fast. We *need* this book." Others, however, gave us puzzled looks or expressed dismay that we would waste time on anything so unimportant to society as companion animals. As they put the matter: "With so many children in the world starving or without health care, it's appalling that people spend so much money on pets." One colleague sarcastically suggested that a better title for the book would be *Eat Your Pet* (we think she was joking, but we do discuss such issues in chapter 23).

Late in 2006, we did not have easy responses to such comments, but we had a hunch that there was more to the pet food story than seemed obvious. And then, in March 2007, Menu Foods, a manufacturer of "wet" (canned and pouched) pet foods based in Canada, announced that a few cats that had eaten its foods had become sick or died from kidney blockage. The company would be recalling 60 million cans and pouches of nearly one hundred different brands of pet foods. Suddenly, we no longer had to justify our interest in writing about pet foods. It was immediately obvious that pet foods were the proverbial canary (we prefer Chihuahua) in the coal mine. Pet foods displayed early warning signs of massive safety problems in the worldwide production and distribution of many other consumer products ranging from toothpaste to prescription drugs and, later, to Chinese infant formulas and American peanut butter.

The recall exposed previously hidden links between pet foods and the human food supply. Pet foods could no longer be considered as a tiny but profitable niche market. Instead, it was evident that pet foods are part of a global network for producing food for people and for farm animals, as well as for cats and dogs. We all share *one* interconnected food supply.

This means that anyone who cares about the safety and quality of food for people, pets, or other animals also needs to care about how pet foods are made, used, and monitored. Indeed, the implications of the recall are so profound that one of us (Nestle) ended up telling its story in a separate book, *Pet Food Politics: The Chihuahua in the Coal Mine* (University of California Press, 2008).

WHAT ARE PET FOODS?

Let's begin by visiting the pet food aisle of a good-sized supermarket. In the summer of 2008, for example, the Wegmans supermarket in Ithaca, New York, devoted both sides of an entire 120-foot aisle to pet foods and products. We estimated that this took up 13 percent of the store's center-aisle space, roughly the same proportion devoted to sodas. The shelves rose six feet above the floor, and each was packed with cans, pouches, and bags of foods, treats, and chews in sizes ranging from three-ounce cans of cat food to forty-pound bags of dog kibble. We counted out the number of four-foot sections, multiplied them by the number of shelves, and came up with 328 linear feet of shelf space devoted to cat foods, and 395 feet to dog foods—more than 700 linear feet of supermarket real estate devoted to these products.

As is true of most pet food aisles, dog food takes up more space than cat food. Although Americans own many more cats than dogs—94 million compared to 78 million—dogs eat more than cats, and owners tend to spend more money on food and treats for them.

At the time, Wegmans carried several leading brands produced by major pet food companies, along with its own favorably priced, private-label Bruiser dog food and Buju & Ziggie cat food brands. Choosing from any such array of products is a daunting task. Price is only one of many considerations. Manufacturers design pet foods for a large number of particular purposes, each aimed at a particular market segment.

The most important distinction is between complete-and-balanced foods and snacks or treats. Commercial pet foods share much in common with infant formulas. They provide complete nutrition in one convenient package. If you follow the feeding directions, the food takes care of your pet's requirements for calories and all essential nutrients. In contrast, snacks and treats have some nutritional value but are incomplete and need to be supplemented with foods that contain all of the nutrients required by a cat or dog.

Within the complete-and-balanced category, you can select from among foods that differ in form or price; are targeted to an animal's stage of life, breed, or health condition; meet your expectations for ingredient quality; are consistent with your personal values about diet, nutrition, or the environment; or do or do not contain supplements aimed at relieving disease symptoms. We talk about each of these market segments in subsequent chapters.

Complete-and-balanced pet foods are marketed as dry, semi-moist, or wet. Dry foods sell the best, which should be no surprise. They are relatively inexpensive and easy to store as they do not require refrigeration. Within each of these categories, companies offer products by brand. Within each brand, they offer variations in size, flavor, and other factors targeted to particular market segments. The size differences are obvious; the weights are listed on the packages. You can choose the one that is most convenient or least expensive. Flavors, however, are more complicated. A typical brand might come in beef, seafood, and poultry flavors, for example. Do the choices of form, flavor, and market segment make any difference to the health and happiness of a dog or cat—or do they matter most to its owner? That is what this book is about.

Along with our discussion of the various products, we give our candid opinions of the value of their ingredients and the issues raised by the way they are marketed. We also give you the information you need to form your own opinions about the products and their marketing, and how much these issues matter in deciding what and how much to feed your cat or dog. We invite you to join us on this journey, and hope that you find it as interesting, entertaining, and useful as we did.

The
ORIGINS of
COMMERCIAL
PET FOODS

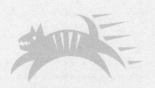

What Pets Ate

To UNDERSTAND WHAT pet foods are all about, it helps to know what dogs and cats are supposed to eat, what they used to be fed, and how modern science determines what they are fed now. We are fortunate to live at a time when we know as much as we do about the nutritional needs of dogs and cats. We have good information about these needs from four quite different sources: the evolutionary origins of dogs and cats, their anatomy and physiology, experiments conducted to define their nutrient requirements and, not least, the experience and observations of pet owners, pet breeders, and veterinarians.

We will have more to say about the anatomical, experimental, and experiential evidence in later chapters, but here is a quick summary. The digestive tract of dogs is typical of omnivores, meaning that dogs are able to extract nutritional value from any food animal or plant. Like humans, dogs have a digestive tract that is about six times the length of their bodies. Dogs will eat *anything*. We too are omnivores but tend to be fussier about which parts of animals or plants we eat.

In contrast, cats are carnivores. Their digestive tracts are only about four times their body length and adapted to extract nutrients efficiently from devoured animals.

Even so, cats are also able to digest carbohydrates (starches and sugars), fats, and proteins from plants. We address the question of whether cats can or should eat grains in the context of vegetarian diets in chapter 19.

Next, experimentation: research studies in the twentieth century revealed the specific nutrient requirements of dogs and cats. Oddly, those studies had two purposes, neither of which had anything to do with pets: to define human nutritional requirements, and to identify the most efficient feed for farm animals. Researchers accomplished both goals. But as a bonus they also produced the information needed to establish standards for the nutrient content of pet foods.

Human history provides further experiential evidence. Humans have thousands of years of experience with feeding dogs and cats. Think of the situation this way: We have been so successful in promoting the nutritional health of pet dogs and cats that they survive to the present day and in large numbers. Unlike many of their close relatives, they did not go extinct. And now, let's look at what evolution has to say about the nutrient needs of these animals.

EVOLUTION: DOGS AND THEIR DIETS

It makes no difference who studies dog evolution or by what method. Ancient fossils and modern genetics give the same result: dogs descended from wolves. Although wolves have inhabited earth for 40 million years or more, dogs are evolutionary newcomers. Fossils indicate that animals resembling modern dogs first appeared in East Asia a mere 12,000 to 14,000 years ago. Genetics may push the date back to 15,000 years ago, or perhaps a bit earlier, but let's play it safe and say the critical period was 12,000 years ago at about the same time that humans were beginning to establish agricultural settlements.

The fossil history and genetic evidence constitute scientific facts. Beyond these facts, scientists do not have a clue as to how dogs evolved from wolves or how or when they developed into hundreds of breeds readily distinguishable by sight and, to a growing extent, by genetic analysis. In the absence of facts, we have speculation. Some speculators propose that people adopted wild wolves, tamed them, and bred them for docility, loyalty, and other desirable domestic traits. Others suggest that wolves sought out human company—and the food that came with it—and happily tamed themselves. No matter. After 12,000 years of domestication, dogs may still resemble their wolf ancestors in some ways but in other ways they are quite different. In adapting to people, for example, some dogs came to prefer the company of humans to that of other dogs, a situation impossible to imagine for wolves. The domesticated dog is a different animal—genetically, physiologically, and psychologically—from a wolf in the wild, and its dietary needs and habits are also quite different.

Wolves, for example, are carnivores that eat every bit of their prey: flesh, bones, blood, intestines, other organs, and wastes. These parts of the animal, which we usually consider inedible offal, are excellent sources of vitamins and minerals as well as of proteins, fats, and calories. In the wild, the carnivore diet of wolves promotes growth and reproduction quite efficiently. But dogs, like humans, evolved as *omnivores;* they can eat and take advantage of a much broader range of foods—anything that comes their way.

During the 7,000-year period from 12,000 to 5,000 years ago, we can only guess at what dogs ate. One reasonable guess is that dogs gathered around the garbage dumps of early agricultural settlements and ate whatever they could hunt, scavenge, or beg from humans. Written records begin in Egypt about 5,000 years ago, and even the earliest provide evidence for human contact with dogs. Papyrus fragments, tomb paintings, building decorations, and statues show that the ancient Egyptians kept many kinds of dogs, some for hunting but also as house pets. These materials depict clearly recognizable breeds of dogs—salukis, other medium-sized dogs with straight ears, and basset hounds. They show dogs hunting, on leashes, and with given names. Although we do not know exactly what the ancient Egyptians fed their dogs, we do know that at least one palace employed a "messenger for dogs' food."

But we can speculate that for at least the last 5,000 years, dogs flourished on the highly nutritious parts of animals that humans found unpalatable as well as on food garbage that humans threw away. Once dogs became house pets, however, human disgust restricted their diets. Dogs no longer had access to the nutrients present in animal intestines, other organs, and bones. If dogs were to grow and reproduce, they had to obtain the nutrients they needed from other food sources. As we will see, they did.

EVOLUTION: CATS AND THEIR DIETS

The question of when cats and people began their close association turns out to be one of great interest to geneticists as well as to archeologists. Cat geneticists—yes, such people exist—have traced the origins of today's domestic cats to wild ancestral cats that lived 100,000 to 200,000 years ago. As for domestication, archeologists say that happened at least 9,500 years ago. At a grave site in Cyprus dating from that era, archeologists found a skeleton of a cat and a human buried just three feet apart. They were not surprised by this finding. By that time, humans lived in communities where they raised agricultural crops. With crops come mice, and archeologists have uncovered masses of mouse skeletons at ancient agricultural settlements. With mice come cats.

The best guess as to how cats were tamed in those early settlements seems quite plausible: humans stored grain, mice found grain, cats found mice, cats had kittens, and children adore kittens. This arrangement between cats and humans worked well for both. Cats took care of mice. Humans sheltered cats. As evidence, consider the number of domestic house cats now alive on earth—perhaps half a billion. In sharp contrast, the populations of most of the thirty-six surviving species of wild cats have declined to the point of near extinction.

As is the case with dogs, we know little about the extent of cat domestication until the ancient Egyptians depicted cats on papyrus, wall paintings, statues, and other art objects, and buried these objects in tombs that remained undiscovered for millennia. From this evidence, it seems clear that the Egyptians of 5,000 or 6,000 years ago viewed cats as religious objects. Images of cats appear on amulets, seated figures, heads, mummy cases, columns, scarabs, and jewelry from that era. Later artifacts depict cats in hunting scenes as well as living indoors, under chairs, on laps, wearing collars, and drinking milk and eating fish.

The precise role of cats in ancient Egyptian society is not easy to fathom, but it must have been an important one. The Egyptians buried mummified cats in their own separate tombs, and in staggering numbers.

The burials were discovered in the late nineteenth century when farmers came across a tomb containing the mummified remains of about 80,000 cats and kittens. They sold some of the mummified cats as souvenirs but used most of them—at least nineteen tons' worth—as fertilizer. A small collection of mummified skulls from that tomb are still preserved in the British Museum.

Following the Egyptian era, cats had plenty of time to become thoroughly domesticated to the ways of humans. They also became indispensable as a means to keep mice under control. Travelers on land and sea took cats with them, thereby enabling archeologists to track the gradual migration of cats from Egypt to Greece to India and to China. Italian coins and pottery demonstrate that cats must have been introduced into southern Italy by 400 BC. Some of the coins show cats being fed meat, birds, or cakes. Sicilian writings from the first century BC talk about the specific foods fed to cats kept by priests. The priests fed the cats grains as well as meat—wheat flour mixed with wheat kernels soaked in milk, along with choice Nile fish.

Such evidence indicates that dogs, cats, and humans have had a mutually beneficial existence for millennia. The animals hunted, scrounged food, and ate whatever humans threw away or were willing to spare. They survived, grew, and reproduced, and did so without the help of commercial pet food. In the light of history, commercial pet food is a thoroughly modern invention, made possible when the industrial revolution brought large numbers of people into cities to work, created systems for the manufacture and distribution of consumer goods, and promoted a consumer culture based on demands for convenience.

EARLY FEEDING PRACTICES

That dogs and cats survived to the present day makes perfect sense. Mice are an excellent source of nutrition for cats, and food waste is just fine for dogs if the foods are varied enough. Owners and breeders were close observers of their animals and could figure out if the animals' diets were inadequate. Long before anyone knew anything about body needs for vitamins, minerals, and other essential nutrients, dog owners and breeders understood that the diets of their animals had to follow what we now understand as basic principles of nutrition: balance, variety, and moderation.

Let's start with moderation, which refers to energy (calorie) balance. Dogs and cats should not be overfed to the point where they get fat. Today's concerns about pet obesity (chapter 15) are nothing new. Throughout the 1800s, for example, books on dog care cautioned owners not to overfeed their animals, to limit the number of daily feedings, and "never to present more to a dog than he will eat with a good appetite." In the early 1900s, Anna Comstock, an assistant professor of nature study at Cornell, worried that most dogs are fed too often and advised: "Do not pay attention when your dog begs for food, since to yield would most likely ruin his health." A century later, this is still good advice.

The principles of balance and variety derive from our understanding of food composition. Plant and animal foods contain a great many nutrients but in different amounts. Because each food has its own unique complement of nutrients and some foods have more of any one nutrient than others, mixing foods compensates for possible shortages. Early owners and breeders could see that dogs did better when fed more than one kind of food. An 1858 guide to dog care, for example, pointed out that while wild dogs (wolves) ate meat, domestic dogs also needed other foods:

> The natural food of the dog is flesh, and it is found that those in a wild state prefer it to every other kind of nutriment, but . . . [s]tag-hounds, fox-hounds, harriers, and beagles, are generally fed on oatmeal . . . [T]he meal should be made into porridge, with the addition of a little milk, and occasionally the kitchen offal, such as remnants of butchers' meat, broth, and soups, the raspings and refuse of bakers' shops, or hard, coarse, sea-biscuit (sold as dog-biscuit), well soaked and boiled with bullocks' liver or horseflesh.

Besides meat and oatmeal, dogs needed vegetables (for vitamins, as we now know). An 1860 book for owners of hunting dogs said: "It is well to observe that vegetables of almost any kind, as potatoes, carrots, parsnips, and even cabbages, may be added . . . to the dog's great advantage.

In the 1880s, kennels fed mixtures of oatmeal and horsemeat to their charges. Horses had a high mortality rate and their meat was cheap and widely available for this purpose. In 1900, a how-to book about managing dog diseases summarized decades of published advice:

> Sheep-heads, trotters, and ox-noses form a highly nutritious and valuable food, especially for invalid dogs; boiled down, they form a glutinous jelly, of which dogs are particularly fond. Whatever kind of flesh-meat is used, meal should form the basis, and none is better than the coarse Scotch oatmeal, thoroughly cooked . . . The dog has a natural fondness for bones, independently of which they are of great value to him. One should always be allowed at least once or twice a week.

Such advice made it clear that a close relationship with a butcher was essential for feeding dogs properly. Owners were advised not only to feed ox-noses and the heads of sheep to their dogs, but to do so often: "For a person who keeps several dogs, there is no better mode than to let the butcher regularly supply him with sheep heads, which will cost a mere trifle, at the rate of one for each dog every second day." The heads of sheep were so commonly used as food for dogs in the nineteenth century that books provided recipes for cooking them. Here, for example, is a recipe for puppy food from 1859:

> In the fourth week get a sheep's head, boil it in a quart of water till the meat comes completely to pieces, then carefully take away every particle of bone, and break up the meat into fragments no larger than a small horse-bean; mix all up with the broth, thicken this to the consistence of cream with fine wheat flour, boil for a quarter of an hour, then cool and give alternately with the milk.

This would make a nutritious food, especially with a few vegetables and bones tossed into the soup, but seems rather inconvenient for modern kitchens.

And what about cats? Much less has been written about the early feeding practices of cat owners. Although the principles of balance, variety, and moderation also apply to the diets of cats, owners did not need to be concerned about them. Cats that ate mice and an occasional bird took good care of their own nutritional needs. Their independence meant that owners were unlikely to see what the cats were eating. Early advice about what was best to feed house cats tended to reflect the owners' personal experience rather than any kind of systematic observation. An 1898 book about the care of angora cats, for example, advised a diet of milk and oatmeal, a fare that would not be nutritionally adequate without the addition of a mouse or two. Well into the 1900s, books about cat care assumed that owners were preparing food for their animals: "[In] my own cattery we have horse-flesh delivered three times a week and two cods'-heads each day. . . . Cods'-heads must be well boiled and boned, and mixed with scalded biscuits or bread. . . . Once a week, when possible, have two chilled rabbits. Cook them well."

Faced with the daily chore of cooking and boning sheep heads, cods' heads, or chilled rabbits, anyone might be grateful for the convenience of commercial pet food. By 1900, biscuits had become a common food for dogs, and dry and canned foods for dogs and cats would soon find a ready market. Although the origins of commercial pet foods date back two hundred years or more, the pet food industry, in the form we know it today, only began in the early part of the twentieth century. Modern pet foods required the development of canning technology, but they also were based on increasing knowledge of the specific nutritional requirements of dogs and cats.

3

What Pets Need

TODAY THE NUTRIENT needs of dogs and cats, and the ways in which these needs differ from those of humans, are well established. Indeed, the nutritional details are so well known that we can safely say that more is known about the nutrient requirements of pets than of people. We know this as a direct result of experiments using dogs as subjects. The digestive physiology of dogs is so similar to that of humans that dogs could be used to determine nutritional principles that applied to humans as well. Cats, with their shorter digestive tracts, differ too much from humans to be used in those kinds of studies. Instead, information about the nutritional needs of cats came later as the result of research studies designed specifically for that purpose.

NUTRITIONAL SIMILARITIES

One great marvel of animal physiology is that all animals—including humans—have similar nutrient requirements despite their diversity in size, shape, ecological niche, and dietary habits. Animals, from the smallest to the largest, require nearly the same collection of fifty or so nutrients—sources of energy (calories), vitamins, minerals, amino acids, and fatty acids—for their growth, reproduction, and survival. Like humans, other animals obtain required nutrients through the foods they eat: plants as well as prey animals.

Plants constitute the basis of animal life. Small animals eat plants. Wolves and cats eat smaller animals and get plant nutrients that way. Plants can supply all of the essential nutrients that animals need with only one exception—vitamin B_{12}. That exceptional vitamin is made by bacteria. Smaller animals eat bacteria along with grass and feed, and incorporate vitamin B_{12} into their tissues. Animals further up the food chain (like us) get vitamin B_{12} when we eat animal-derived foods.

Bacteria are the source of vitamin B_{12} but that is not all they are. They also produce additional nutrients required by animals—biotin and vitamin K, for example. Perhaps more important, they help with the digestion of plant fiber. In chapter 18, we examine the benefits of certain kinds of bacteria on digestive function in the context of the increasingly popular "probiotic" supplements and food products marketed to dogs and cats.

Bacteria are so important that the digestive systems of animals are specialized to promote their proliferation. Cows, for example, have rumens—digestive organs adapted as fermentation vats. In them, bacteria ferment grasses into fatty acids used for energy, and make some of the vitamins and amino acids (building blocks of protein) that cattle need for growth and reproduction. Other ruminant animals—sheep, deer, and goats—do the same. As for nonruminants, horses and rabbits have large intestines adapted for bacterial fermentation. Some rodents eat their own bacteria-laden feces and get many vitamins that way. Dogs will do this too, if given half a chance. Dogs, cats, and people house billions of intestinal bacteria. These make all the vitamin K we need and help convert fiber into usable nutrients.

During the process of digestion, animals break down the carbohydrates, proteins, and fats in foods into units—sugars, amino acids, and fatty acids—small enough to be absorbed into the body. These are used to build body parts or to produce energy. That is why dogs and cats are able to eat the same kinds of foods we do. With only a few exceptions, pets require the same nutrients we do, digest food in the same way, and do just fine on diets similar to ours. These similarities may be one reason why cats and dogs make such easy companions.

As we mentioned earlier, the wild ancestors of domestic dogs and cats were relatively strict carnivores that ate all parts of their prey. But in the thousands of years that cats and dogs have been adapting to the ways of humans, these animals have evolved to prefer and to be able to use a much greater variety of foods. Commercial pet foods may seem far removed from the ancestral diets of wild cats and dogs, but the modern progeny of those animals survive and reproduce quite well on such products.

NUTRIENT REQUIREMENTS

We mentioned that dogs were used as experimental animals to study human nutrition. Dogs have been used for this purpose since the eighteenth century and were only recently replaced by rats and mice. Studies using dogs, for example, were performed to explain the metabolism of the vitamin niacin and its role in the human disease pellagra. That disease, now virtually eliminated, was the scourge of the rural South in the early part of the twentieth century among people eating diets based mainly on corn. Corn contains niacin, but in a form that makes it rather unavailable. And although niacin can be made from a common amino acid, tryptophan, corn happens to be unusually low in tryptophan. Dogs fed corn-based diets developed black tongue, a disease characterized by loss of appetite and weight, an inflamed tongue, and foul-smelling feces. By 1937, feeding experiments demonstrated that both pellagra and black tongue were due to niacin deficiency. The studies also demonstrated that dogs could make enough niacin when they ate protein-rich foods containing tryptophan. Such studies helped to identify niacin as an essential nutrient for dogs and humans. In the United States today, niacin is added to white flour as well as to commercial pet foods.

In order to perform such studies, investigators fed the dogs mixtures of highly purified ingredients—proteins, fats, carbohydrates, vitamins, and minerals—for long periods of time. The use of purified diets revealed much of what we know today about vitamin and mineral deficiencies. Such diets are, however, too expensive and inconvenient to use for studying the effects of supplements or food ingredients on the health of dogs or cats. Studies using purified diets also were conducted before concerns about animal welfare led to greater controls over research on dogs and cats. For these reasons, it is unlikely that most of those early nutrition studies could be repeated today. We grapple with the ethics of doing this kind of research on cats and dogs in chapter 25.

NUTRITIONAL EXCEPTIONS

We said that the requirements of people and pets are similar, as indeed they are in most respects. Research using purified diets in dogs has led to much greater understanding of the nutritional differences between cats, dogs, and people. Fortunately, we only have to deal with seven special cases:

1. Dogs and cats make their own vitamin C. People do not and must obtain vitamin C from food plants.
2. Dogs and people are able to synthesize the vitamin niacin from the amino acid tryptophan. Cats cannot do this and require ready-made niacin.
3. Humans and dogs can convert beta-carotene, a precursor of vitamin A, to the active vitamin. Cats cannot and require ready-made vitamin A from animals or supplements.
4. Human skin contains a precursor of vitamin D that is activated by sunlight. But this precursor is present in low levels in the skin of dogs and cats.
5. Dogs and people make arachidonic acid, a fatty acid precursor of hormones and other body chemicals, from an essential fatty acid, linoleic acid; cats do not make quite enough to support pregnancy or the growth of kittens.
6. Most mammals can synthesize enough of the amino acid arginine to meet their needs; dogs and cats must obtain some arginine from food proteins.
7. Cats need a food source of taurine, an amino acid essential for normal vision, nervous system development, heart health, and reproduction. Dogs make some taurine from sulfur-containing amino acids and do not need any extra un-

less their protein intake is especially low. We humans make enough taurine on our own and do not need supplements.

Because these exceptions can be difficult to keep straight, we summarize them in table 1. One of the great benefits of commercial pet foods is that they are formulated to take care of these nutritional details without anyone having to worry about them.

Table 1
UNIQUE NUTRIENT REQUIREMENTS OF HUMANS, DOGS, AND CATS[a]

NUTRIENT REQUIRED	HUMANS	DOGS	CATS
Vitamin C	Yes	No	No
Niacin (a vitamin)	Yes[b]	Yes[b]	Yes
Preformed vitamin A	No	No	Yes
Preformed vitamin D[c]	No	Yes	Yes
Arachidonic acid (a fatty acid)	No	No	Yes
Arginine (an amino acid)	No	Yes	Yes
Taurine (a nonprotein amino acid)	No	No	Yes

a Other essential nutrients are the same for cats, dogs, and humans.

b Humans and dogs make some niacin from tryptophan.

c Humans require vitamin D when they do not get enough sunlight exposure; dogs and cats do not make enough vitamin D unless they are outdoors most of the time.

FROM SCIENCE TO FEEDING ADVICE

By the early 1940s, purified-diet research had identified most essential vitamins and minerals, their food sources, and many of their roles in human and animal physiology. The new science, however, did not always translate into sensible feeding advice. Then, as now, self-proclaimed experts gave conflicting instructions about the best way to feed cats and dogs. Some argued, for example, that large numbers of dogs suffer from malnutrition because they do not get enough meat, whereas others said that too much meat induces calcium deficiency. A rather relaxed 1939 guide to dog feeding considered bones nonessential mineral supplements, said dogs should not be permitted to scavenge food, and advised owners to take their choice on the raw food question ("the notion that the raw-meat eater is a dangerous dog is pure fallacy"). By the 1940s, obesity had already been identified as a serious problem for pets: "It is more than likely that among house-pet dogs . . . many have died from being fed too much than for any other reason."

Some makers of pet foods were aware of the emerging information about vitamin and mineral requirements, and quickly incorporated the new knowledge into their marketing campaigns. Advertisements for Puss 'n Boots (then owned by Quaker Oats) invoked nutrition to convince owners of the special value of this product:

> Many cat owners have assumed that any piece of fish will meet his needs. Biologists tell us that is a mistake. . . . When *whole* fish is properly prepared for cat food, nature's balance of vital elements remains intact. . . . The fillets contain proteins. The liver and glands yield vitamins. The bone structure supplies calcium. . . . Each part of the fish contributes nutritive elements, but only the *whole* fish represents the nutritive whole.

In part to settle some of the questions about pet feeding, but also to standardize the nutrient content of commercial products, the National Research Council (NRC) convened a committee to establish guidelines for the nutritional requirements of dogs. This committee's first report in 1953 marked the beginning of the modern era of pet feeding based on science.

INTRODUCING THE NRC: RECOMMENDED ALLOWANCES

Since 1953, NRC reports have summarized the scientific basis of pet feeding, defined minimal nutrient requirements, and translated the science into recommendations that govern the nutrient content of food products made for dogs and cats. Because the NRC establishes the basis of what goes into pet foods, it is worth knowing how this group works. The NRC is one of four units that together constitute the National Academies, a group chartered originally by President Abraham Lincoln in 1863 "to investigate, examine, experiment, and report on any subject of science or art" when requested to do so by the government.

The NRC established its Committee on Animal Nutrition in 1928. This committee remained relatively inactive until World War II when the need to increase production of farm animals for food became a national priority. At that point, this committee went into action. It reviewed research on the nutritional requirements of farm animals and published brochures on the nutrient needs of pigs, chickens, sheep, beef cattle, dairy cattle, and horses. Later, it appointed subcommittees to update these publications and to prepare new reports on additional animal species—dogs and cats among them.

The NRC's first technical report on the *Nutrient Requirements of Dogs* appeared in 1953. The subcommittee responsible for this report consisted of distinguished physiologists and nutrition scientists—mostly from universities, but some from industry—who had used dogs to study vitamin and mineral requirements. The names of those scientists are still recognizable to nutrition students and practitioners. For example, Morgan Hall, the building that currently houses the nutrition science department at the University of California, Berkeley, is named after one of the original members of the dog subcommittee, Agnes Fay Morgan. From the beginning, the dog subcommittees defined the minimal levels of nutrients required to support growth and reproduction. They also established standards of adequate intake of specific nutrients—recommended allowances—that generally were higher than minimal requirements.

Subcommittees revised the dog report every few years based on the availability of new research, the particular research interests of the scientists who prepared the reports, and the ways in which the reports were expected to be used. With each of the successive revisions in 1962, 1972, 1974, and 1985 (and most recently in 2006), the dog subcommittees expanded the number of nutrients for which they defined minimum requirements and adjusted the recommended allowances in response to more recent research and practice.

The NRC recommended allowances are supposed to be based entirely on the science, but nutrition science is often inconsistent or incomplete and, therefore, requires interpretation. Interpretation depends on the viewpoint of the interpreter. Differences in interpretation explain why the NRC issued two reports so close together in 1972 and 1974, events that illustrate how difficult it is to make scientific judgments independent of other considerations. At issue was the level of protein dogs should be eating. Unlike earlier reports, the 1972 version included a separate section warning of the dangers of high-protein diets:

> Difficulties associated with high protein diets have become more commonplace since the introduction of dog foods composed almost entirely of meat and meat by-products. . . . Optimal levels of dietary protein for some physiological states of the dog are not completely defined, but it is clear that diets containing as much as twice the minimum required amount of protein can have serious consequences, irrespective of vitamin and mineral supplementation, if fed over long periods. . . . Diets high in protein contribute to renal disease. . . . There is no evidence proving that animal protein is an essential constituent of a dog's diet.

Aren't dogs supposed to eat high-protein diets? To a pet food company advertising its products as high in animal protein ("the natural food for dogs"), advice against using such foods set off alarm bells. Liggett & Myers, the tobacco company that then owned Alpo, one of the bestselling all-meat products on the market, threatened to sue the NRC. Although the controversial statements were backed up by citations to several research studies, the NRC asked the subcommittee to review them again. The subcommittee spent two years doing so, and issued a revised report in 1974—with the offending section deleted. A cover letter from the chair of the NRC Committee on Animal Nutrition introduced the report with a letter that included this most unusual paragraph:

> In this revision the Subcommittee refrained from discussing the possible problems relating to the effects of high-protein diets pending the availability of more definitive studies in the future.

Based on the accumulated professional experience of some of its members, however, the Subcommittee, as well as the Committee on Animal Nutrition, continues to share a general belief that prolonged intake of high-protein diets can be harmful to dogs. The Subcommittee believes that any adverse effects of this nature can be avoided by general adherence to the guidelines on dietary protein levels recommended in the report.

Subsequent NRC reports say nothing further about upper limits on the amounts of protein or meat to be fed to dogs. Although this incident might appear to be a flagrant example of the intrusion of commercial considerations into science, the "more definitive" studies that came later failed to show harm from high-protein diets except, perhaps, to older dogs with kidney disease.

As for cats: the NRC first described the minimum nutrient needs of cats in 1972 as part of its larger report, *Nutrient Requirements of Laboratory Animals*. The writer of the cat section, Stanley Gershoff, was a university researcher who had used cats in nutritional studies at his laboratory at Harvard. The NRC's first separate report on cat nutrition did not appear until 1978. Although that subcommittee was chaired by Duane Ullrey, a distinguished comparative animal nutritionist from Michigan State University, the other members all worked for pet food companies. Pet food companies had a vested interest in determining what nutrients to put into cat food and much of the practical work on cat nutrition had been performed by in-house company researchers. Only later, as more university researchers became interested in cat nutrition, was the NRC able to appoint them to committees. By 1986 the subcommittee working on cat nutrition consisted almost entirely of scientists affiliated with universities.

In 2006, the NRC combined the dog and cat publications into one report, *Nutrient Requirements of Dogs and Cats*. This report is a joint effort of government and industry; the subcommittee's expenses were paid by the National Institutes of Health, the Food and Drug Administration, and the Pet Food Institute, a trade association of pet food manufacturers. For anyone interested in the nutritional content of pet food, this report is the Bible, comparable in its scope, comprehensiveness, and authority to the *Dietary Reference Intakes* for humans produced by the Institute of Medicine, also a unit of the National Academies. The NRC's 2006 report:

- Reviewed research on the basic anatomy and digestive physiology of dogs and cats.
- Described the formulation and processing of dry and wet pet foods and treats.
- Listed the nutrient composition of common pet food ingredients.
- Evaluated the safety and effectiveness of pet food additives and supplements.
- Recommended allowances for intake of more than forty nutrients for growing pregnant, lactating, and adult dogs and cats.

The European Pet Food Industry Federation (FEDIAF) published a similar report in 2008. From the standpoint of science, the information in these reports is as good as it gets. Because the NRC report is lengthy and highly technical, its scientists have summarized the most practical information in pamphlets designed for dog and cat owners. Unlike most NRC publications, these are available on the Internet at no cost (see appendix 6 for addresses). We recommend them highly.

INTRODUCING AAFCO: NUTRIENT PROFILES

To understand anything about what goes into pet foods, you have to know about AAFCO—the American Association of Feed Control Officials—a group formed in 1909 to reconcile inconsistencies in state laws governing what went into feed for farm animals and, therefore, dogs and cats. We will have more to say more about AAFCO in later chapters. Here, we discuss its development of "nutrient profiles," standards for the nutrient content of pet foods.

AAFCO did not do anything special about pet foods until 1956, when it established its first pet food committee. That committee, composed of state feed control officials with advisors from pet food companies and trade associations, issued its first report on pet food labeling in 1961 and its first set of "model regulations" for pet food contents and labels—those that it hoped states would adopt as laws—in 1968.

Although the NRC's recommended allowances represent the gold standard for the nutrient needs of cats and dogs based on research, they are not recipes for making commercial foods. For one thing, they are based largely on experiments using purified nutrients, not foods. But pet foods are typically made from foods or food ingredients (except for supplementary vitamins and minerals). For another, the NRC's recommended allowances in the mid-1980s were set at levels designed to meet minimum nutrient requirements for dogs and cats, levels that did not account for variations in bioavailability—how well food ingredients are digested, absorbed, and metabolized—or losses of nutrients that occur when pet foods are cooked.

AAFCO set about developing nutrient profiles that take such factors into consideration. It began with the NRC minimum nutrient requirements based on purified diets. It then converted the requirements to practical minimum and maximum nutrient standards (profiles) for dog and cat foods made from "nonpurified ingredients," meaning real foods. Over the years, AAFCO established profiles for thirty-six nutrients for dogs; these cover the needs for protein, fat, linoleic acid, amino acids, minerals, and vitamins. For cats, it has defined profiles for forty-two nutrients to deal with their more complicated nutritional requirements.

AAFCO profiles also suggest maximum levels of certain nutrients—fat-soluble vitamins and some minerals—that might prove toxic if consumed in excess. When a pet food is made with ingredients that meet the complete set of AAFCO nutrient profiles for a dog or cat, it qualifies for the designation, "complete and balanced." In 2009, AAFCO profiles were still based on the 1985 recommendations for dogs and the 1986 recommendations for cats, but committees were revising the profiles to make them consistent with the NRC's more recent 2006 report. For the first time, the NRC 2006 report defined recommended allowances that exceeded minimum requirements; these came closer to AAFCO's nutrient profiles. When AAFCO revises its profiles to conform to the NRC 2006 publication, the allowances and profiles are likely to be much the same and to establish more uniform standards for the nutrient content of pet foods.

With these details in mind, we can now examine the universe of pet foods in the United States—how they were invented, the kinds of products that are now available, the companies that make the products, and the ways in which pet food contents are determined and monitored.

4

Inventing Commercial Pet Foods

EVERYONE WHO WRITES about the origins of the commercial pet food industry invariably begins with James Spratt and his legendary dog biscuits. Spratt was an American inventor and peddler of lightning rods who obtained the first patent for dog biscuits in England in 1861. In one version of the legend, Spratt had a flash of inspiration when his ship docked near London and he observed the crew throwing leftover biscuits to hordes of eager dogs. In another, Spratt was already in London when he was "offered some inedible, discarded ship biscuits for his dog and thereupon decided his pet was worthy of more consideration." No matter. In whatever way Spratt got into this business, he did not invent dog biscuits. His 1861 patent application merely claimed "Improvements in the preparation of food for hogs, dogs, cats, and poultry, and in apparatus for the same." If he invented anything, it was the marketing potential of his patent. With it, Spratt founded a successful pet food and supply business that lasted well into the twentieth century.

By 1861, dog biscuits had been in commerce for a long time. They evolved from the hardtack biscuits fed to British sailors on long ocean voyages—thick crackers of flour, water, and salt baked to jaw-breaking firmness. Dependence on milled flour as the main or only source of nutrients explains why the British navy suffered so terribly from generalized malnutrition as well as scurvy from lack of vitamin C. Even in those early days, milling removed much of the nutrient-rich germ and bran from wheat flour. The addition of fats, meat, oatmeal, and vegetables to the basic recipe increased nutrient balance and variety and vastly improved the nutritional value of hardtack for sailors as well as for dogs.

Decades before Spratt acquired his patent, companies produced nutritionally enhanced biscuits intended for dogs and advertised these products in magazines intended for hunters. In 1792, for example, *Sporting* described a visit to the manufacturing plant of one Mr. Smith, whose dog biscuits the magazine recommended. Advertisements for Mr. Smith's biscuits appeared in *Sporting* well into the 1820s, invariably accompanied by testimonials such as this one from a man whose dog, Emerald, won the Ashdown Cup: "I must say it is the best food for greyhounds I have ever tried."

By the 1850s, dog biscuits were so widely marketed that they were listed in catalogs of British trade items, and guidebooks to London identified shops where they could be purchased. Apparently, their ready availability made them useful for purposes beyond feeding dogs—adulteration of coffee, for example. In 1855, a London coffee merchant felt the "duty to caution our friends and the public against the present unjust and iniquitous system pursued by many grocers in adulterating their coffee with roasted beans, dog biscuit, chicory, and tan." His place, of course, did no such thing.

Spratt took full advantage of the rising popularity of commercial dog food. He acquired a second patent in 1868, this time for "improved preparations of food for horses, cattle, game, poultry and other domestic animals." Advertisements for Spratt's Patent Meat Fibrine Dog Cakes often included testimonials like this one from J.H. Murchison of London in 1873: "Having used Spratt's Patent Biscuits in large quantities for some years . . . I consider them the best food for dogs. I must add that my kennels have been singularly free from disease, particularly considering the large number of dogs I have had there." By the late 1870s, dog biscuits were marketed so aggressively that British huntsmen complained about the "impudence" of biscuit sellers who attempted to gain access to their exclusive society in order to peddle such wares.

Spratt also made biscuits for cats, and these elicited their own testimonials. One satisfied cat owner wrote in 1876: "I have tried Spratt's Patent Cat Food with a great number of cats . . . and have nearly always found it [to] agree; and at a cat show it would, I believe, be both handy and cleanly." Another compared Spratt's to other commercial products: "Of the solid foods sold . . . the least generally said the better . . . some of it is simply rubbish; the chief efforts of the vendors being the extraction of cash. . . . The only exception is Spratt's Cat Food."

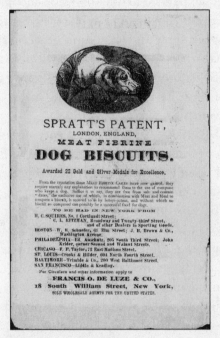

FIGURE 1
Advertisement for Spratt's Patent Dog Biscuits, 1880.

Source: Catalog of the Westminster Kennel Club April 27–29, 1880.
Courtesy of the Library of the American Kennel Club.

In the 1870s, Spratt began to sell his products in the United States, especially through publications and exhibitions targeting kennel clubs and dog shows. After his death in 1880, the company moved part of the business to America, where its offices in New York continued to file patents for improved biscuits. The advertisement from that year shown in figure 1 emphasizes that the cakes are salt-free and contain patented "dates" that ensure the success of this food. Another, in 1881, touted the addition of a special variety of beets to the formula: "the only one that bears the enormous heat necessary for perfect baking, whilst retaining the essential vegetable quality uninjured, and in its highest condition for the dog."

Spratt's soon established a factory in Newark, New Jersey, where the company manufactured biscuits branded with "Spratt's" and "Trade Mark X" in enormous ovens said to be fifty feet long and twelve feet wide. In England, Spratt's expanded to offer one-stop shopping for anything a pet owner might need: supplies and appliances; boarding, quarantine, and shipping services; show and exhibition services; and informational brochures and magazines—much like modern pet supply stores. The company marketed its products at the 1904 World's Fair in St. Louis, Missouri, in what must have been a stunning display; the walls of the exhibition space were tiled with dog biscuits.

But by the early 1900s, Spratt's had plenty of competition. Many companies made dog biscuits and advertised them with testimonials. Indeed, commercial biscuits were so widely available by 1915 that owners were advised to give them to dogs three or four times a week. And by the 1930s, dog biscuits came much as they do today, in multiple sizes and shapes—square, oval, bone-shaped, cubes, pellets, kibbled—and with any number of ingredients found in modern pet foods and treats: meat, meat by-products, cereal grains, ground bone, dried milk, bean meals, cod-liver oil, fish meal, molasses, salt, and yeast.

Today, vitamin and mineral mixes have replaced cod liver oil and yeast, but little else has changed. The marketing of the old biscuits also seems thoroughly modern. In 1930, for example, the Chappel company advertised Ken-L-Biskit as "scientifically prepared . . . entirely different from any other dog biscuit ever made," and as containing "all of the food elements vital to the dog in just the right proportion." By the early 1940s, pet food marketers were taking full advantage of the new knowledge of vitamin and mineral requirements in their promotional materials:

> If your dog is listless and sullen . . . chances are his diet's to blame! Any dog, to be alert and happy, needs essential food

elements. . . . Milk-Bone contains vitamins A, B, D, E, and G [*sic*]. It's made of wholesome ingredients including: nourishing milk, high protein beef meat meal . . . fortified cod liver oil, irradiated yeast . . . wheat germ, ground whole wheat, soy bean oil meal . . . Give Milk-Bone to *your* dog. Make it a regular part of his diet—starting today!

CANNED ("WET") PET FOODS

Until the early 1900s, commercial pet foods were almost exclusively produced in the form of dry biscuits or cakes, largely because no other means of preservation existed. Although meat canning was invented in the 1840s, metal cans were too expensive to use until the early 1900s. Even then, the canning of pet food encountered numerous technical problems; these problems had to be solved before such products could be widely sold. The historian Katherine Grier, whose accounts of the origin of pet food are exceptionally thoughtful and well documented, identifies the Kennel Food Supply Company of Fairfield, Connecticut, as the first dog food canner in the United States, based on advertisements it placed in kennel magazines in 1916.

From the beginning, what went into pet foods is much like what goes into pet foods today and whether the contents are good, bad, or inconsequential for pet health depends much on point of view. Grier refers to the earliest canned pet foods as "packaged industrial food scrap." Canned pet foods were invented to feed cats and dogs of course, but the basic rationale for their creation—a rationale that still applies—was to find something to do with the waste left over from meatpacking and feed milling operations. It was no accident that feed companies like Ralston Purina developed pet food lines or that the first large canner of dog foods, Chappel Bros., owned a horse slaughtering plant in Rockford, Illinois.

Animal by-products were—and still are—prime drivers of pet food production. The remains from processing animals for human food production have always been fed to dogs, but large slaughterhouses raise the disposal problem to a monumental scale. At best, humans consider only about half the weight of a food animal to be edible, meaning that the slaughter of a single steer or horse produces hundreds of pounds of skin, bones, organs, and other parts that humans will not eat. These parts have excellent nutritional value and it seemed obvious that turning them into pet food made better economic sense than dumping them into the nearest river or landfill.

The history of the development of pet food companies has much to teach us about the modern pet food industry. Chappel Bros., for example, started out as a supplier of horses to the U.S. government during World War I. When the war ended, Chappel exported horse meat to France but also sought a domestic use for it. The company bought a slaughterhouse and a canning plant, and spent several years figuring out how to overcome technical problems. Once those were solved, Chappel was ready to begin selling Ken-L-Ration canned dog food in 1923. The company had a ready supply of horses from those put out of work by the increasing popularity of automobiles and the mechanization of farming. When that supply of horses was depleted, Chappel headed west and rounded up wild horses. By the 1930s, canned dog foods—based on horse and other meats—were well established products widely distributed through grocery stores. In 1932, the A&P chain offered three cans of Calo dog food for 25 cents. In comparison, sirloin steak was 37 cents per pound and a whole chicken cost 23 cents in those early days of the Great Depression.

A 1935 advertisement for Ken-L-Ration offered a choice of horse meat (yellow label) or beef meat (white label), but the beef brands had too much competition and did not do well. During the 1930s, horses were not the only animals hunted specifically for pet foods. Enterprising hunters went after whales and sea lions expressly for this purpose. Canned foods with these and other ingredients were marketed for cats as well as dogs. The first canned food specifically for cats, Puss 'n Boots, was introduced in 1934 but its ingredients were much the same as those in dog foods.

In 1939, the U.S. Department of Agriculture (USDA) observed that many kinds of canned pet foods were marketed as complete rations, even though their composition varied widely. The ingredients in canned foods added water but were otherwise much the same as those in dry foods: meat, meat by-products, fish, cereals, vegetables, bone, yeast, cod-liver oil, and charcoal. Prior to the onset of World War II, sales of canned pet foods exceeded those of the dry foods. The war changed that balance. Restrictions on the use of cans for pet food and on the amount of animal protein such products could contain discouraged the manufacture of wet foods. Although sales eventually returned to prewar levels, dry foods proved more convenient and popular in the long run.

During the 1940s, horse meat remained a major ingredient in canned foods. This can be seen in the large collection of historic but undated pet food labels posted by Katherine Grier on the Internet. Many of the labels indicate horse meat as the leading or only ingredient. In figure 2, we provide an example of a label from the 1940s. This Alpo ("Al-Po") label lists horsemeat, meat by-products, and horse heart or liver as principal ingredients, with sodium nitrite as a preservative, along with a statement that sounds thoroughly modern: "no cereal fillers" (see chapter 7).

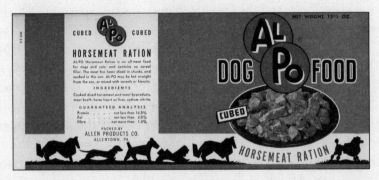

FIGURE 2
Alpo dog food label, 1940s.

Source: IPC Dennison Company Collection, East Tennesee State University
Archives of Appalachia, Johnson City, Tennessee.

Horse meat continued to be used for pet feeding despite increasing public discomfort with the idea of slaughtering horses for food either for humans or pets. During World War II, New York City required permits from sellers of horse meat and insisted that they dye the meat with a coloring agent to prevent its diversion into the human food supply. In 1952, the *New York Times* investigated a fraud in which horse meat was sold illegally as beef. Remarkable facts emerged in this investigation: half a million horses were slaughtered annually; each horse produced about 550 pounds of dressed meat; altogether, horses yielded 275 million pounds of meat annually; and—if you can even imagine this—93 percent of horse meat production went into pet foods. The remaining 7 percent was shipped to Europe as "very nice meat" for humans.

But some American humans also ate horse meat. This became obvious in California. Although this state did not allow horse meat to be sold for human consumption, stores ostensibly selling it to feed dogs and cats could not keep up with the demand. As the price of beef rose, so did the number of two-footed customers. This situation was much like the raw milk situation today. In states where raw milk can only be sold to feed pets, nobody knows who really uses it. Then, the sellers of horse meat complained that while Europeans consider horse meat a delicacy Americans have "this mental thing" against eating horses.

Indeed, "this mental thing" led states to enact laws banning the sale of horse meat. Texas was the first state to enact such a law in 1949, making us wonder whether beef ranchers might have had something to do with that action. In 1971, Congress passed the Wild Free-Roaming Horses and Burros Act, which protected wild horses on public lands and prevented companies from rounding them up for slaughter. This legislation reduced the amount of horse meat available and increased its price. The higher cost coupled with public pressure to stop killing horses induced pet food companies to replace horse meat with that from other animals, particularly beef. Today, although horse meat continues to be permitted for use in pet foods, no company of which we are aware uses it and we have never seen it listed as an ingredient on a product sold in grocery or pet supply stores. Otherwise, the ingredients of today's canned pet foods look much like those from the middle of the last century with only a couple of additional exceptions. Nitrates are no longer used as preservatives because they were linked to cancer in the 1970s. And vitamin and mineral mixes have replaced cod-liver oil and yeast as sources of certain vitamins.

Pet Foods as an Industry

Since the days of James Spratt, the pet industry has grown into an important economic force in the United States. If you live with a dog or cat, you may think of your animal as a cherished companion, but from a business standpoint your pet is the rationale for a lucrative marketing opportunity. An impressive majority—62 percent—of American households include at least one pet, most likely a cat or dog, but also fish, birds, and more exotic creatures. This book considers only cats and dogs mostly because of their economic impact. According to a 2009–10 pet owners survey by the American Pet Products Association (APPA), 39 percent of American households owned at least one dog and 33 percent owned at least one cat (some owned both dogs and cats). These households represented a population of 94 million cats and 78 million dogs—all of them needing to be housed, cared for, and fed.

The industry that emerged to meet the needs of pets and their owners includes the manufacturers, marketers, and sellers of supplies (including food), the performers of services (including breeding and veterinary), and the trade associations, publications, and lobbyists that represent and serve those groups. According to the APPA, Americans spent more than $45 billion on their pets in 2009, up $2 billion just from the previous year, and more than twice the amount spent ten years earlier. This, says the APPA, makes pets and pet services the eighth largest retail business in the United States—larger than either the movie or music businesses.

Pet foods account for the largest single category of spending on pets—estimated at $17.4 billion in 2009. This amount exceeds the expenditures for veterinary care (about $12 billion), veterinary drugs and supplies ($10 billion), the cost of the animals ($2 billion), and other unspecified services ($3 billion). Of the $17.4 billion, 95 percent goes for dog and cat foods. This means that foods for dogs and cats constitute a $16.5 billion industry, one with a value greater than the gross national product of nearly 60 percent of the world's countries.

The APPA conducts surveys to find out how much money individual pet owners spend on their dogs and cats each year. If you are an average pet owner, you say your largest expenses are for veterinary surgery and routine care, boarding your animals during vacations, and food, vitamins, and treats—in that order. Altogether, pet owners in 2009 said they spent an average of about $1,500 on dogs but much less on cats, just a little over $1,000 (appendix 1 gives the details).

Impressive as these amounts are, they could be underestimates. They do not account for services such as dog walking, medical insurance, or photography. But it is difficult to know whether they are underestimates or overestimates. Pet owners say they spend just $200 for food each year for each pet. If you multiply that amount by the number of cats and dogs in the United States, the total adds up to $35 billion, a figure more than twice the $17 billion earned by commercial dog and cat food companies. The gap could mean that many owners feed their pets table scraps or cook for them. Whatever its explanation, pet food companies view the gap as leaving plenty of room to expand sales.

THE PET FOOD INDUSTRY: EMERGENCE

By 1953, as we have explained, the pet food industry was already well established and pets so much a part of American life that the National Research Council found it useful to issue its first recommended allowances for dog food. In the years following World War II, pet ownership flourished and so did pet foods. Appendix 2 outlines some of the more important events in the emergence of the pet food industry from 1953 to the present.

The growth of the industry was slow at first but by 1970 had reached a milestone—$1 billion in sales—at which point it exceeded the market for ready-to-eat cereals, frozen vegetables, and canned soups. From then on, sales increased steadily as shown in figure 3. The increase in growth was stimulated by the hefty profit margins on pet foods, said to be 12–20 percent before taxes in those days. Nevertheless, investment analysts worried about long-term profitability. Some observed "a positive irrationality in the pet food business that is disturbing. . . . The industry is beset by frequent introductions of unneeded products, fierce price wars, and an abundance of costly promotions that consumers love but managers hate."

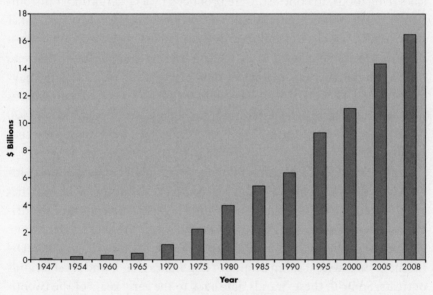

Figure 3
Growth of pet food sales, 1947–2008.

Sources: **1947–1975:** Morton Research Corporation, The Pet Food Industry, An Economic, Marketing, and Financial Investigation, 1977; **1980–1990:** JC Maxwell, Wheat First Securities Business Trends Analysts, 1992; **1995–2000:** Mintel Marketing Intelligence, Pet Food, US 2001; **2005–2008:** Global Market Information Data Base, Euromonitor International, 2008.

Investment experts were troubled by two trends: shifting patterns of pet ownership and increasing consolidation of the industry. During the

1980s, the number of cats in American households exceeded the number of dogs for the first time—a trend explained by the increase in one-person households and in families with two wage-earners. Cats do not need to be walked. They require less attention and fewer toys than dogs. But they are of much less interest to the pet food industry; they do not eat as much as dogs. Even though Americans own 16 million more cats than dogs, cat foods account for just 40 percent of total pet food sales. Dog foods brought in about $9.9 billion in sales in 2009, compared to about $6.5 billion for cats (the rest went for foods for other kinds of pets).

Consolidation occurred early in the industry, especially for cat foods. By 1970, only six companies—Quaker Oats, Carnation, Heinz, Lorillard, Ralston Purina, and Borden—accounted for 78 percent of all cat food sales. Dog foods, in contrast, were produced by a larger number of companies, many of them quite small. The top six—Liggett & Myers, Quaker Oats, Mars, Associated Products, Ralston Purina, and General Foods—took in just 43 percent of sales. Of the leading companies of that era, only Mars remains as a major pet food player. Even so, Mars's primary brand in the 1970s, Kal Kan, no longer exists as it evolved into what is now called Pedigree. The remaining leading makers of pet foods in 1970 either dropped out of the business or sold their pet food brands to other companies.

Indeed, pet food companies during the last half century played Monopoly by switching brands from one company to another. The switches are so confusing that we thought it would be instructive to trace the origins of one company's current pet food holdings. We picked Del Monte as an example because it owns a classic brand, Milk-Bone. In 2009, Del Monte owned at least seven brands of dog and cat foods and seven brands of treats. Some of these brands date back to the early years of the twentieth century, as shown in figure 4.

Milk-Bone biscuits, or something like them, were manufactured by the F.H. Bennett company in the early 1900s. Wheatsworth acquired F.H. Bennett in 1926 and sold it to Nabisco in 1931. In the 1990s, in a series of mergers and acquisitions involving the cigarette companies R.J. Reynolds (which owned Nabisco) and Philip Morris (which owned Kraft Foods), Milk-Bone ended up with Kraft Foods, which, in turn, sold it to Del Monte in 2006.

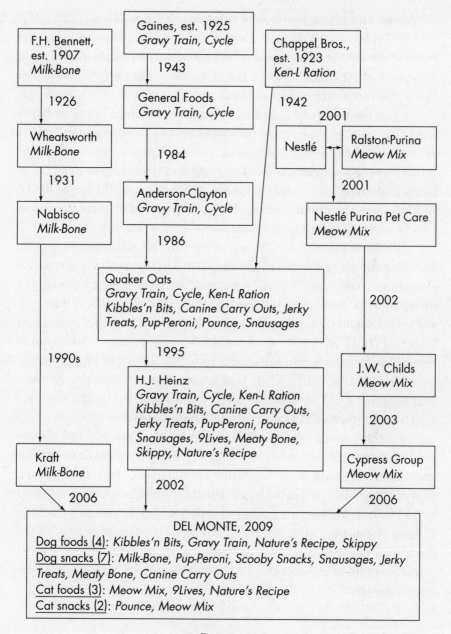

FIGURE 4
The origins of Del Monte's pet food holdings, July 2009.

Meow Mix also has a venerable history. It belonged to Ralston Purina, which merged in 2001 with Nestlé's Friskies' business to form Nestlé Purina PetCare. As an antitrust condition of the merger, Meow Mix had to be sold off; it quickly passed through two private equity companies before Del Monte acquired it in 2006.

Notice the number of cigarette companies involved in the early pet food business. Pet foods must have been part of the companies' efforts to diversify their product mix as well as to improve their image. Liggett & Myers bought Alpo in 1964 and sold it in 1980. Also in 1964, Lorillard bought the Usen Canning Company, the maker of Tabby Cat foods. In 1968, Loews acquired Lorillard but quickly got rid of its cat food business by selling it to Lipton in 1969.

Milk-Bone played only the tiniest part in the astonishing cigarette company drama recounted in the 1990 bestseller and subsequent movie *Barbarians at the Gate*. The drama started with the sale of Nabisco, the owner of Milk-Bone, to R.J. Reynolds in 1985, creating RJR Nabisco. In 1989, Philip Morris combined General Foods and Kraft to form Kraft General Foods. As a result of subsequent leveraged buyouts and acquisitions, Nabisco, Kraft, and Milk-Bone ended up as part of Philip Morris, later called Altria. When Altria began the process of divesting Kraft, it sold Milk-Bone to Del Monte in 2006. In this sense, pet foods closely reflect trends typical of the larger business community.

One final point: what continues to drive the expansion of the pet food industry is its impressive profitability. Here is an example of what one current pet food company, Hill's Pet Nutrition, does for its owner, Colgate-Palmolive. Worldwide sales of Hill's pet products amounted to $2.1 billion in 2008, an amount that accounted for just 14 percent of Colgate-Palmolive's sales of consumer products—but 18 percent of the company's operating profits. Hill's pet foods are said to command gross profit margins of 55–60 percent, a phenomenon we explain in subsequent chapters.

WHO'S WHO IN THE PET FOOD INDUSTRY

Today's pet food industry includes the makers and sellers of foods, treats, and supplements, but also the suppliers of raw materials (including meat and grain processors) and ingredients. Some pet food ingredients are imported and represent a significant component of United States trade. In 2006, pet food manufacturers employed 14,500 people in the United States.

The Sellers

If you want to buy commercial pet food, you can find dog or cat food just about anywhere. Even so, 50 percent of the dog food and 60 percent of the cat food sold in the United States is purchased at supermarkets or Walmart and other big-box stores. Pet superstores sell about 19 percent of the dog food and 16 percent of the cat food. Recently, drug stores and other nongrocery retailers have started to sell pet foods along with foods for humans and you can now pick them up along with shampoo and toothpaste; such places now account for sales percentages similar to those in pet superstores: 19 and 13 percent of dog and cat food, respectively. Pet shops and veterinary clinics account for less than 10 percent of sales each.

The Manufacturers

Virtually all (98 percent) of the makers of dog and cat foods belong to a trade association, the Pet Food Institute (PFI), "the voice of U.S. pet food manufacturers," devoted to education of the public and professionals and lobbying of Congress and state and federal agencies. In 2009 its members include twenty-nine companies that manufacture pet foods and fifty-nine affiliated companies that supply ingredients, equipment, or service to the industry. Most pet food used in the United States is made domestically. Only a small amount is imported. In 2008, for example, about $131 million worth of pet food was imported from China.

Although most large pet food companies maintain their own manufacturing facilities, many pet food brands are made by contract manufacturers—co-packers—who cook up products for small and large brands and those sold under private labels. The extent of the contract manufacturing segment was revealed during the 2007 pet food recalls when the public learned that one factory belonging to a Canadian co-packer, Menu Foods, manufactured products sold under ninety-five brand names.

Doane, a large contract manufacturer acquired by Mars in 2006, makes Walmart's Ol' Roy dry foods along with about two hundred other private-label brands. Del Monte manufactures cans and pouches of the Walmart brands, Ol' Roy and Special Kitty. In 2009, other co-packers were Chenango Valley Pet Foods in New York State and American Nutrition in Ogden, Utah. Some manufacturers specialize in treats, such as Hampshire Pet Products in Joplin, Missouri. Co-packers are able to produce ready-made pet food formulas or to design foods to meet customers' specifications. If you want to have your own brand made, no problem. At a conference of pet food ingredient suppliers in 2008, we asked a contract manufacturer what we would need to do to have his company make a line of pet foods for us. His answer: "Just bring money."

The Marketers

We cannot even guess the number of companies that market pet foods or treats in the United States. People in the industry tell us that hundreds of companies market complete-and-balanced foods, food supplements, treats, and nutritional supplements for dogs and cats. Many of these are small operations. All are supposed to register in the states in which they are located, but no central registry keeps track of them.

As we discussed earlier, the pet food industry is becoming increasingly consolidated. In the early 2000s, the top five pet food companies— "Big Pet Food"—controlled 74 percent of the market; by the end of 2008, they controlled 80 percent. Table 2 summarizes the current state of pet food marketing in the United States. Purina PetCare is the dominant player by far, controlling 34 percent of all sales of dog and cat foods. Its parent company is Nestlé, the Swiss multinational corporation (no relation to Marion Nestle, alas). Nestlé particularly dominates sales of cat foods; it controls 70 percent of the canned cat food market and 53 percent of the dry cat food market. In 2008, Mars, through acquisitions of Doane Pet Care, S&M Nu Tec (Greenies), and Nutro, held 18 percent of the U.S. pet food market.

The next three leading companies controlled shares of about 9 or

Table 2

LEADING PET FOOD MARKETERS IN THE UNITED STATES, 2009

RANK	COMPANY	MARKET SHARE, %*	PET FOOD BRANDS, 2009	
#			DOG	CAT
1	Nestlé Purina PetCare	34	Alpo, Beneful, Dog Chow, Mighty Dog, Pro Plan, Puppy Chow, Chef Michael's, Purina Moist & Meaty, Purina One, Purina Veterinary Diets, Beggin' Strips, Cheweez, T Bonz	Cat Chow, Deli-Cat, Fancy Feast, Friskies, Kit 'N Kaboodle, Kitten Chow, Purina One, Pro Plan, Purina Veterinary Diets, Whisker Lickin's
2	Mars Petcare (Mars Inc.)	18	Cesar, Pedigree, Greenies, Goodlife Recipe, Nutro, Royal Canin, Wholemeals	Whiskas, Sheba, Goodlife Recipe, Nutro, Royal Canin, Temptations
3	Hill's Pet Nutrition (Colgate-Palmolive)	10	Hill's Science Diet, Hill's Prescription Diet	Hill's Science Diet, Hill's Prescription Diet
4	The Iams Company (Procter & Gamble)	9	Iams, Eukanuba	Iams, Eukanuba
5	Del Monte Foods	9	Kibbles 'n Bits, Gravy Train, Nature's Recipe, Skippy, Milk-Bone, Pup-Peroni, Scooby Snacks/Snausages, Jerky Treats, Meaty Bone, Canine Carry Outs	Meow Mix, 9Lives, Nature's Recipe, Pounce, Meow Mix
6	Other	20	Smaller company and private-label brands	

* Sources: Packaged Facts. *Pet Food in the U.S.: Dog Food,* January 2009: and company websites.

10 percent each. Private-label brands accounted for about 11 percent of total sales, but analysts guess that Walmart's Ol' Roy dog food and Special Kitty cat food accounted for nearly one-third of all such sales. Walmart is privately held and does not have to disclose sales figures for specific brands, but a company official told us that Ol' Roy sales amounted to about $1 billion in 2008. If this is true, Walmart's share of private-label brands is higher than one-third. Smaller companies trying to establish a niche in this crowded market have tended to concentrate on alternative foods (premium, organic, natural) or special diets (kosher, vegetarian, raw). Together, such "natural" products comprise the fastest growing segments of the pet food market, but their fraction of total sales remains below 10 percent in total.

Nestlé Purina PetCare may overpower other pet food companies in the United States, but Mars owns the largest share of the worldwide market. In 2008, the global market for dog and cat food was about $49 billion, as shown in table 3. This means that the United States accounted for one-third of worldwide sales, and Europe as a whole for slightly less ($15 billion). Latin America was the third largest market, accounting for sales of about $6 billion. Canada sold $800 million (Canadian) of dog food alone, 70 percent produced by just four companies: Nestlé Purina, Effem Foods (Mars), Del Monte, and Procter & Gamble.

Table 3
THE FIVE LEADING INTERNATIONAL PET FOOD COMPANIES, 2009*

#	COMPANY, COUNTRY	MARKET SHARE, %	RETAIL SALES, $ BILLIONS
1	Mars Inc., U.S.	26	12
2	Nestlé SA, Switzerland	24	11
3	Procter & Gamble, U.S.	6	3
4	Colgate-Palmolive, U.S.	6	3
5	Del Monte, U.S.	4	2

* Figures rounded off. Source: Global Market Information Database, *Global Market for Pet Food and Pet Care Products* (Chicago: Euromonitor International, 2009).

THE BRANDS

Finally, we get to the brands of dog and cat foods that you might pick up at a grocery store. In table 4, we summarize the results of a survey that asked consumers what brands they buy. The table lists their top five choices of brands of dog and cat foods.

Table 4
LEADING PURCHASES OF PET FOODS REPORTED BY SURVEY RESPONDENTS, 2006

DRY FOOD BRAND (PARENT COMPANY)	% BUYING BRAND	CANNED FOOD BRAND (PARENT COMPANY)	% BUYING BRAND
DOG FOODS			
Pedigree (Mars)	17	Alpo (Nestlé Purina)	27
Ol' Roy (Wal-Mart)	12	Mighty Dog (Nestlé Purina)	13
Kibbles and Bits (Del Monte)	11	Iams (Procter & Gamble)	6
Purina Dog Chow (Nestlé Purina)	11	Hill's Science Diet (Colgate-Palmolive)	5
Iams (Procter & Gamble)	10	Eukanuba (Procter & Gamble)	3
CAT FOODS			
Friskies (Nestlé Purina)	17	Friskies (Nestlé Purina)	39
Purina Cat Chow (Nestlé Purina)	16	9Lives (Del Monte)	29
Meow Mix (Del Monte)	13	Fancy Feast (Nestlé Purina)	30
Iams (Procter & Gamble)	11	Whiskas (Mars)	15
Whiskas (Mars)	7	Iams (Procter & Gamble)	4

Source: Mintel Reports, *Pet Food and Supplies, US* (Chicago: Mintel International Group, August 2008).

Taken together, the information in tables 2–4 provides a broad overview of pet foods as an industry. In researching this book, we were fortunate to have access to libraries that purchased industry research reports containing such details. If we had to buy them on our own, the cost to us would range from $2,500 to $5,000 each. That alone is a barrier to access to information. We have drawn the sales and other figures we quote from multiple sources; they are necessarily rough estimates. This industry puts up other barriers, as well. As we found out through personal experience, it is exceptionally secretive about the way it operates.

A CLOSED SOCIETY

In researching this book, we found ourselves warmly welcomed into some corners of the pet food world but denied access to others, often for reasons that seemed absurdly contrived. In the fall of 2006, for example, we applied to attend a meeting of the Pet Food Institute (PFI). The PFI website provided separate application forms for members and nonmembers, with separate fees for the two categories. We filled out the nonmember forms, sent checks for the nonmember fees, and made airline and hotel reservations well in advance of the meeting. Just before the meeting, we realized we had never received our credentials and called the Institute to ask about them. Oops. Hadn't anyone told us? We were not eligible to attend because we were not members. The nonmember application form? A mistake, apparently. It disappeared from the website the very next day, but reappeared two years later.

A Purina Nutrition Forum did permit us to attend but did not invite us on the participants' tour of Purina's manufacturing facilities. An oversight? When we asked to see the facilities, we were told "not possible." We asked if we could visit other research facilities. No, because of the "competitive nature of the business." One of us (Nestle) personally knows an international vice-president of Purina's parent company, Nestlé. Could he arrange a visit? Unfortunately, not possible.

In contrast, we were invited to—and one of us (Nesheim) did—visit the factory of Chenango Valley Pet Foods, a large private label manufacturer in upstate New York. That gave us a much better idea of how dry pet foods are made. One of us (again, Nesheim) also spent several days visiting Hill's research and canning facilities in Kansas. And both of us were welcomed into Bravo's raw-food manufacturing facility in Connecticut. After hearing of our frustration at lack of access, a friend who holds a senior position at Mars arranged for us to visit the Waltham Centre for Pet Nutrition in England, where the company conducts research on cats and dogs. We were impressed with how well all of these facilities were organized and managed. Their managers must have known they had nothing to hide.

One last story: In 2008, at a Chicago forum run by the trade magazine *Petfood Industry,* we met a representative from Summit Ridge Farms, a pet testing facility in Pennsylvania. She told us that the facility often had visitors and there would be no problem arranging a tour. We quickly arranged a date. A few days before our scheduled arrival, we received an email message from the company's president, Michael R. Panasevich, canceling it: "As a supplier to the pet food industry, my interest would not be served and I would not be able to divulge any additional information concerning our services . . . my clients expect the utmost confidentiality and our reputation depends upon keeping anonymous from any and all public forums and media."

We had no plans to engage in industrial espionage, and were taken aback by these rebuffs. We suspect that some of the secrecy must come from the desire to protect testing facilities from unwanted attention from animal welfare advocates. But companies also would rather not have the public know how pet food is made, and what goes into it. The reasons for this are the subject of the next chapter.

WHAT'S in THOSE PACKAGES?

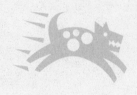

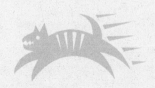

Pet Foods: Wet and Dry

INGREDIENTS IN COMMERCIAL pet foods come in three categories: more or less unprocessed fresh meats and grains, rendered meats and by-products cooked to remove their fat, and food additives—thickeners, preservatives, vitamins, and minerals that come premade or premixed. In this chapter, we go behind the scenes and describe where these ingredients come from and how they are combined into the finished pet food products.

Because the processes for making dry and semi-moist or wet pet foods are so different, dry and wet products are usually made in different factories. That is why manufacturing plants so often co-pack many different brands. Once a factory is set up to make a particular kind of pet food, it can alter the formulas, shapes, and sizes of the products to suit the demands of particular brands. Menu Foods, the Canadian pet food co-packer of canned and pouched foods that was involved in the 2007 recalls, used 1,300 recipes to make 5,000 different lines of dog and cat foods at its plants.

The ingredient at fault in that recall was melamine-laced wheat flour posing as wheat gluten. Menu Foods obtained the false wheat gluten from an American company that imported it from China. If wheat gluten came from China, where do other pet food ingredients come from?

Soon after Menu Foods issued its first recall, we met a pet food company official who agreed to answer that question. His company, which is owned by one of the leading Big Pet Food makers, makes "alternative" products with no by-products, no antibiotics or hormones, and no artificial additives. At the time we met, the company was actively seeking domestic suppliers for its ingredients. But in what he viewed as "testimony to the sad state of our food system," local sources simply did not exist. By this he meant that pet food companies typically bought ingredients from the cheapest sources they could find, regardless of other considerations. He agreed to reveal the source of each of the ingredients listed on the labels of several of his company's complete-and-balanced foods, provided that we did not reveal his name, the name of his company, or the names of the companies that supplied the ingredients in its foods. Even so, the information is instructive, as shown in table 5.

Table 5
SOURCE OF INGREDIENTS IN ONE
"ALTERNATIVE" CAT FOOD, 2007

INGREDIENT	SOURCE
Ocean fish	North American flagships
Chicken	A U.S. poultry supplier
Fish broth	North American flagships
Chicken liver	A U.S. poultry supplier
Brown rice	U.S.
Potato protein	The Netherlands
Carrots	U.S.
Potatoes	U.S., The Netherlands
Minerals	U.S., Canada, Mexico, Brazil
Locust bean gum	Spain, Italy, Portugal
Guar gum	India, Pakistan, Indonesia
Salt	U.S.
Taurine	China, Thailand, Japan
Vitamins	Germany, Switzerland, Denmark, China

Feed your cat this food and it is participating in an international feast. This particular company advertises that its officials personally know the people who produce its meat, poultry, and fish ingredients and that they get the ingredients from very few sources. At that time, the company bought taurine and some vitamins from Chinese suppliers. This company's other products were even more international; their ingredients came from France, Great Britain, Korea, and Switzerland, as well as the other countries listed in the table. As our informant put the matter, finding and monitoring these sources turned out to be a challenge. One constructive outcome of the recalls was to force his and other companies to do a better job of tracking the sources of their ingredients.

With international ingredients in hand, let's take a look at how pet food manufacturers make dry, semi-moist, and wet products.

DRY (10–12 PERCENT WATER)

Dry foods and treats come in many sizes and shapes—baked biscuits, ground meal, pellets, and kibbles—and these are made by distinct processes. In the old days, dog biscuits were baked and dry foods were produced as meal or pellets. Today, with the exception of dog biscuits, which are still largely baked, dry pet foods are extruded. If you have ever used or seen a pasta maker, you know just how this works. You mix ("precondition") ingredients to the right consistency, and force the mix through shaping dies. High moisture ingredients like chicken can be incorporated into dry foods at this preconditioning step; the moisture is removed later on.

Preconditioning and extrusion establish the desired size, shape, and texture of the dry food. Because the processes involve heat and pressure, extrusion cooks the food, kills contaminating microorganisms, and gelatinizes the starch so it is easier to digest. After extrusion, the kibbles are dried. Now the fun begins. The maker sprays the kibbles with additional fat, protein digests, flavor additives, and antioxidants, and gives them another round of drying. At last, the dry foods are packaged, labeled, and shipped.

Although this description makes the manufacturing process sound relatively straightforward, it is not. Kibbles are governed by the requirements of two masters: nutrition and marketing. The ingredients must meet

AAFCO profiles. And they must be formed into shapes, textures, colors, and sizes that please pet owners, who, after all, do the buying. The physical characteristics of dry foods have hardly anything to do with nutritional quality or how eagerly a dog or cat might eat the product. Instead, the form has everything to do with selling the product to pet owners. Dogs and cats could not care less, but people love buying foods in attractive shapes and colors for their pets. The cute shapes and colors are there for *your* pleasure.

SEMI-MOIST (25–35 PERCENT WATER)

Semi-moist foods are the old-style, hamburger-like patties and today's "chubs," tubes of soft, sliceable pet food. These foods are made in extruders in much the same way as dry foods. Because their moisture content is higher, semi-moist foods are more susceptible to microbial contamination; they have to be loaded with preservatives to inhibit the growth of molds and bacteria. To keep the moisture evenly distributed, these foods also contain sugary "humectants" such as glycerin, high fructose corn syrup, maltodextrins (small starches), honey, and table sugars. Some dog foods use propylene glycol as a moisturizer, but this substance can be toxic to cats and is not used in cat food. Chubs have to be wrapped tightly to seal in the moisture, which is why the newer kinds are wrapped in plastic casings. Although popular when first introduced, semi-moist products made up less than 1 percent of pet food sales in 2009.

WET (74–82 PERCENT WATER)

Wet foods are sold in sealed cans or pouches, and making them is no different than canning any other kind of food. Food canning is a science and an art. The science has to do with combining the right ingredients in the right proportions, and sterilizing the final product so it doesn't spoil or make pets sick. The art comes in preparing the ingredients so they will look, smell, and taste good—to owners as well as pets—once the can is opened. Canned pet foods usually begin with relatively low-grade meat trimmings that are reconstituted into pieces that look like chunks of meat. This requires suspending meat particles in gels, heating them so they coagulate into chunks, or using extruded vegetable protein to simulate meat. Some "premium" or "superpremium" pet foods contain actual chunks of meat, but many do not.

With or without actual meat chunks, premium and nonpremium foods must meet the same AAFCO nutrient profiles. But surely the harsh canning and extrusion processes destroy nutrients? Indeed they do, particularly the more fragile nutrients like vitamin C. Heat-induced loss of vitamin C is one reason why nutritionists are always telling humans to eat fresh fruits and vegetables. But dogs and cats don't need vitamin C in their food; they make vitamin C in their own bodies. AAFCO profiles are set high to compensate for nutrient losses that do matter, and pet food makers usually adhere to the profiles.

But back to the canning: canners measure out the slurry into cans, pouches, or trays, seal the packages, and heat ("retort") the packages to temperatures high enough to kill bacteria and their spores. Retorted products are sterile, safe to feed to cats or dogs, and ready to be labeled, packed, and shipped. Because this technology is complicated and requires expensive machinery, it is easier for small manufacturers (and, sometimes, big ones) to contract with co-packers to do the canning.

One final point: manufacturers of dry or wet foods have to be able to track the separate food batches. The lot codes on product labels help them do this. In the 2007 recalls (or in any recall for that matter), when consumers called the companies to complain that pet foods were making their cats or dogs sick, the companies could trace the complaints to particular lot numbers. Menu Foods realized that the wheat gluten it had just obtained from a new supplier must have been at fault because it was the only ingredient that had changed from previous lots.

FORMULATING PET FOOD RECIPES

The job of the pet food formulator—the recipe developer—is to figure out how to combine ingredients that meet AAFCO nutrient profiles in a form that pets are willing to eat and owners are willing to buy. As one pet food maker told us, the finished product has to taste nasty enough for dogs and cats to eat, but look and smell good enough to please owners. And the ingredients cannot cost so much that the product will be too expensive to sell. The formula is the key to all this. Formulators used to work out the details by hand. Today, they use sophisticated computer programs—linear programming—to calculate how much of every ingredient is needed to provide the necessary nutrients at the lowest possible cost.

Formulators begin with a list of specifications for nutrient levels (minimums as well as upper limits), flavor components, and special ingredients. Their computer programs include information about the nutrient composition of pet food ingredients; this comes from standard tables of food composition or from the companies' own information. The programs combine data on nutrient content with information about current costs to produce "least cost" recipes that meet the specifications. Formulators also must deal with moisture and other constraints that affect the texture of the finished products.

But formulators also have to deal with marketing demands. Marketers, for example, like to have meat appear first on the ingredient list, which shows that it is the predominant ingredient by weight. Or they might want a supplement added so the product label can carry a health claim. Vitamins and minerals cause no particular formulation challenges because they are added as a mix in amounts that compensate for losses in processing. This leaves the principal problem in formulating pet foods: combining ingredients to supply protein and calorie needs.

Although the actual recipes for pet foods are closely guarded trade secrets, it is not difficult to make some educated guesses about them. In chapter 10, we explain how to read pet food labels using a Whiskas dry cat food as an example. That food, typical of commercial kibbles, has a relatively uncomplicated formula that includes just four major ingredients that supply calories and protein—corn, chicken by-product meal, corn gluten meal, and animal fat. Should you wish, you can construct a recipe by using the ingredient list and information from the guaranteed analysis section of the food label, which lists protein (30 percent), fat (12 percent), fiber (4.5 percent), moisture (12.0 percent), calcium (1 percent), phosphorus (0.8 percent), and taurine (0.1 percent).

The first step is to find out how much protein and fat are in the principal ingredients. These can be looked up in the handy food composition tables in the 2006 National Research Council report, as summarized in table 6.

Table 6
COMPOSITION OF PROTEIN AND FAT IN WHISKAS DRY CAT FOOD INGREDIENTS, % BY WEIGHT

INGREDIENT	% PROTEIN	% FAT
Corn	9	4
Chicken by-product meal	59	14
Corn gluten meal	56	2
Animal fat	0	100

Source: National Research Council, *Nutrient Requirements of Dogs and Cats* (Washington, DC: National Academies Press, 2006).

While a computer program could figure out in seconds how to combine these ingredients to meet the guaranteed analysis in the proper order on the ingredient list, we did this by trial and error. After several attempts, we came up with the recipe shown in table 7:

Table 7
A GUESS AT THE FORMULA FOR WHISKAS DRY CAT FOOD, % DRY INGREDIENTS BY WEIGHT*

INGREDIENT	AMOUNT, %	PROTEIN PROVIDED BY THE INGREDIENT, %	FAT PROVIDED BY THE INGREDIENT, %
Corn	44	4	2
Chicken by-product meal	30	18	4
Corn gluten meal	15	8	Trace
Animal fat	6	0	6
Minor ingredients: vitamins, minerals flavors	5	1	0
Totals	100	31	12

* Based on the order of appearance in the ingredient list. Protein and fat content derived from nutrient composition tables.

This formula is unlikely to be exactly the same as that of the Whiskas recipe but we think it probably comes close. We are guessing that the lesser ingredients on the ingredient list amount to about 5 percent. You can put together your own formula for meeting AAFCO's nutrient profiles using common household ingredients, as we explain in chapter 21.

The Ingredients

FEDERAL FEED LAWS and AAFCO model regulations call for pet food labels to list all of the ingredients in the product in descending order by weight. But companies do not have to list the amounts of the ingredients, and these also are well-kept trade secrets. We have just shown how to extract a recipe for a pet food from its label. To understand the significance of the other ingredients, we need to make two assumptions. The first is that the most important sources of calories and protein in pet foods are likely to be among the first five ingredients on the list. Second, let's assume that anything that comes after salt on the list is likely to be present in very small amounts—just a pinch or two. To see how this works, let's take a look at the ingredient contents of the dry Whiskas cat food we discuss further in chapter 10.

Ingredients: Ground yellow corn, chicken by-product meal, corn gluten meal, animal fat (preserved with BHA/BHT), natural poultry flavor, wheat flour, rice, brewer's dried yeast, salt, potassium chloride, choline chloride, wheat gluten, turkey by-product meal, caramel color, calcium carbonate, dl-methionine, taurine, minerals (zinc sulfate, copper sulfate, manganese sulfate, potassium iodide), whitefish meal, vitamins (dl-alpha tocopherol acetate [source of vitamin E], folic acid, vitamin A acetate, niacin, vitamin B_{12} supplement, riboflavin supplement [vitamin B_2], vitamin D_3 supplement, d-calcium pantothenate, thiamine mononitrate [vitamin B_1], biotin, pyridoxine hydrochloride [vitamin B_6], red #3, ethoxyquin (a preservative).

Despite the length of this list and the hopelessly confusing parentheses and brackets, this product is typical and not unusually complicated. Its first ingredient—the one present in greatest amount—is ground yellow corn. The next two ingredients are chicken by-product meal and corn gluten meal. These make this product a corn-based food with chicken by-products added. Salt is the ninth ingredient on this list and is a reasonable point at which to divide the items by weight.

THE SALT DIVIDER

The amount of salt in pet foods is a mystery; its amount is not usually listed on package labels. Salt is sodium chloride (40 percent sodium, 60 percent chloride). Although AAFCO profiles deal with both components, excess chloride is rarely a problem. Most attention focuses on sodium because too much of it raises the risk of high blood pressure and its consequences—heart disease, stroke, and kidney disease—in animals as well as people. The AAFCO profile is set at 0.3 percent sodium by weight for dog foods and 0.2 percent by weight for cat foods. Meat ingredients, such as poultry by-product meal, also contribute some sodium, but the amount in grains and vegetables is low. One survey of more than ninety commercial dry dog foods found their average sodium content to be 0.4 percent, a bit higher than the AAFCO standard but not excessive. This 0.4 percent sodium translates to 1 percent salt.

Not knowing the amount of salt can be a problem when pets with heart problems are supposed to be on reduced-salt diets. Tobi, a dog belonging to some friends of ours, had a heart condition. Tobi's veterinarian told our friends to give him foods with a sodium content of less than 0.5 percent. This surprised us, as it translates to 1.25 percent salt—higher than the AAFCO profile and the average amount in pet foods. Our friends wanted to know the salt content of the Royal Canin foods they were using. They wrote the company, and soon heard from the Royal Canin consumer representative: 0.25 percent sodium, an amount well below both the veterinarian's recommendation and the AAFCO profile. They would not need to buy special foods, but their veterinarian had no way to know that.

Because most pet foods use similar formulas, our rule of thumb is that any ingredient that follows salt on the list must make up less than 1 percent of the diet. This has to be true for ingredients like vitamins and trace minerals because only tiny amounts are needed. But turkey by-product meal is the fourth ingredient after salt on the Whiskas ingredient list. Just a pinch of an ingredient is all a pet food maker needs to assure you that its product comes with "tantalizing turkey flavor." Salt is a convenient marker of quantity, and we use it here to distinguish the major ingredients by weight (before the salt) from the minor (after the salt).

AAFCO INGREDIENT DEFINITIONS

The ingredients in commercial pet foods are not random. They are governed by AAFCO model regulations. These call for *every* ingredient in a pet food to be listed on its label, and every ingredient on the label to conform to a specific definition, one approved by AAFCO and recognized by the FDA. The requirement for conformity to definitions is reassuring. Although pet owners may argue about the quality of permitted ingredients, the AAFCO requirements mean that pet food makers may not dump just anything into formulas just because that anything might have some nutritional value. And most states follow AAFCO guidelines, or something like them, for ingredient definitions and labeling.

We learned the importance of AAFCO definitions when we were asked by the Canadian Broadcasting Corporation (CBC) to review a script for an investigative report on pet food that it aired in the wake of the 2007 recalls. In one part of the script, the CBC announcer is speaking with a Canadian veterinarian:

CBC: Old boots, wood shavings, and motor oil. Add some vitamins and minerals and this brew could actually pass a nutrient test. . . . By regulation, pet food labels list the key nutrient values—like protein, fat, and fiber. But it turns out these regulations have big enough holes to drive just about anything through. Old leather work boots can be a source of protein. . . .

VETERINARIAN: Now we need fiber.

CBC: Wood shavings.

VETERINARIAN: The next essential ingredient is fat.

CBC: Crankcase oil is a fatty ingredient. . . . It's a poisonous mixture but our Old Boots pet food meets the required government regulations for the key elements—protein, fat and fiber.

Is this frightening scenario even remotely possible? No way, at least not in the United States. Although the accusation holds a grain of truth, it is only a tiny grain: AAFCO does have an approved definition for leather as an ingredient in pet food:

> **Hydrolyzed leather meal** is produced from leather scrap that is treated with steam for not less than 33 minutes at a pressure not less than 125 pounds per square inch and further processed to contain not more than 10 percent moisture, not less than 60 percent crude protein, not more than 6 percent crude fiber, not more than 2.75 percent chromium, and with not less than 80 percent of its crude protein digestible by the pepsin digestibility method.

This definition firmly excludes indigestible leather processed into boots. We have never seen hydrolyzed leather meal listed on a pet food label, and we doubt state feed control officials would allow it. The requirement for approved AAFCO definitions also firmly excludes the other ingredients. AAFCO does not have an approved definition for either wood shavings or crankcase oil. The FDA considers neither substance to be GRAS (generally recognized as safe), which means that neither is allowed as an ingredient in animal feed. Furthermore, AAFCO requires ingredients to be listed by their common names, and we simply cannot imagine a pet food company listing wood shavings and crankcase oil on its product labels, or any customer buying a food with those items listed on the label. Although we repeatedly pointed out that this scenario was highly unrealistic, the CBC aired the program early in 2008 with the segment unchanged. Journalism like this sows further confusion and is not helpful to owners and their pets.

At a *Pet Food Industry* forum in April 2008, we told this story to Sue Tasa, the official in charge of employee training for Pet Food Express stores in the San Francisco Bay Area. She used to be a sales representative for Hill's Science Diet and immediately recognized the scenario. She told us that she had given similar "Old Shoes" pitches to convince veterinarians and consumers that Science Diet contained higher quality ingredients than your run-of-the-mill supermarket pet food. She and her colleagues argued that a mixture of old shoes, wood chips, and crankcase oil met pet food labeling requirements.

We can think of plenty of reasons to criticize commercial pet food but this isn't one of them. Legitimate concerns about the quality of the ingredients in pet foods are worth bringing to public attention but not this way. With that, let's take a look at what really is in pet food.

BEFORE THE SALT: MAJOR INGREDIENTS

The most important sources of calories and nutrients in pet foods are real foods—the ones that start out as animals and plants with recognizable names. Meat, poultry, fish, grains, vegetables, and, occasionally, fruits invariably appear at the top of pet food ingredient lists.

Animal-Based Ingredients (Fresh)

AAFCO definitions precisely describe the ingredients permitted—and not permitted—in foods for farm animals and pets. AAFCO publishes these definitions in its *Official Publication,* and the 2009 edition includes more than one hundred pages describing approved ingredients, ranging from Alfalfa to Yeast. Animal-based ingredients come in two categories: fresh and rendered. "Fresh" refers to parts of animals used just as they are. "Rendered" means cooked and processed into meals. Here are some official AAFCO definitions for fresh ingredients:

Meat is the clean flesh derived from slaughtered mammals and is limited to that part of the striate muscle which is skeletal or that which is found in the tongue, in the diaphragm, in the heart, or in the esophagus; with or without the accompanying and overlying fat and portions of the skin, sinew, nerve, and blood vessels which normally accompany the flesh.

Poultry is the clean combination of flesh and skin, with or without accompanying bone, derived from the parts or whole carcasses of poultry or a combination thereof, exclusive of feathers, heads, feet, and entrails.

If the meat or poultry comes from just one source, AAFCO says it can be named after that source: lamb, beef, venison, chicken, turkey. These definitions make it clear that meat and poultry ingredients in pet food include parts of animals that are rarely if ever marketed for human consumption. For people, "chicken" means legs, thighs, and breasts or pieces used for chicken nuggets. For pets, however, "chicken" usually means mechanically deboned necks, wings, or racks or frames (the parts of the body left over after most of the meat is removed). Mechanical deboning produces a slurry of leftover meat, fat, and pieces of bone. The livers of food animals have their own definition: "**Animal liver:** if it bears a name descriptive of its kind, it must correspond thereto." Hence: bison liver, chicken liver.

Animal By-products (Fresh)

Although you might consider the backs, necks, racks, and livers of animals to be by-products—and we certainly do—AAFCO does not. It distinguishes, although not always clearly, between fresh meat and poultry and fresh by-products:

Meat by-products are the non-rendered, clean parts, other than meat, derived from slaughtered animals. It includes, but is not limited to, lungs, spleen, kidneys, brain, livers, blood, bone, partially defatted low temperature fatty tissue, and stomachs and intestines freed of their contents. It does not include hair, horns, teeth, and hoofs.

Poultry by-products must consist of non-rendered clean parts of carcasses of slaughtered poultry such as heads, feet, viscera, free from fecal content and foreign matter except in such trace amounts as might occur unavoidably in good factory practice.

If you find the distinction between the animal's meat and its by-products difficult to discern, we do too. We have come to view virtually all pet food ingredients as by-products of human food production. But we understand why the distinction matters. The very idea of by-products can induce queasiness in the strongest of stomachs. Try these approved AAFCO definitions, for example:

Blood meal is produced from clean, fresh animal blood, exclusive of all extraneous materials such as hair, stomach belchings, and urine, except as might occur unavoidably in good manufacturing practices.

Poultry hatchery by-product is a mixture of eggshells, infertile and unhatched eggs, and culled chicks which have been cooked, dried, and ground, with or without removal of part of the fat.

You might be appalled at the idea of feeding such things to your dog or cat or even to your neighboring farmer's pig, but be assured that we have never seen either of these last two ingredients on pet food labels. However you feel, the animals themselves are unlikely to mind. Meat and poultry by-products are highly nutritious and fully capable of supporting animal health. And before rejecting by-products out of hand, consider the ecological implications: if farm animals or pets do not eat animal by-products, those valuable nutrients will go to waste.

Animal Meals (Rendered)

But let's move on to the second class of animal ingredients, the meat meals. AAFCO defines meat or poultry meals as the rendered (cooked to remove the fat and water), dried, and ground products of the original animals.

> **Poultry meal** is the dry rendered product from a combination of clean flesh and skin with or without accompanying bone, derived from parts of whole carcasses of poultry or a combination thereof, exclusive of feathers, heads, feet and entrails.

In practice, poultry meals are made from the backs, necks, and other parts that remain after most of the flesh is removed. Meat or poultry by-product meals are the same, but the starting materials are by-products. Our Whiskas example contains two such ingredients—chicken and turkey by-product meals—in this category:

> **Poultry by-product meal** consists of the ground, rendered, clean parts of the carcass of slaughtered poultry, such as necks, feet, undeveloped eggs, and intestines, exclusive of feathers, except in such amounts as might occur unavoidably in good processing practices.

As with the fresh ingredients, AAFCO allows by-product meals made from one source to be called by that source: chicken by-product meal, for example. Although poultry by-product meal may sound unappetizing, it is rich in nutrients. It contains about 60 percent protein, 14 percent fat, and 15 percent minerals by weight (the rest is water). As we discuss in the next chapter, there is much pressure to produce this material. About 9 billion chickens are slaughtered each year in the United States, providing a vast source of poultry by-products. As pet food companies can easily demonstrate, dogs and cats have no objection to eating rendered meals and by-product meals. Pets like eating foods made with them, and can digest rendered materials quite efficiently.

How nutritious are rendered meals? George Fahey, a researcher at the University of Illinois, says that in his experience poultry by-product meals can be highly nutritious but vary in nutritional value. Some, for example, have more feathers than others and need to be cooked longer to make their nutrients digestible. In one experiment, he compared the benefits of two diets, one of fresh poultry made up of necks, backs, and viscera, to one of poultry by-product meal made from the same parts. The protein in the poultry by-product meal was somewhat less available than the protein in the fresh diet (81 percent compared to 89 percent), but fat was well digested in both. When he repeated the study with beef and beef by-product meals, he found no difference in protein availability. Animal by-products, he says, are good sources of digestible nutrients. Other studies also support this conclusion.

Fish and Fish Meal

AAFCO does not define "fish," but when you see terms in ingredient lists like Tuna, Whitefish, or Ocean Fish, they mostly refer to fish "racks" left over after a gutted fish is filleted or sushi meat is removed, with or without the heads. Fish meals are another matter:

> **Fish meal** is the clean, dried, ground tissue of undecomposed whole fish or fish cuttings, either or both, with or without the extraction of part of the oil.

Fish meal, in contrast to meat and poultry meals, mostly comes from fish caught specifically for that purpose (menhaden, for example) or from "by-catch" fish inadvertently caught by companies fishing for other kinds. The parts left over from processing fish for human consumption also go into fish meals like tuna meal.

If the notion of catching fish to feed farm animals and pets makes you concerned about the environmental waste involved in this practice, pet food is the least of the problems. "Only" 10 percent of the global supply of forage fish is used to feed pets. In comparison, pigs and poultry consume more than 20 percent each. And weirdly, the largest percentage of fish meal goes to feed farmed fish. All of this puts pet food manufacturers into fierce competition for a share of this scarce resource. Ingredient suppliers tell us that as the oceans become even more overfished, menhaden and by-catch fish will become too expensive to feed to pets.

Let's end this part of the discussion with two more examples of typical animal by-product ingredients:

Animal fat is obtained from the tissues of mammals and/or poultry in the commercial processes of rendering or extracting.

As in the case with the by-product meals, if it comes from one source it can be named for the source, which is why you sometimes see poultry fat or chicken fat on food labels.

Animal digest is a material which results from the chemical and/or enzymatic hydrolysis of clean and undecomposed animal tissue.

This last ingredient, unsavory as it may sound, is a key flavoring agent typically sprayed onto dry pet foods to make them taste more like animal flesh so cats and dogs will want to eat them. Animal fat provides calories and the kinds of fatty acids pets need. The Whiskas label notes that animal fat is preserved with BHA and BHT. We discuss these preservatives later in this chapter.

Plenty of research demonstrates that cats and dogs like to eat, can digest, and can use by-product meals, unappealing as they may be for human use. The nutritional value of the meals depends on the parts of the animals that are used and how the materials are rendered. Pet food company officials tell us that since the 2007 recalls, they are working closely with suppliers to obtain better quality ingredients—not so much because they are better for pets but very much because they will be more acceptable to pet food buyers. Rendering, as we discuss in the next chapter, is an important issue in pet food marketing.

Grains and Grain Meals

Although animal by-products are the most common sources of protein in wet pet foods, grain ingredients—mostly corn, rice, and wheat, but sometimes barley and sorghum—usually make up the bulk of the weight of dry commercial dog and cat foods. Many of these plant ingredients are also by-products, but of grain rather than animal processing. For example, brewer's rice—also known as broken or chipped rice—consists of the small fragments of rice kernels that separate out from the larger kernels of milled rice.

As mentioned earlier, the first ingredient on the Whiskas label is ground yellow corn. Corn has some protein and fat—9 percent and 4 percent by weight, respectively—but its major constituent is starch, a complex carbohydrate. While nobody thinks of cats as starch eaters, studies have shown that cats can digest most of the starch from corn, rice, wheat, rye, oats, and sorghum (we say more about the issue of grain feeding in chapter 19). Grinding, cooking, and extrusion improve the digestibility of plant starches, which is exactly how dry pet foods are made. Extrusion heats and gelatinizes the starches, making them more digestible.

Plants have lower proportions of protein than animals so plant-based pet foods need a protein boost, which is where meat and poultry by-product meals come in. Soybeans are a plant exception. The percentage of protein in cooked soybeans is close to that of meat and the percentage is even higher—48 percent—in soybean meal, the residue remaining after the oil is extracted from whole soybeans. Soy flour is finely powdered soybean meal and equally rich in protein. But soybean ingredients do not appear on pet food labels very often. Soybeans tend to produce more poop and gas than owners like (we deal with this problem in chapter 12). We have seen soy ingredients in Ol' Roy dry dog food and Wegmans dry cat food and in canned foods that use soy protein isolate or textured soy to simulate meat chunks. Because soybeans are high in fiber, foods advertised as "low residue" tend to avoid it.

Corn gluten meal is a frequent source of protein in pet foods, and is the third ingredient in the Whiskas product. It is 55 percent protein, and is made by removing the germ and bran and repeatedly washing away the starch.

"Fillers": Binders and Thickeners

Ingredients in either wet or dry pet foods do not naturally stick together, so companies add substances to bind and thicken. These, including grains, are sometimes pejoratively referred to as "fillers," although some have substantial nutritional value. We do not view nutrient-rich grain ingredients as fillers. The Whiskas cat food lists two such ingredients: wheat flour (before the salt) and wheat gluten (after the salt). Wheat flour is 10 percent protein but wheat and rice glutens can be as much as 75 percent protein. These glutens are precisely the ingredients that were adulterated with melamine and caused pets to become ill in 2007.

Pet foods also need some texture and this is the reason you see guar gum, carrageenan, dried kelp, and beet pulp on ingredient lists, usually before the salt. These are gelatinous carbohydrates extracted respectively from guar beans, red seaweed, kelp, and sugar beets. They are mostly soluble fiber and do not have much nutritional value. Hence: fillers.

AFTER THE SALT: MINOR INGREDIENTS

Ingredients that follow salt on the list are added in tiny amounts. Most vitamins and minerals, for example, are required in milligram quantities, which is why nutritionists refer to them collectively as micronutrients. Anything that follows vitamins and minerals on the ingredient list will be present in even fewer milligrams. In the Whiskas ingredient list, whitefish meal appears in the midst of the minerals and vitamins. Don't count on it—or turkey by-product meal—to provide much nutritional value in this product. That is why we so enjoy reading the labels of products like "Prairie Homestyle Beef Stew for Dogs" (Nature's Variety). Here's what follows the mineral mix in its exceptionally long ingredient list: rosemary, artichokes, cranberries, pumpkin, tomato, blueberries, broccoli, cabbage, kale. These sound delicious but we doubt that a can could contain more than a blueberry at most.

Vitamins and Minerals

The Whiskas label lists twelve vitamins. One additional vitamin—vitamin K—is required but not added. Bacteria in the intestines of cats and dogs (and people) make this vitamin in adequate amounts. Vitamins are cheap—many are synthesized in China or other Asian countries—and are typically added as part of a pre-prepared mix of vitamins and minerals. The mix is added to supplement the amounts that are normally present in food ingredients. Usually, vitamins are added at levels three to five times higher than AAFCO profiles to compensate for losses during canning, extrusion, and storage. The AAFCO profile for vitamin A, for example, is 5,000 international units (IU) per kg, but vitamin mixes typically supply 20,000 to 25,000 IU. The AAFCO profile for the vitamin thiamine is one milligram, but a vitamin mix might provide six milligrams.

AAFCO model regulations include recommendations for twelve minerals in foods for both dogs and cats. The mineral mixes contain calcium and potassium in amounts close to that of salt, but other minerals—zinc, manganese, iodine, copper, and selenium—are added in much smaller amounts. The food ingredients provide whatever additional minerals are needed. Minerals are not usually added in excess as they are highly stable and unaffected by cooking, extrusion, light, air, or storage. In great excess, they can be toxic, as happens in occasional manufacturing errors.

Antioxidant Preservatives

Wet pet foods are sterilized during the canning process and have a long shelf life. We bought some canned foods in 2008 stamped with "best by" dates in 2011. Dry and semi-moist foods are expected to stay fresh for up to a year after they are manufactured. AAFCO model regulations do not require manufacturers to put "sell by" or "use before" dates on packages, and such "best by" dates are voluntary or may be required by some state laws. We, of course, think all pet foods should have such dates on them, because it is not unusual for large, opened bags of dry kibble to sit around for a long time. The products do not smell good (to humans) to begin with, and it is sometimes difficult to know if and when they go bad.

The fats sprayed onto dry foods are naturally unstable. So are omega-3 fatty acids. In the presence of light and air, they oxidize and become rancid. Rancidity not only makes them smell and taste bad but also destroys some of the activity of vitamins A and D. To prevent fat oxidation, pet food manufacturers add antioxidants, natural or synthetic. The most commonly used natural antioxidants are vitamin E (tocopherols), vitamin C (ascorbic acid), and citric acid. These are indeed natural substances and nobody has concerns about using them, but they do not preserve fats nearly as well as synthetic antioxidants.

Synthetic antioxidants, however, have a bad reputation, so bad that the labels of alternative pet foods often advertise their absence. A can of Azmira Holistic Animal Care Dog Food, for example, says "We refuse to use any artificial colorings, artificial flavorings, or preservatives." This statement refers to the three synthetic antioxidants approved for use in pet foods: BHT, BHA, and ethoxyquin. Our Whiskas dry cat food example contains all three.

The FDA considers BHA and BHT to be GRAS (generally recognized as safe) in the amounts commonly used. Ethoxyquin is another matter. The FDA has approved the use of ethoxyquin in animal feed, but not in foods for humans (except for certain spices). But the Coast Guard requires it to be used as a preservative during transport of fish meal, and at quite high levels: 400 parts per million (ppm) if the fish meal contains less than 12 percent fat, and 1,000 ppm if it contains more. The Coast Guard has reason to be concerned about fish meal oxidation. Fish meal is so highly susceptible to oxidation that it can heat up, burst into flame, and set ships on fire. Ethoxyquin prevents such disasters. Why ethoxyquin rather than natural antioxidants? It is cheaper and works better. But this means that pet foods containing fish meal are likely to contain traces of ethoxyquin, even if that antioxidant does not appear in the ingredient list.

In the 1980s, the FDA heard reports that ethoxyquin caused pets to develop a long list of problems—itchy skin, lethargy, kidney problems, reproductive disorders, and cancer. It conducted a safety review of ethoxyquin in 1989. The FDA was particularly interested in a study in which dogs were fed ethoxyquin at doses up to 100 milligrams per kilogram (mg/kg) of the animals' body weight. Such high doses caused visible signs of toxicity. But much lower doses, 10 mg/kg of body weight, also caused dogs to develop "mild" cellular changes in their livers and kidneys. The FDA said that a daily intake of 3 mg/kg of body weight caused no observable effects. The FDA translated this dose into an amount in feed that its scientists considered safe: 150 ppm. Quick explanation: mg/kg is the same as ppm but mg/kg is usually used to describe amounts in the body whereas ppm is used for amounts in feed.

Subsequently, Monsanto, the maker of ethoxyquin, reported the results of a five-year study in dogs. Lactating dogs (but no others) fed foods containing amounts of ethoxyquin higher than 150 ppm exhibited a reddish brown pigment in their livers and higher-than-normal levels of liver enzymes in their blood, indicating possible liver damage. The FDA said the damage could have occurred because the lactating dogs were consuming three times as much food as other dogs and, therefore, three times as much ethoxyquin—amounts that were higher than the 150 ppm "safe" level.

In 1997, even though Monsanto's studies showed no problems with ethoxyquin at levels commonly consumed, the FDA asked pet food makers to voluntarily halve the amount of ethoxyquin in their products to no more than 75 ppm. The FDA said: "If new information becomes available that questions the safety of ethoxyquin at 75 ppm in dog food, or shows it to be an effective antioxidant at levels below 75 ppm, CVM [the FDA's Center for Veterinary Medicine] will consider further action." As of mid-2009, the FDA has said nothing further on the subject.

Given this history, it is not surprising that ethoxyquin is viewed with suspicion by Internet commentators, and that concerns about it spill over to BHA and BHT:

> Potentially cancer-causing agents such as BHA, BHT, and ethoxyquin are permitted at relatively low levels. The use of these chemicals in pet foods has not been thoroughly studied, and long-term build-up of these agents may ultimately be harmful. . . . Ethoxyquin has never been tested for safety in cats.

Some authors of books about pet feeding also take a dim view of these substances: "Look for natural preservatives . . . Stay away from BHA,

BHT, and ethoxyquin." In contrast, Donald Strombeck, the author of the popular book *Home-Prepared Diets,* views ethoxyquin as far superior to other antioxidants: "Ethoxyquin is safe as well as effective. . . . Ethoxyquin, more so than any other antioxidant, has anticancer properties. . . . Ethoxyquin can bind carcinogenic chemicals and can bind to enzymes that convert inert chemicals into ones causing cancer."

No doubt as a result of the fuss about it, we do not see ethoxyquin on very many ingredient lists these days. Companies using synthetic antioxidants are mostly using mixtures of BHT and BHA. But pet food makers are increasingly switching to natural antioxidants such as vitamin E (or mixtures of vitamin E tocopherols), even though these may not preserve shelf life as well as the synthetic antioxidants. In September 2009, Whiskas products on store shelves listed ethoxyquin as an ingredient, but the Whiskas labels on the company's Internet site listed BHA, BHT, and tocopherols, suggesting that the company might be planning to phase out use of ethoxyquin at some point.

The Rendered Ingredients

MUCH CONCERN ABOUT what goes into pet foods centers on the use of rendered ingredients. These are worth a closer look. As we already have mentioned, a driving force behind the development of pet foods was the desire to find profitable uses for the by-products of human food production. In 1941, when the United States housed a dog population of 15 million (as opposed to today's 78 million), one veterinarian estimated that more than 37 million acres of land were required to produce food for them. We have no idea where he got this figure or if it is even remotely correct, but it makes an important point. Every one of America's 172 million cats and dogs needs to be fed and their food must come from somewhere. Commercial pet foods do more than just feed cats and dogs. They help to solve the substantial environmental problem created by the waste of human food production.

Consider the numbers of animals slaughtered in the United States for food in 2008: about 3 million sheep, 35 million cattle, 117 million pigs, 264 million turkeys, and 9 *billion* chickens. We do not eat much of the organs and bones—the offal—of these animals even though many of these by-products are just as nutritious as the parts we do eat. By-products account for 49 percent of the weight of cattle, 44 percent of pigs, and 37 percent of chickens. We guess that animal by-products easily add up to 54 *billion* pounds a year in the United States alone. Small amounts of animal waste can be composted, but quantities like this overwhelm any disposal system. None of the obvious disposal options—incineration, burial, and dumping in landfills—is adequate to the task. All are environmentally hazardous, and all are wasteful of useful nutrients.

Instead, practically all slaughterhouse waste is sent to rendering plants to be turned into meals that can be fed to farm animals or pets. The rendering industry takes raw meat and bones from animal slaughter and cooks them to a high temperature that destroys microbes and yields a range of animal by-products: meat-and-bone meal, meat meal and meat by-product meal, poultry meal and poultry by-product meal, blood meal, animal fats, and "tankage" (residues from carcasses, exclusive of hair, hooves, horns, and digestive tract contents). Meat-and-bone meal is rich in protein and bone minerals, especially calcium and phosphorus. By-products are used in commercial feeds for cattle, sheep, pigs, chickens, turkeys, and farmed fish, as well as for pets. The amounts used in pet food are anything but trivial. According to industry statistics, fully one-fourth of rendered animal by-products ends up in pet foods.

The point of the Canadian television program discussed in the previous chapter was to alert the public to the unsavory and potentially unhealthful nature of rendered animal products in pet foods. The idea of pets eating parts of animals that we would not dream of eating can be disturbing. But pets, as we have explained, have always been fed animal by-products and carcass waste, rendered and not (recall those sheep's heads). Only two things have changed since the invention of commercial pet foods: the role of pets in human life and the scale of the rendering operation. Today, many pets are kept indoors where their eating habits are intimately observed. You might be disgusted by the former practice of feeding dogs on butchered horse entrails, but that eating occasion took place outside the home, where you didn't have to look at it.

In researching this book, we gradually came to view rendering as a significant public service. We think it is better—ecologically and nutritionally—to render animal wastes rather than to bury them in landfills, burn them in incinerators, use them as fertilizer, or even, as one critic of the pet food industry suggests (and is actually happening in some places), turn them into biofuels.

Rendered animal meals are highly nutritious feeds for farm animals and pets. Rather than forbidding them, we think it would be much better to set standards for what goes into rendered ingredients. If rendered animal wastes are treated properly and do not contain toxic elements, they ought to be good for the health of the animals that eat them. If such standards existed, concerned pet owners might find it more acceptable to feed rendered by-products to their cats and dogs.

But what about what goes into rendered materials now? The most alarming suspicions are that meat-and-bone meal could be derived from maimed or sick animals, including cows dying of mad cow disease or—even worse in the opinion of many pet lovers—euthanized pets. Let's hold our noses and examine these unsavory possibilities.

DO PETS EAT THE REMAINS OF MAD COWS?

Although it is not impossible that the remains of cows with mad cow disease (bovine spongiform encephalopathy, or BSE) could be rendered into pet food ingredients, we think the probability is now extremely low. Before we explain why, we need to explain what we mean by "not impossible." For this, we must return to AAFCO definitions. Some AAFCO-approved definitions of ingredients derived from animals begin with asterisks:

> *Meat Meal is the rendered product from mammal tissues, including bone, exclusive of any added blood, hair, hoof, horn, hide trimmings, manure, stomach and rumen contents, except in such amounts as may occur unavoidably in good processing practices.

The asterisk refers to this warning statement: "*Use of this ingredient, from mammalian origins, is restricted to non-ruminant feeds unless specifically exempted. . . . Feeds containing prohibited material must bear the following label statement: 'Do not feed to cattle or other ruminants.'"

Cows are ruminants. Dogs and cats are not. Ingredients marked with asterisks are permitted in pet food. Meat meals made from cattle and cow by-products display asterisks because they could transmit mad cow disease, so called because it makes cows behave peculiarly. This disease, which is similar to scrapie in sheep and Creutzfeld-Jakob disease in people, is invariably fatal; it progressively destroys the brain and nervous system. In the 1990s, an epidemic of BSE among cattle in Great Britain led to the destruction of about five million cows and caused the death of about 150 people unlucky enough to have eaten meat from cows sick with the disease. Dogs did not "catch" BSE, but some cats did. The British epidemic involved the death of eighty-nine cats that presumably ate pet foods made from by-products taken from cows sick with BSE.

BSE is an unusual disease. It and its human, cat, and other variants are believed to be caused by abnormally folded proteins—"prions"—in the brain and nervous system. The BSE epidemic still lacks a full explanation, but here is one of the more prevalent ideas about its origin: cows "caught" prions from inadequately rendered meat-and-bone meal made from sheep infected with scrapie, and sheep prions transformed into prion proteins that could infect cows. More cows got sick when they were fed inadequately rendered meat-and-bone meals from infected cows. Prions, it turns out, are not destroyed by the usual methods for rendering slaughterhouse waste. Once the British government banned the feeding of rendered sheep and cow meals to cows, the epidemic ended. Few cases have been found in cows, and none in cats, in Great Britain since 2001.

In the United States, two agencies deal with BSE—the FDA and USDA. The FDA banned the feeding of meat meals derived from mammals to ruminants in 1997. But it continued to allow mammalian meals to be fed to nonruminants—pigs and chickens, as well as dogs and cats—although with some restrictions. The meat meals must come from countries free of BSE and must not contain brains and spinal cords of animals older than thirty months (those most at risk of BSE). All animals must have passed inspection for human use. But brains and spinal cords can still be rendered into animal feed—and, therefore, pet food—if they come from younger cattle. On its part, the USDA routinely tests for BSE in a fraction of cows headed for slaughter and it restricts imports of older cattle. In May 2008 the USDA banned the slaughter of "downer" cattle, those unable to walk (a symptom of possible BSE). These measures, if followed, should keep high-risk cattle out of rendered meals.

Federal agencies cite these measures as the reason why we have not seen BSE in American cows. With the exception of several older cows imported from Canada, no cases of BSE have been found in the United States, and no variants of BSE have been found among younger cows, people, or cats. But not every cow is tested for BSE, and critics cite numerous examples of violations of bans on imports and the kinds of by-products that go into rendering. In one especially relevant situation, shipments of animal by-products from prohibited countries somehow got into the United States. The FDA said nobody needed to worry; the by-products went into pet food, not into the human food supply. Oh.

That was in 2001. In 2002, the General Accounting Office (now the Government Accountability Office) issued a strong critique of what it viewed as glaring gaps in the oversight system: "While BSE has not been found in the United States, federal actions do not sufficiently ensure that all BSE-infected animals or products are kept out or that if BSE were found, it would be detected promptly and not spread to other cattle through animal feed or enter the human food supply." In 2007, the FDA Science Board wrote that the FDA has been "denied funds that would bring the feed industry into compliance with new regulations. . . . To this day, the BSE research program . . . remains seriously underfunded."

So where does that leave us with pets? Dogs have not yet been found with prion diseases, although many other animals get them. Beyond prions, we are not aware of any other infectious particles or organisms that can survive the rendering process. We cannot be 100 percent certain that rendered ingredients are free of prions, but we think they probably are. If prions from mad cows were getting into cat food, some cats would have shown symptoms by now. To our knowledge, no U.S. cats have been reported with variants of mad cow disease. Nevertheless, we wish federal agencies required much broader testing for this disease, and did a better job of controlling the parts of animals that go into rendered materials. This is a food safety issue that affects people and farm animals, as well as pets, and is another reason for our contention that we have only one food supply.

DO PETS EAT PETS IN PET FOOD?

It would never have occurred to us to ask this question except that the Internet is full of warnings that commercial pet foods contain the rendered remains of euthanized cats and dogs. One source of this idea is a popular book by the journalist Ann Martin.

> As this third edition of *Food Pets Die For* goes to press, cats and dogs from shelters and veterinary clinics throughout the United States and Canada are still being rendered to make a protein source called "meat meal." Rendering plants then sell this meat meal to pet food manufacturers. It is still legal to render dog and cat carcasses, along with a variety of other animal remains . . . to make a protein source for pet food.

Yes this is still legal, but could it really be happening? While rendering pet carcasses into meat meal most certainly occurred in the past, we think it increasingly unlikely that this practice continues in the United States. Let's start with some unarguable facts. Most meat meals are made from the by-products of animals used to produce human food. And yes, about half of all livestock that die from disease or other causes in the United States—more than three billion pounds annually—also end up in rendering plants. So do the carcasses of roadkill as well as those of dogs and cats. But these deceased animals are not necessarily rendered together. In a somewhat less than comforting statement, the industry says that its typical practice is to render slaughterhouse by-products into animal feed but to render other dead animals into fertilizer.

Like farm animal by-products, dead pets confront society with a difficult disposal problem. One deceased pet is relatively easy to bury. Our small lot in upstate New York came with a gravestone marking the place where a previous owner laid Rusty to rest on May 16, 1966. Rusty, to judge by the portrait etched into the stone, was an especially cheerful cocker spaniel, and we keep his memorial site free of debris and planted with flowers.

But the number of dogs and cats that die and require disposal each year would overwhelm anyone's backyard. The total is not known, but one hint comes from the American Society for the Prevention of Cruelty to Animals (ASPCA), which reports five to nine *million* dogs and cats euthanized annually by its shelters alone. This number, enormous as it is, does not account for pets that die at home of natural causes, under the care of a veterinarian, or in animal hospitals. What happens to the remains of these pets, as we soon discovered, is something nobody likes to talk about.

Considerable evidence suggests that dead pets used to be—and perhaps still are—rendered into meat meals or fertilizers. In the early 2000s, reporters in several cities became aware that dead pets were sent to rendering plants. In St. Louis, for example, a local television station filmed a truck pulling up to a rendering plant. The truck sign said, "Serving the Pet Food Industry." For more than thirty years—as a public service— this company had been accepting euthanized dogs and cats from local shelters and delivering them to be rendered. The resulting uproar ended that service, causing the city to send the dead animals to a landfill until it could build an incinerator. As recently as 2004, Los Angeles sent 112,000 dead cats and dogs to rendering plants. In commenting on this practice, one editorial writer said:

> Gruesome, definitely. News, hardly. The grim practice of rendering animals is not new, as anyone who grew up on the farm can attest. Rendering animals, large and small, is a highly efficient and environmentally sound way to recover useful protein, fats, gelatins and other products, not to mention recovering a few bucks. They don't send horses to the glue factory for nothing.

At about that time, the FDA's Center for Veterinary Medicine weighed in on the controversy with a report on the pentobarbital content of dog food. Pentobarbital is the drug most often used for euthanizing dogs, cats, cattle, and horses. If euthanized animals are rendered, this drug could get into animal feed and pet food. The FDA tested dog foods for pentobarbital and found it in many samples, but at extremely low levels (the highest was 0.032 ppm). The foods most likely to contain pentobarbital indeed were those with rendered ingredients such as meat meals and animal fat as the main ingredients.

The FDA concluded that the amounts of pentobarbital were too low to cause harm to pets eating those foods. Fine, but that's not really the question. What we want to know is whether the pentobarbital came from euthanized pets. To answer this question, FDA scientists tested foods and feed for mitochondrial DNA characteristic of dogs and cats as well as of cows, pigs, sheep, goats, deer, elk, and horses. Among thirty-one samples, they identified DNA from cows and pigs in twenty-seven. But they did not find dog or cat DNA in even one sample. The testing, the FDA said, was sensitive enough to detect five pounds of rendered remains in fifty tons of finished feed. On this basis, the FDA scientists concluded that "the source of pentobarbital in dog food is something other than proteins from rendered pet remains." We are hugely relieved by this result, even though it tells us that some euthanized animals end up as feed, not fertilizer.

As you might imagine, trying to get a handle on the pet rendering situation is not easy. We began by asking representatives of health departments in several cities to tell us how they dispose of dead pets and roadkill. Most simply did not know. One health official in California, who for obvious reasons requested anonymity, said:

> After exploring and rejecting various possibilities like the County Hospital cafeteria and the school lunch program, we determined that the animals are kept in cold storage at the animal control site and shelter. Once a week they are picked up by a truck from a rendering company, in this case, Koefran Industries in Sacramento. About what happens next, it is outside my county and we know nothing, nothing. . . .

An Internet search for Koefran Industries made it clear that this company collects dead animals from any number of California counties, but then what? The company runs an incinerator facility as well as a rendering plant. We called Koefran and asked what they did with the pet remains they collected from shelters. These, we were told, were either cremated or disposed of by group burial.

We also asked shelter representatives what happened to their deceased charges. Officials of the Humane Society told us that they thought most euthanized pets were cremated. An SPCA no-kill animal shelter in Ithaca, New York, sends its remains to a facility at the Cornell University veterinary school, where animal carcasses and wastes are steam sterilized, treated with lye, and sent to a wastewater plant to be converted to methane gas for generating electricity.

A representative of another rendering company told us that his company used to accept the remains of pets years ago—the company was located right next to an animal shelter—but has not done so since the early 1980s. Pet food companies insist that their meat by-products do not contain rendered pets. Overall, we do not see much evidence that the practice continues. Like the situation with BSE, it is possible that some pets are rendered into pet foods, but we see few signs of this happening and we think it increasingly unlikely. Score this as a win for pet advocates.

As for the alternatives, conversion to methane requires expensive equipment and neither incineration nor landfills are environmentally sound solutions to the disposal problem. Among other troubling effects, dumping euthanized carcasses in landfills can poison wildlife. Deaths among eagles and other birds feeding on landfill carcasses have been ascribed to the pentobarbital used to kill the animals. For owners who are disgusted by the mere idea of pets eating pets, alternative pet foods offer a welcome choice. As we will see, the "yuck factor" plays a big role in modern pet food marketing. Marketers know that some pet owners do not want to feed anything to their dogs and cats that they would not themselves be willing to eat. As we demonstrate in chapter 12, the makers of certain premium and alternative pet foods use the absence of rendered ingredients as a marketing tool. They advertise their products as made with "no rendered meats or fats" and "no animal by-products." If a product says that on a label, can you believe it? We address that issue next.

Who Sets Pet Food Rules?

THE PET FOOD industry is fond of saying that pet foods are better regulated than human foods. The Pet Food Institute says: "Pet foods are one of the most highly regulated food products. They are required by law to provide on their labels more information than most human foods . . . regulation of pet foods is the same as human foods."

Well, not quite. In our judgment, the regulation of pet foods is severely constrained by the lack of genuine federal authority. Oversight of pet foods is shared—not always smoothly—among three entities: the FDA, the feed control officials in individual states, and the Association of American Feed Control Officials (AAFCO). It is not easy to explain how oversight works in practice because the system is so complicated. The FDA has some, but not much, authority over pet food. States devise their own rules. AAFCO, an organization of state and FDA officials in partnership with industry, develops model regulations for states to use: these, however, are voluntary unless incorporated into state law. The three groups work together to develop and enforce uniform standards throughout the country, and most officials involved in these groups think the system works pretty well. We have our doubts.

THE FDA'S ROLE

The FDA's authority over pet foods comes from the Federal Food, Drug, and Cosmetic Act, which defines food as "articles used for food or drink for man or other animals. . . ." Since ingredients in farm feeds could leave residues in meat and milk and get into the human food supply, the law gives the FDA the authority to regulate ingredients in animal feed as well as those in pet foods. The FDA exerts its authority through the rules laid out in the 1977 Code of Federal Regulations. These deal in extraordinary detail with, among other such matters, the misbranding (meaning mislabeling) of feed for farm animals. Besides specifying minute details of font sizes and the location of information on package labels, the code requires feed labels to properly identify only three items: (1) the product, (2) the name and address of the manufacturer, and (3) the name of every ingredient in the product "in descending order of predominance by weight." Federal rules leave everything else to the discretion of the states. Although entirely unmentioned in the code, pet food labels are expected to follow the rules for those for animal feed.

The FDA's job is to enforce federal regulations but its role in pet food oversight is rather limited. In carrying out its multiple missions, the FDA clearly distinguishes oversight of food for people from that of farm animals and pets; it oversees foods for these groups through two distinct units. The FDA's Center for Food Safety and Applied Nutrition (CFSAN) regulates human food, whereas the Center for Veterinary Medicine (CVM) is in charge of animal feed and pet food. The CVM monitors feed contaminants, oversees the labeling of feed contents, and approves the safety of feed additives. In general, the CVM applies the same rules to pet foods as it does to animal feed.

THE STATES' ROLE

Individual states conduct much of the day-to-day regulation of pet foods. About half the states have adopted AAFCO model regulations and incorporated their provisions into the feed laws. This means, of course, that half the states have *not* adopted the model standards. But the nonadopted states expect pet food companies to follow the AAFCO models anyway.

As long as companies do, they can market their products anywhere in the United States without getting into trouble with federal or state feed control officials. Although AAFCO views the laws of the states that have adopted the model regulations as "fairly uniform," they are not uniform and cannot be. For one thing, as AAFCO president Ricky Schroeder explained to us in 2008, the organization is continually tinkering with the model regulations. Constant tinkering means that no state law can keep up with the changes and none ever completely conforms to the AAFCO models. The inconsistencies cause problems for pet food companies, particularly when companies make claims for the health benefits of their products that fall under state or federal "regulatory discretion." Regulatory discretion (as we explain later) leaves it up to the states or the FDA to decide on a case-by-case basis whether a particular rule is worth the trouble to enforce.

Pet food manufacturers complain about the inconsistencies in requirements and enforcement levels from one state to another. Some states, such as Colorado, Kentucky, New Mexico, and Texas, are vigilant in enforcing state standards for farm animal feed and pet foods. Others, such as California, Florida, and Nevada, are reputed to be less vigilant. Some state regulators conduct laboratory tests on pet food samples to make sure the contents are consistent with label guarantees; others do not. The New York State Department of Agriculture and Markets, for example, has an impressive laboratory that analyzes about five hundred samples of animal feeds and pet foods annually, but this level of oversight is unusual.

AAFCO'S ROLE

As we mentioned earlier, state officials responsible for enforcing the feed laws got together to form AAFCO in 1909. A principal motive for forming the association was to resolve some of the problems caused by the lack of uniformity in state regulations. AAFCO was and is a voluntary, nonprofit corporation. Its membership consists of state and federal officials in charge of implementing feed laws, and researchers who conduct studies on animal feeds. Of the three entities—the FDA, the states, and AAFCO—AAFCO is the only one that deals with pet foods directly. It does so through its long-standing pet food committee, first appointed in 1956.

The pet food committee of AAFCO began issuing reports in 1961 and produced the first set of model regulations in 1968. These called for the ingredients to be listed in descending order by weight, for foods to be named in certain ways, and for other food labeling provisions that are now generally accepted. The committee added "complete and balanced" to the model regulations in 1970 to indicate that the nutrient contents of pet foods met the recommendations of the National Research Council. It added feeding protocols to demonstrate the nutritional adequacy of pet foods in 1982 and introduced its own more generous nutrient profiles in 1994.

During this half century, the AAFCO model regulations gained more and more supporters. The regulations were endorsed by the American Feed Industry Association, the National Grain and Feed Association, and the Pet Food Institute, and, as noted, were adopted by about half the states. In developing and tweaking the model regulations, AAFCO works closely with the FDA, and an FDA official sits on the AAFCO board of directors in an advisory capacity.

AAFCO also works closely with the pet food industry. In 2009, the pet food committee consisted of ten members, three of them FDA officials and the others state feed control officials. Like other AAFCO committees, the pet food committee has its own trade advisory group. AAFCO says, "It is the general practice of AAFCO to invite representatives of industry/trade associations and consumer groups to serve as advisors." These representatives are "to be available to answer questions relevant to animal nutrition, analytical expertise, industry practices or other pertinent questions." Advisors sit in on committee meetings, but are not supposed to vote. For the pet food committee, advisors outnumber the actual committee members; the ten advisors and four alternates mainly represent industry and veterinary groups such as the Pet Food Institute, the American Pet Products Association, and the Canadian Veterinary Medical Association. Since 2008, as a consequence of the 2007 pet food recalls, the advisory group includes a consumer representative from the organization Defend Our Pets, which advocates for more rigorous oversight of pet foods.

DOES THE SYSTEM WORK?

From an outsider's point of view (ours, in this instance), the framework for regulation of pet foods seems to be exceptionally messy, with responsibilities divided between federal and state agencies, each with its own conflicting or nonexistent rules and regulations. AAFCO attempts to mediate between federal and state authorities and the pet food industry. The resulting gaps and overlaps in regulatory authority have become more evident as the pet food industry has evolved from a small sideline of large companies producing animal feed to an exceedingly profitable enterprise on its own.

The lack of federal authority to resolve regulatory inconsistencies was thoroughly exposed by the 2007 pet food recalls. The FDA, for example, could not order companies to recall pet foods containing melamine-tainted ingredients. Recalls were voluntary and entirely up to the discretion of the manufacturer. Pet owners demanded greater federal involvement in pet food regulation and Congress responded, to some extent. Late in 2007, Congress directed the FDA to consult with AAFCO, veterinary medical associations, animal health organizations, and pet food manufacturers—precisely the membership of the Pet Food Committee and its advisors—to establish federal standards for ingredient definitions, content standards, and labeling requirements. Although these directives sound much like business as usual, the legislation appeared to recognize for the first time that pet foods differ from animal feed and that more specific federal authority over their contents and labels would be helpful, if not essential. But nothing much happened until 2009, when Congress considered bills giving the FDA greater authority over food safety.

The 2007 legislation also directed the FDA's parent agency, the Department of Health and Human Services, to establish an early warning and surveillance system for identifying episodes of adulteration and outbreaks of illness associated with pet food. This made sense. Pet food companies issue recalls on a regular basis, and the FDA regularly sends warning notices to pet food companies about potentially dangerous products.

In 2008 alone, the FDA warned about illnesses in dogs caused by Chinese chicken jerky, announced voluntary recalls by Mars Petcare of products contaminated with *Salmonella*, seized foods at a PETCO distribution center infested by rodents and other pests, and ordered an Evangers plant in Illinois to correct potentially dangerous processing failures before it would be allowed to send canned foods into interstate commerce. Such incidents show no signs of stopping.

One in particular illustrates why a better system of pet food oversight is needed, if for no other purpose than to restore trust. In May 2009, Nutro Products (Mars) announced a voluntary recall of several lines of dry cat foods because their vitamin pre-mix contained incorrect levels of zinc and potassium as the result of a manufacturing error. This would not have attracted much notice except that it occurred after two years of consumer complaints that cats were getting sick or dying after eating Nutro Foods. Just because a cat gets sick after eating a food does not necessarily mean that the food is responsible for the illness. But when neither Nutro nor the FDA appeared to investigate, more than eight hundred cat owners filed complaints with ConsumerAffairs.com, a web-based group that solicits information about such problems.

ConsumerAffairs.com filed a Freedom-of-Information Act request for FDA documents related to Nutro complaints, but reported that the FDA refused to release them because doing so would "interfere with enforcement proceedings." At that point, as the *San Francisco Chronicle* pet columnist Christie Keith put it, "what had been a fairly low-level story . . . suddenly became one of the hottest pet topics on the Internet among pet lovers already sensitized to food safety issues from the pet food recalls of two years earlier." Although an independent group tested Nutro foods and claimed that zinc levels exceeded 2,100 mg/kg (the AAFCO profile is just 75 mg/kg), Nutro continued to deny that anything was seriously wrong with its products, and the FDA remained silent. Pet owners could only conclude that neither government nor industry was looking out for their interests. Christie Keith again: "There's a much bigger story here. The FDA works for us. We pay its bills. And it's supposed to ensure the safety of the American food and drug supply for both people and animals."

As we argue throughout this book, we only have one food supply and it must be safe for all eaters. A food safety system that protects pets should also protect people, and vice versa. A better system would be similar to the one for humans run by the Centers for Disease Control and Prevention, and would nudge pet food regulation closer to that of human food. The 2007 legislation did not give the FDA the power to recall tainted products. Instead, it called for the FDA to work with pet food companies and interested organizations to enhance the quality and speed of communication with the public during a recall. When we asked FDA officials why Congress hadn't passed a stronger law, they told us that this was the best that could be expected in the 2007 political climate. Legislation introduced under the new administration in 2009 was expected to improve food safety. Pet foods, like human foods, are subject to politics.

COMMERCIAL PET FOODS:
The MARKET

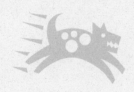

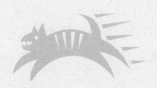

What's on Those Labels?

READING A PET food label is no simple task. Pet food labels do not look like the labels on food products meant for humans. For one thing, they follow the rules for animal feed, not human food. This, as we explain in appendix 3, is a result of the messy history of feed regulations, federal laws overseen by the FDA, model regulations developed by AAFCO, and laws passed by individual states. Pet food companies also put things on labels that are not necessarily covered by rules and regulations. Fortunately, most companies design their labels to be consistent with guidelines produced by AAFCO.

The labeling guidelines take up an astonishing sixty-four pages of very fine print in AAFCO's 2009 *Official Publication,* but even that is not enough room to explain the rules. In 2008, AAFCO published a separate looseleaf binder packed with examples meant to explain how to interpret the labeling guidelines. These guidelines specify the font, placement, and order in which information appears on the label as well as items of much greater interest, such as what is actually in the food and its nutrient content. All of this is so difficult to understand that the FDA publishes its own guide to pet food labels.

Even so, hardly anyone can make sense of them. Surveys report that just 49 percent of pet owners and an even smaller percentage of veterinarians (39 percent) think the nutrition information on pet food labels is easy to understand. We are surprised that the percentages are so high. Figuring out what the labels mean is no task for the fainthearted, as we now explain.

In 2008, we bought a package of Whiskas Meaty Selections™ dry cat food, a bestselling brand, to use as an example of a label that conforms to AAFCO guidelines. Its front panel is shown in figure 5. The label displays several of the required elements: what the product is, what kind of pet is supposed to eat it (Food for Cats & Kittens), and the package weight (net wt 1 lb, 454 grams). On this label, the name and address of the manufacturer (Masterfoods, a Division of Mars, Vernon, CA) appear on the back of the package, as shown in figure 6.

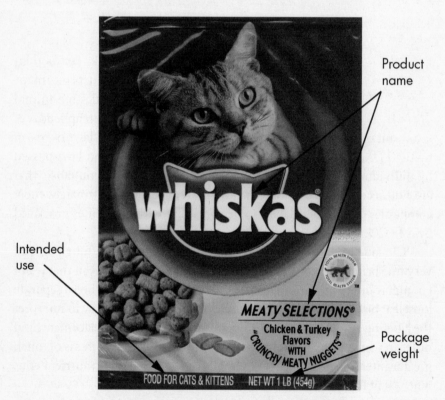

FIGURE 5
This package design conforms to AAFCO labeling guidelines.

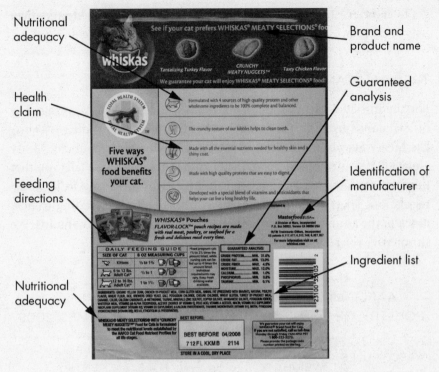

FIGURE 6

The back panel of this package complies with specific AAFCO guidelines.

Beyond these minor details, the labeling issues get much more complicated. AAFCO model regulations call for five components to be on package labels:

- The brand and product name
- A statement of guaranteed analysis
- A statement of nutritional adequacy
- Feeding directions
- The list of ingredients in descending order by weight

The Whiskas label also displays claims for the product's health benefits. AAFCO model regulations do not say much about health claims, but they are a key factor in marketing. In some situations, but not this one, AAFCO also calls for labels to list the calorie content of the products. We get to calories later in chapter 15. We have already discussed ingredient lists in chapter 7. Here, we examine the first four label elements.

THE BRAND AND PRODUCT NAME

For the initiated, the names of pet foods are deep with meaning. The official name given on the front panel of the Whiskas product is Whiskas Meaty Selection Chicken and Turkey Flavors with Crunchy Meaty Nuggets. If you are in on the AAFCO guidelines, the name tells you that this food contains practically no meat, chicken, or turkey. AAFCO model regulations specify the precise wording of the name according to how much of the animal-based ingredients the product actually contains. We summarize the rules in table 8.

Table 8

AAFCO MODEL REGULATIONS FOR USE OF ANIMAL, POULTRY, OR FISH INGREDIENTS IN PET FOOD NAMES, 2009

AAFCO RULES	MINIMUM INGREDIENT WEIGHT, %	TYPICAL LABEL STATEMENTS
The 100% rule	100% (except for minor additives and water used in processing)	All-tuna cat food; all-beef dog food; 100% venison
The 95% rule	At least 95% (70% if water is used for processing)	Tuna cat food; beef dog food
The 25% rule	At least 25% (10% if water is used for processing); requires descriptor that implies the presence of other ingredients	Chicken dinner (or entrée, recipe, or formula)
The 3% rule	At least 3%; requires "with" or "contains"	Contains tuna; made with real beef
The flavor rule	Source must be given in the ingredient list	Meaty; chicken flavor

From the name alone, you can tell that the flavor rule applies (meaty chicken and turkey flavors, meaty nuggets). To know the source of the flavors, you must go to the ingredient list. As we have seen, the flavors in this product come from chicken by-product meal, natural poultry flavor, and turkey by-product meal. Chicken and turkey meat comprise less than 3 percent of the total ingredients. Otherwise, the name would say "contains" or "made with." Poultry by-product meal does not count as chicken or turkey meat.

Our example is a dry food, but canned pet foods are about 80 percent water, which means that only about 20 percent is real food (some water comes with the meat itself). A product labeled "100 percent Venison," for example, is just that: venison and water and, perhaps, trace amounts of preservatives, flavorings, or spices. Canned 95 percent turkey must contain at least 70 percent turkey. Under the 25 percent rule, a canned chicken dinner must contain chicken as 10 percent of the total product weight. The moral: read the ingredient list.

THE GUARANTEED ANALYSIS

The AAFCO label guidelines say pet foods must list the guaranteed content—minimum or maximum—for "crude" protein, fat, and fiber, and water. Crude, in this context, does not, as you might think, refer to the quality of the ingredients; it refers to the testing method. The particular requirements of the guaranteed analysis have existed virtually unchanged for the last century. By the 1920s, most state feed laws required such lists on feed sacks.

The guaranteed analysis gives you some idea of the nutritional adequacy of the product. This idea, for the most part, appears to be reasonably close to reality. In an analysis of 2,200 wet and dry pet foods made by two hundred companies, investigators found that the measured contents of guaranteed nutrients differed from the guaranteed analysis by an average of no more than 1.5 percent. Although this difference is trivial, the range of differences was not. At the extremes of protein measurement, for example, some samples had 14 percent less than the guarantee, while others had 34 percent more. Such findings make us think that a better nutrition labeling system is essential, along with better oversight.

The guaranteed analysis tells you nothing about the sources of the protein, fat, and fiber (for that information you must check the ingredient list), and does not mean much except by comparison to standards of nutrient intake. These, as we have explained, come from two sources:

the National Research Council's (NRC) research-based recommended allowances for the levels of nutrients a pet requires for health, and AAFCO's practice-based nutrient profiles for growth, reproduction, and adult maintenance. The Whiskas Meaty Selections is designed for cats at *all life stages*. Since it is difficult to see in the figure, we reproduce its guaranteed analysis in table 9:

Table 9
GUARANTEED ANALYSIS, WHISKAS MEATY SELECTIONS

SUBSTANCE	MINIMUM OR MAXIMUM	% BY WEIGHT
Crude protein[a]	Minimum	31.0
Crude fat[a]	Minimum[b]	13.0
Crude fiber[a]	Maximum	4.5
Moisture[a]	Maximum[c]	12.0
Calcium	Minimum	1.0
Phosphorus	Minimum	0.8
Taurine	Minimum	0.1

a. Required by AAFCO model regulations; other guarantees are voluntary. b. A maximum guarantee also is required when the label says a product is "lean," "lite," or contains less fat. c. The maximum moisture allowed is 78% except for stews, gravies, and sauces; moisture is low in dry foods like this one.

Crude protein

"Crude" measurements give an indication of the amounts of nutrients present based on certain analytical methods. The method for measuring protein, for example, does not really measure protein; it measures the nitrogen content and compensates for the amount of nitrogen in an average protein (this was the situation that created the pet food recalls of 2007; melamine is 67 percent nitrogen and appears on testing to be protein). An average protein is about 16 percent nitrogen by weight. To estimate the amount of protein in a food, you multiply its amount of nitrogen by 6.25 (which is 100/16). Hence: crude.

For the Whiskas cat food, Mars guarantees that protein makes up at least 31 percent of the weight. Is this high or low? To figure this out, you need to consult the NRC's recommended allowances for the protein requirements of cats of various ages and compare them to AAFCO's more generous nutrient profiles. As shown in table 10, the NRC says adult cats need diets containing 20 percent protein. To this amount, AAFCO adds a safety factor that takes into consideration the cat's ability to digest, absorb, and use the protein, and the needs of most cats in the population. Like the Meaty Whiskas, products formulated for all life stages must use the *highest* AAFCO amount, in this case the one for cats that are growing, reproducing, and lactating—30 percent. Whiskas makes it 31 percent protein.

Table 10
RECOMMENDED PROTEIN ALLOWANCES FOR
CATS, % DRY INGREDIENTS BY WEIGHT

LIFE STAGE	NRC RECOMMENDED ALLOWANCE	AAFCO NUTRIENT PROFILE
Kittens after weaning	22.5	30.0
Adult maintenance	20.0	26.0
Pregnant adult cats	21.3	30.0
Lactating adult cats	30.0	30.0

Sources: National Research Council, *Nutrient Requirements of Dogs and Cats* (Washington, DC: National Academies Press, 2006). *AAFCO Official Publication,* 2009. Both recommendations are for a diet with 4,000 calories per kilogram of food (about 1,800 calories per pound).

The amount of protein in this product may be more than sufficient, but what about its quality? For proteins, quality refers to the balance of constituent amino acids. Proteins are made up of twenty amino acids, about half of which dogs, cats, and humans make on their own. Because the others have to be eaten, they are called *essential.* Human requirements for essential amino acids are the same as those for pets, with only one exception: the amino acid arginine. Pets need it in their diets; we don't.

Quality refers to how well the proportions of essential amino acids in a protein match the amino acid needs of the animal to which it is fed. In general, meat proteins have an amino acid composition more like the animals that are eating them; their quality is considered higher. But the essential amino acids in corn, wheat, rice, and soybeans are exactly the same as the essential amino acids in chicken or beef. It is just that plants don't have as much of some of them. That is why manufacturers sometimes add essential amino acids—most often lysine and methionine—to the formulas of pet foods made largely from grains.

In an animal's body, proteins are major components of muscles, bones, enzymes, and hormones. They have the same kinds of functions in plants. When your dog eats meat or grains, digestive enzymes in its intestine disassemble proteins into their constituent amino acids. These are quickly absorbed and used to make body proteins or, if in excess, broken down to release energy.

Getting pets (or humans) to eat enough protein is no big deal. A mixture of protein sources—even from plants—provides plenty of amino acids, essential and not. In general, cats need more protein for their weight than dogs, perhaps because they use protein less efficiently. Just as with cat foods, dog foods formulated to meet the needs of all life stages have a guaranteed protein analysis that exceeds the NRC recommendations and reflects the highest AAFCO standard for the protein needs of a dog producing milk for her puppies.

Crude Fat

Dogs and cats can digest fats of any kind quite well and often prefer foods that taste fatty. Crude fat measures the amount of fatty components extractable from food by certain solvents. This measure gives the total amount of fat but says nothing about its type—whether it is saturated, unsaturated, or polyunsaturated, or omega-3 or omega-6.

All food fats—no exceptions—are mixtures of saturated, unsaturated, and polyunsaturated fatty acids. The differences are in the proportions. Meat fats have more saturated fatty acids; vegetable fats are more polyunsaturated. The degree of saturation matters because in humans diets high in saturated fats raise levels of blood cholesterol and increase the risk for coronary heart disease. Saturated fats also raise the level of blood cholesterol in dogs, but do not appear to promote heart disease to the same extent. This may be because dogs make more of the good kind of cholesterol (HDL) and are better at removing cholesterol from arteries than we are. Cats have a similar tolerance for high-fat diets. Fats provide more than twice the calories per weight of food than either protein or carbohydrate. Both cats and dogs can put on weight if they eat high-fat diets, especially if they are sedentary, a problem we take up in chapter 15.

Whether a fat is omega-3 or omega-6 also matters. We—people, dogs, and cats—require both. In the omega-6 series, we require linoleic acid. If pets do not eat enough linoleic acid, they develop skin and coat problems. Cats require an additional fatty acid in the omega-6 series: arachidonic acid. Most animals, including dogs and humans, are able to make arachidonic acid from linoleic acid, but cats perform this conversion too slowly to meet their needs.

In the omega-3 series, we—dogs, cats, humans—appear to require alpha-linolenic acid (ALA), although our need for it is less well established than for linoleic acid. In the body, ALA is converted to a longer chain fatty acid, abbreviated EPA, which in turn is converted to an even longer chain fatty acid known as DHA (ALA → EPA → DHA). The ratio of omega-6 to omega-3 fatty acids matters because too much omega-6 may inhibit the conversion of ALA to DHA, which explains some of the interest in adding omega-3 fatty acids to human foods as well as pet foods. The NRC included a recommended allowance for ALA in its 2006 report, but so little information is available on the amount needed by cats and dogs that AAFCO has not yet created a profile for it. Although, as we discuss later (chapters 14 and 15), we think more needs to be learned about requirements for omega-3 fatty acids, pet food manufacturers are adding them to more and more products, usually in the form of fish oil or flaxseed.

Cats appear to need more fat in their food than do dogs. The NRC fat allowance for adult dogs is 5.5 percent of the dry ingredients in a food; for cats it is 9.0 percent. The AAFCO profile is also 9.0 percent. But animals can tolerate much more fat than that. The NRC says a safe upper limit is 33 percent fat. A diet containing this much fat, however, would be very high in calories. Although high-calorie diets are just the thing for hard-working Alaskan sled dogs, such diets greatly exceed the needs of a sedentary house cat.

Crude Fiber

Fiber is a term that loosely describes the indigestible carbohydrates in a food. Crude fiber measures indigestible carbohydrates, but does not indicate their source. The source matters. Recall the Canadian Old Boots scenario. Dogs and cats can digest the carbohydrates in grains, but they cannot get much nutritional value from wood chips. The point of the crude fiber maximum is to reveal poorly digestible ingredients in animal feeds. The Whiskas example guarantees a maximum of 4.5 percent crude fiber, which is not much. Pet food manufacturers deliberately increase the fiber content for products intended for inactive dogs and cats or those on diets. A Hill's "Light Adult" dry cat food, for example, guarantees a maximum of 10 percent crude fiber. In general, high-fiber products are lower in calories.

The Voluntary Guarantees

AAFCO allows pet food companies to list additional nutrient guarantees for which it has not established profiles. These are voluntary, but must be marked with an asterisk referring to a disclaimer: "*Not recognized as an essential nutrient by the AAFCO Cat [or Dog] Food Nutrient Profiles." The Whiskas cat food lists added calcium, phosphorus, and taurine in the voluntary category, but some products list many more. A Nutro dog food (Ultra Chicken, Salmon, and Lamb Formula), for example, lists linoleic acid, zinc, selenium, vitamin E, ascorbic acid [vitamin C], DHA, alpha-linolenic acid, l-carnitine, and taurine. Because complete-and-balanced pet foods are required to meet AAFCO profiles—and, therefore, all nutrient requirements—without the voluntary additions, there is really only one reason for adding extra nutrients: marketing. We will discuss how extra nutrients are marketed in later chapters. For the moment, we comment only on the additions to the Whiskas formula.

Calcium and phosphorus: For the most part, dogs and cats require slightly more calcium in the diet than they do phosphorus. The AAFCO profiles for all life stages are 1.0 percent (calcium) and 0.8 percent (phosphorus) in the dry ingredients, a ratio close to 1 to 1. These minerals are needed for growth, bone formation, and milk production in cats and dogs. Adult animals require only one-third to one-half as much calcium and phosphorus for their weight as do growing and lactating animals. In the wild, dogs and cats got their minerals in about the right proportion by eating the bones and organs of their prey.

The usual sources of calcium and phosphorus in pet foods are meat or poultry by-product meals, bone meal, and calcium phosphates or carbonates. The by-product meals contain bone mixed in with tissues as the source of these minerals; their ratio of calcium to phosphorus is about 1 to 1. Meat without bone, however, is too low in calcium. Beef hearts and kidneys contain 7 milligrams calcium per 100 grams but 200 milligrams of phosphorus: the phosphorus to calcium ratio approaches 30 to 1, which is much too high. A dog or cat fed only meat will get too little calcium for proper bone formation. This is one reason why pet food companies and veterinarians caution against feeding animals all-meat diets (raw or cooked) or homemade diets. We agree that adequate calcium is an important concern but view it as one relatively easy to address (see chapter 21).

Taurine: The Meaty Whiskas cat food lists a guaranteed analysis for taurine to emphasize that it meets the AAFCO standard for this nutrient. Taurine is an amino acid, but one that is not a component of body proteins. It is made in the body from amino acids that contain sulfur (methionine and cystine), but cats, especially young ones, do not make enough taurine and need to have it added to their diets. Without it, they develop vision and heart problems and do not grow well. Dogs do a better job of making their own taurine. They do not need more as long as the protein in their diets contains enough methionine and cystine, which most proteins do. People do not need added taurine either, despite the popularity of sports drinks containing it. Cats eating diets that meet AAFCO profiles are getting plenty of taurine and do not need more.

In general, pet foods that meet AAFCO profiles fully meet the nutrient needs of cats and dogs, and adding higher levels of nutrients is not especially useful. The addition of ascorbic acid (vitamin C), for example, is quite unnecessary; dogs and cats make their own. As we discuss in the next chapter, the amounts of extra nutrients added voluntarily are usually quite small, sometimes extremely small. When you see voluntary guarantees, think *marketing*.

THE STATEMENT OF NUTRITIONAL ADEQUACY

The entire point of pet foods is convenience—one-stop nutrition. Complete-and-balanced foods provide all the nutrients needed by a dog or cat in one package; you do not have to think twice about your pet's nutrient needs. Giving your dog or cat a pet food might appear to violate the "variety" principle of nutrition, but manufacturers usually put a variety of ingredients into their products. These ingredients are selected to meet the complete nutritional needs of a dog or cat for one or all stages of life. A pet food label that says "complete and balanced for puppies" indicates that the food is specifically formulated for that life stage. A label statement that the product is "complete and balanced for all life stages" means that the food will support the life of a dog or cat of any age as well as one that is reproducing or lactating.

As we mentioned earlier, pet foods are like infant formulas. Like human babies, dogs and cats are completely dependent on these products for their complete nutritional needs. And just like infant formulas, pet foods must be carefully formulated, manufactured, and monitored. If a critical nutrient turns out to be present in an inappropriate amount, formula-fed infants and pets eating pet foods will not thrive (such errors do happen, but rarely). So let's give credit to AAFCO for setting standards for products that meet a pet's complete nutritional needs in a form that is convenient and relatively inexpensive.

For the most part, pet food companies take great care to make sure that dogs and cats will grow, reproduce, and stay healthy eating their products as the sole source of nutrition. AAFCO requires companies to demonstrate that the products really do support pet growth, maintenance, reproduction, and lactation—or all of those life stages—but gives them three ways to do this. Companies can demonstrate nutritional adequacy by

- Formulating foods to meet AAFCO nutrient profiles.
- Testing the foods on cats and dogs through feeding studies.

- Using the product "family" method: making foods with formulas similar to those shown to be nutritionally adequate in feeding studies.

In our view, these methods are anything but equivalent. The testing method is far superior to the profile methods, as we now explain.

AAFCO Nutrient Profiles

The Whiskas product uses the profile method for establishing nutritional adequacy. Its label says: "Whiskas Meaty Selections with 'Crunchy Meaty Nuggets' Food for Cats is formulated to meet the nutritional levels established by the AAFCO Cat Food Nutrient Profiles for all life stages." This statement tells you that the manufacturer did not feed this food to cats in a feeding trial. Instead, Mars's formulators mixed ingredients that together provided the same level of nutrients called for by AAFCO nutrient profiles for all life stages.

Cat and dog foods labeled for all life stages must contain the highest levels of nutrients recommended by AAFCO for any life stage, and commercial pet foods usually contain those higher levels or exceed them. If a label says that the food is suitable for a particular life stage—kittens or puppies, for example—the nutrient levels must meet the AAFCO profile for *all* life stages.

All of this sounds fine in theory, but some aspects of the nutrient profile method concern us. In 1994, two leading researchers on cat nutrition, James Morris and Quinton Rogers, criticized the use of AAFCO profiles as standards for nutrient adequacy. Their principal objection had to do with the lack of information about the availability of nutrients from ingredients in pet foods—how well cats and dogs can use what they eat. The profile method does not address that consideration except by adding nutrients at levels higher than NRC recommendations. The amounts may be adequate, but the nutrients won't do the pets any good if they can't digest or absorb them. That is why we—and many others—believe that feeding studies are necessary to demonstrate nutritional adequacy.

Feeding Studies

Purina Dog Chow demonstrates nutritional adequacy through feeding studies. Its label says: "Animal feeding tests using Association of American Feed Control Officials (AAFCO) procedures substantiate that Purina Dog Chow provides complete and balanced nutrition for all life stages of dogs." This statement tells you that the company carried out—or contracted out—actual feeding trials with this product, that the experiments followed protocols specified by AAFCO, and that the animals successfully grew and reproduced eating just that food.

In chapter 25, we discuss the ethics of research using dogs and cats, but for now let's simply describe the experiments. AAFCO's protocols require the use of only eight dogs or cats. Eight is not many for statistical purposes, but should be enough to expose real problems if they exist. To support a claim that a cat food is complete and balanced for all life stages, companies are required to conduct a lengthy feeding trial in two stages. The first phase, designed to demonstrate that a food "supports reproduction and lactation," begins with eight cats ("queens") fed the product to be tested from the time they become pregnant until their kittens are six weeks old. A comparison control group of at least eight queens goes through the same protocol eating a product that has already been tested. For the claim, "supports growth," kittens no more than nine weeks old are fed the test foods for ten weeks. Feeding trials for dog foods are conducted according to a similar protocol.

For "adult maintenance," companies must feed the product to eight adult dogs or cats for at least twenty-six weeks. The feeding protocols govern the amount of weight that the animals are allowed to lose—no more than 15 percent during the trial for an individual animal, and not more than 10 percent overall for the group—and also specify standards for other measures of adequate feeding. Finally, a veterinarian must monitor the health of the animals at all times.

Feeding trials constitute the gold standard of proof that a pet food really does maintain health or can support growth and reproduction—at least during the time and under the specific conditions of the experiment. We think feeding trials answer questions about whether the vitamins in pet foods are destroyed by cooking and extrusion or whether rendering of by-product meals reduces their nutritional value. Yes, these processes destroy some nutrients (so does cooking), but feeding trials demonstrate that the foods are adequate to keep animals alive and in good health during the trial period.

While it makes sense to think that foods formulated to the same nutritional criteria should support the life of cats and dogs just as well as foods that have been tested in feeding trials, we think feeding trials give a greater degree of confidence in the nutritional adequacy of the food. Some support for this view comes from the 2007 pet food recalls. Menu Foods discovered the problem with its foods because the cats participating in the company's routine taste trials formed crystals in their urinary tracts and kidneys that later turned out to be made from melamine and one of its by-products, cyanuric acid. Taste testing is not the same as nutritional adequacy testing, but makes the same point. If companies do not test the food, they are unlikely to find problems with it. If we are skeptical of nutrient profiles, we are even more so of the "product family" method for verifying them.

Nutrient Profile "Families"

The third method for demonstrating nutritional adequacy is through association or line extension. Once a product has been tested in a feeding trial and demonstrated to be nutritionally adequate, any other products made by the same manufacturer using similar ingredients are assumed to work just as well. This is a gray area of pet food oversight, as this method of demonstrating nutrient adequacy requires no special designation on the label. You have no way of knowing whether the food itself has been tested or whether it makes this claim as a family member. We think pet food labels should say which is which.

THE FEEDING DIRECTIONS

The Whiskas product provides directions for feeding according to the weight of the cat. You are supposed to feed a kitten from one-third of a cup to one and three-quarters cups of a food, a five-fold range. A twelve-to-sixteen pound adult cat gets 1.0 to 1.5 cups. She gets more if she is pregnant. If she is nursing kittens, you may feed her up to four times the amount listed. Obviously, as the label understates: "Individual requirements may vary."

Since pet foods are formulated to contain the amounts of nutrients and calories needed, and the amounts needed are roughly proportional to an animal's weight, the feeding directions are a good starting point. But the recommended amounts vary so greatly that you have to do some experimenting. If you are feeding too much food, your pet will gain weight. If the amount is too low, your dog or cat may complain more than is usual, and will be losing weight.

The question of how much to feed is as difficult to answer for pets as it is for humans. Larger dogs and cats need more food than smaller dogs and cats. More active—athletic and working—dogs need much more food for their weight than the sedentary types. Young, growing animals need more food for their weight than do young adult animals, and young animals in general need more food than older animals. Gestation and lactation also increase food requirements.

The feeding directions refer to the specific food. Treats and table foods are extras. If you give your dog or cat more than an occasional treat or table tidbit, these must be subtracted from the recommended amounts (we have more to say about the extras in chapter 16).

One final label caveat: if you are depending on commercial food to feed your pet, be sure you are buying complete-and-balanced formulas. The labels will always say so, but sometimes you have to look twice. In a shop in Berkeley, California, we bought a can of Tripett Original Formula Green Beef Tripe Dog Food, *for all life stages* (our emphasis). The label makes the product look complete and balanced, but it isn't. It is a food supplement. But the only way you would know this is to read the feeding directions: "Tripett is intended to be supplemented with good quality dry or raw food." We repeat: read labels carefully. And now it's time to take a look at what's out there in the pet food marketplace.

The Pet Food Marketplace:
Segments

COMMERCIAL PET FOODS make life easy for owners who can simply open a bag or can of food and not have to worry about their pet's nutritional needs. In return for this convenience, pet foods earn a handsome profit for their manufacturers and sellers. This win-win deal works well for all concerned. It has turned pet foods into a lively industry, one that generates serious money. But serious money means that much is at stake and this industry is highly competitive. Pet owners have many choices about how to feed their pets and commercial companies have to work hard to convince customers to buy their brands rather than those of competitors.

Pet foods—like infant formulas—pose an especially difficult marketing challenge. Nutritionally, they are all alike. Close examination of the label and ingredient list of just about any pet food brand reveals only the subtlest differences. This means that the job of pet food marketers is to figure out how to differentiate their products so pet owners will think there is something special about them. Luckily for marketers, increasing prosperity and changing demographics have led people to consider dogs and cats as important sources of emotional support. The resulting "humanization" of pets—the viewing of dogs and cats as part of the family—opens up new possibilities for brand differentiation and selling points.

PET HUMANIZATION

Much has been written about the increasing humanization of pets, not only in the popular press but also in academic journals. Many people no longer view pets as possessions or "just" animals. According to one survey, 69 percent of pet owners consider pets to be members of the family, and many other surveys document the obvious: people care deeply for their cats and dogs, and are willing to spare no expense to pamper, indulge, or care for them. The editor of the Modern Love column in the *New York Times* made just this point when he wrote that "a small but entrenched segment of the population has come to the conclusion that the companionship of pets (particularly dogs) yields greater satisfaction, loyalty, depth of love and ease of relationship than a boyfriend, girlfriend, husband, wife or child."

Pet humanization explains some of the results of a survey conducted by the American Animal Hospital Association. Most respondents (83 percent) said they thought of themselves as their pets' Mom or Dad, and 60 percent said they told their pets they loved them at least once a day. More than 70 percent said they would go into debt for their pets' health and well-being. To the pet industry, the unqualified love that characterizes the relationship of humans to their pets presents an unparalleled marketing opportunity:

> As a vastly lucrative business, the marketing of pets and pet-related products rests on an emotional bond between consumers and their animal companions. . . . These creatures give unconditional love in return. No matter how nasty we people act toward each other—no matter how dumb our beliefs, how bad our attitudes, or how uncivil our interpersonal behavior—our pets are always glad to see us.

Pets, according to people who study such things, may or may not improve their owner's health (the evidence on that question is mixed) but they definitely do good things for them in other ways: *hedonic,* as providers of emotional intimacy and pleasure; *social,* as indicators of status: *altruistic,* as means to express ethical or spiritual values; and *economic,* as generators of income. For these reasons, the industry considers humanization to be the single most important trend fueling the growth in the global pet food market. Marketers can—and do—use hedonic, social, and altruistic values as the basis of income-generating campaigns to promote their particular products to doting pet owners. They use economic values to promote their products to retailers and veterinarians.

Companies state these approaches explicitly. Del Monte, for example, has taken a special interest in a particular group of cat-loving women who make up just one-third of cat owners but account for half the expenditures on cat food. The company's researchers conduct focus groups, home observations, brainstorming sessions, and interview tapings to provide a basis for reaching this and other groups of pet enthusiasts. Del Monte plans its marketing strategies to take full advantage of pet owners' "irrationality" about what they are willing to spend on their cats and dogs. Overall, advertisers spent $502 million on marketing of pet and pet care products in 2008, exclusively through what the advertising industry calls "measured media"—radio, television, print, and Internet campaigns run through advertising agencies and, therefore, countable. Measured media underestimates the real costs of marketing, as it does not include the amounts spent on other channels such as websites, store product placements, trade shows like Pet Expo, or, as we discuss in chapter 24, support of veterinary education.

MARKETING PET FOOD

One strategy for selling $17 billion worth of dog and cat food a year is to introduce new products to entice consumer interest. In 2008, pet food companies introduced 270 new product lines into the U.S. marketplace. Because dog and cat foods come in multiple sizes, flavors, and packages, the actual number of new items, referred to in the trade as stockkeeping units or SKUs, was 1,483. Worldwide, marketers introduced 669 new pet foods during just the first nine months of 2008 for a total of 2,553 SKUs. About 70 percent of the new products were dog foods and 26 percent were cat foods. Nearly two-thirds went to "mature" country markets while the rest went to developing countries where sales of commercial pet foods are growing rapidly.

To sell new and old pet foods, the companies mostly use traditional advertising channels—radio, television, and print—and buy the messages and time from advertising agencies. How much companies spend to advertise pet products tends to be one of those well-guarded industry secrets, but a research group, Packaged Facts, has access to this information and reports it occasionally. In 2009, for example, Packaged Facts reported that pet retailers PetSmart and PETCO spent about $45 million and $18 million, respectively, on advertising for everything in their stores, including pet foods.

Table 11

MEASURED ADVERTISING EXPENDITURES OF THREE LEADING U.S. PET FOOD MANUFACTURERS, 2008, $ MILLIONS

PET FOOD BRAND	PET FOOD ADVERTISING, $ MILLIONS	TOTAL ADVERTISING, ALL PRODUCTS, $ MILLIONS
MARS, INC.		1,037.6
Pedigree	16.0	
Other Mars brands (Cesar, etc.)	22.3	
NESTLÉ PURINA		1,138.8
Fancy Feast	20.1	
Friskies	25.9	
Other Purina brands	102.0	
PROCTER & GAMBLE		4,838.1
Iams	66.4	

Total advertising for pet food and pet care was $501.9 million in 2008. See: "100 Leading National Advertisers," *Advertising Age,* June 22, 2009.

In some years, Packaged Facts breaks out figures spent on pet food advertising. The 2005 total for the United States was $277 million. Just three companies accounted for 90 percent of that amount—Nestlé Purina, Mars, and Iams (Procter & Gamble). Every June, the trade magazine *Ad-*

vertising Age reports the amounts that the one hundred leading national advertisers spend on measured media, the amounts funneled through advertising agencies. These figures usually include amounts spent for a few specific pet foods, and we show examples from 2008 in table 11.

That year, Nestlé Purina spent more than $100 million to advertise Purina pet foods other than Fancy Feast and Friskies, and Mars spent nearly $40 million to advertise its brands. Procter & Gamble is America's leading national advertiser. Its $66 million spending for Iams pales in comparison to the company's $4.8 billion annual advertising budget. The other major company, Colgate-Palmolive, does not appear on the top-100 list because its measured media expenses are extremely low; it markets primarily through veterinarians.

These figures do not include unmeasured methods such as public relations, although such expenses must be considerable. One pet magazine, for example, sent us a copy of a letter it received from a public relations company working for Iams. Iams, it seems, was offering a "media buy" to editors who would agree to reciprocate by "running an editorial piece which: 1) Introduced the advertised product, 2) Touted its benefits, and 3) Quoted some experts in the field." The letter asked, "If we were to give you a page of advertising for this initiative, would you be able to create any form of edit which helped promote this initiative?" We have to assume that someone at Procter & Gamble approved this dubious venture. The editor of this particular magazine declined the offer and we hope others did as well.

Whatever sums the parent companies use to advertise their products are surely viewed as money well spent. Pet foods are small items, but profitable. As we mentioned earlier, Colgate-Palmolive sold $2.1 billion worth of pet food in 2008 (out of $15.3 billion for all its products worldwide). Nestlé Purina racked in sales of $11.5 billion on pet care products in 2008, but this company sold $102 billion worth of all its products that year.

OVERSIGHT OF PET FOOD MARKETING

We must now introduce yet another federal agency involved in the oversight of pet foods: the Federal Trade Commission (FTC). The FTC regulates advertising, but it is not exactly a consumer protection agency. Its primary purpose is to establish a level playing field for companies selling consumer products so they do not unfairly compete with one another. Advertising, in this sense, is a form of competition and the FTC is concerned about how misleading and fraudulent advertising might give one company an advantage over another. Sometimes these concerns benefit consumers. The FTC has a long history of intervention in pet food advertising. In 1940, for example, the FTC said that Ralston Purina must stop telling consumers that its dog chow contained pure beef, pure meat, and meal, when in fact its principal ingredient was meat meal.

In 1969, the FTC issued marketing guides for companies making, selling, and distributing dog and cat foods. These advised pet food companies not to use advertising to erroneously suggest ("misrepresent") that their products meet nutrient needs, provide medicinal or therapeutic benefits, are fit for human consumption, or are better than the products of competitors. Thirty years later, as part of a periodic review of such things, the FTC requested public comment on the need for such guides. Only six groups filed comments in response to this request, five of them arguing that the FTC should keep the guides in place. AAFCO, these groups said, establishes guidelines only for product labels, not advertising, and guidance about the appropriate basis for advertising would be helpful. Only one comment, from the American Pet Products Manufacturers Association (APPMA), called for getting rid of the guides. The APPMA said the guides were confusing, AAFCO model regulations were sufficient, and the makers of dog and cat foods "are compelled to conform to general truth in advertising standards set by FTC for all consumer goods." FTC agreed with APPMA, and the guides are no longer available.

Today, problems with pet food advertisements get taken up by the Better Business Bureau (BBB). In 2007, the bureau objected to a Procter & Gamble claim that four out of five veterinarians recommend Iams to help dogs and cats live longer. The BBB's advertising division said the "healthier longer" claim lacked scientific substantiation. How did the BBB get involved in this issue? Not, as you might hope, through diligent oversight. Instead, the complaint was filed by a competitor, Hill's Science Diet (Colgate-Palmolive).

Does regulation of pet food advertising matter? As we demonstrate in subsequent chapters, we think much pet food advertising is overblown but unlikely to affect the health of cats and dogs (effects on owners' pocketbooks are another matter). That is why we are amused rather than troubled by a letter sent to us by the food writer Anne Mendelson:

> Trying to feed a young and healthy cat on supermarket brands has become more and more a drowning-in-choices proposition. Well, I ignore as much as I can of the lunacies out there. . . . But today when I got back from shopping I found I'd acquired a $1 coupon good for any of the newest "Fancy Feast Elegant Medleys." More specifically, "three new recipes, inspired by the tastes of TUSCANY." To wit: "White Meat Chicken Tuscany," "Yellowfin Tuna Tuscany," and "Tender Turkey Tuscany." I can only wonder what sort of sonnets or canzoni Petrarch and Dante would have written to the scavengings of the local cats if they'd foreseen the future immortality of all things Tuscan.

Tuscan turkey is just marketing hype and pet food buyers ought to be able to judge such things for themselves. But what about more sophisticated kinds of strategies? We now take up sales strategies aimed at specific market segments distinguished by price, the animal's lifestyle, its breed, and its stage of life. In later chapters, we discuss market segmentation by health condition or other special need and by the value systems, health beliefs, and dietary preferences of pet owners.

MARKET SEGMENTATION: BY PRICE

In May 2008, we decided to do some comparative shopping. We dropped into a local PetSmart to see what we would have to pay for a chicken dinner for an adult dog. We had no trouble finding more than a dozen brands, each priced the same as other kinds (such as turkey, beef, or venison dinners) within its line. For comparison, we stopped by Walmart and bought an Ol' Roy chicken dinner, one that is not available anywhere else. Because the cans ranged in weight from 12.5 oz to 13.2 oz, we converted the price we paid to price per ounce. Table 12 summarizes our observations:

Table 12
COMPARATIVE PRICES OF CANNED CHICKEN DINNERS FOR DOGS, MAY 2008

BRAND (COMPANY)	PRODUCT NAME	PRICE, $	PRICE PER OUNCE, CENTS	FIRST FIVE INGREDIENTS[a]
Ol' Roy (Walmart)	Chicken and Rice Hearty Cuts in Gravy	0.44	3.3	*Water,* poultry, meat by-products, wheat flour, chicken
Alpo (Nestlé-Purina)	Prime Cuts in Gravy	0.50	3.8	*Water,* chicken, turkey, liver, meat by-products
Pedigree (Mars)	Chicken and Rice Dinner	0.55	4.2	Chicken, *water,* poultry by-products, brewer's rice, carob bean gum
Iams (Proctor and Gamble)	Savory Dinner with Tender Chicken and Rice	1.05	8.0	*Chicken broth,* chicken, beef by-products, chicken by-products, beef liver
Nutro (Mars)	Chicken, Rice & Oatmeal Formula	1.06	8.5	*Chicken broth,* chicken, beef liver, chicken liver
Purina ONE (Nestlé Purina)	Wholesome Chicken & Brown Rice Entrée	1.14	8.8	Chicken, *water,* liver, meat by-products, brown rice, oat meal
Science Diet (Hills)[b]	Savory Chicken Entrée	1.39	10.7	*Water,* chicken liver, cracked pearled barley, ground whole grain corn, meat by-products
Blue Buffalo	Chicken Dinner with Garden Vegetables and Brown Rice	1.69	13.5	Chicken, *chicken broth,* chicken liver, carrots, peas

a. Source of water *emphasized;* moisture guarantees varied from 76% to 82%.
b. Nutritional adequacy requirements met by testing; all other products met requirements through similarity to AAFCO nutrient profiles.

Although you might correctly observe that these products are not identical and, therefore, not precisely comparable, we think they are comparable enough, especially because their prices varied by a factor of four. The wide price spread makes us wonder what more you get when you pay four times as much for products with similar names. And what might be the reason for paying more for one of two similar-sounding products made by the same manufacturer, in this case, Nestlé-Purina or Mars?

The difference must have to do with the ingredients, no? Table 12 also lists the first five ingredients in each product. Canned dinners contain about 80 percent moisture, so we have italicized the moisture source to emphasize that whatever you pay for such products, you are paying for only about three ounces of "dry" food but ten ounces of water. When chicken comes first on the list you are still paying for water; chicken on its own is about 65 percent water.

If there are differences among the products, perhaps they have to do with the quality of the ingredients? You might think that the source of the meat would make a significant difference. None of these products contains meat meals or poultry meals among the leading five ingredients, so what goes into rendered materials is not an issue here.

All but two of the products on this list—Nutro and Blue Buffalo—list meat or poultry by-products as major ingredients. Recall that by-products are the nonrendered parts of slaughtered animals or birds that humans don't usually eat, such as lungs, spleen, livers, heads, feet, and viscera free of their contents. But people also do not ordinarily eat the parts of birds and animals listed on pet food labels as chicken or beef; these are the mechanically deboned backs, necks, breastbones, and occasionally the wings of poultry or the meaty scraps and organs of animals that are not sold for human consumption. Are necks and breastbones really better than feet or spleens? Liver can be a by-product or a meat, depending on how it is listed. We are not convinced that these subtle differences in the interpretation of "by-products" merit a higher price.

That is why we are skeptical of the value of paying twice as much for the pricier brands from Nestlé Purina, Mars, or any other manufacturer. The first few ingredients in Purina's Alpo do not look all that different to us from those in Purina ONE. Both have chicken, liver, and meat by-products. The main difference seems to be soy protein (Alpo) vs. brown rice and oat meal (Purina ONE), yet the Purina ONE costs twice as much as Alpo. Is the difference worth it? Are chicken backs and liver in Nutro brands worth twice as much as the nonrendered poultry by-products in Pedigree, both made by Mars? The companies' marketing departments are keeping their fingers crossed that you will think so.

What might make a real difference is how the animals were treated before slaughter. Were they raised free of antibiotics or hormones, grass-fed, free-range, or cage-free? Is their meat sourced from a single supplier? If such issues matter to you (and they matter to us), you might be willing to pay more for pet foods that make and substantiate such claims. We discuss some of these foods in the next chapter. In the meantime, because none of the conventional products listed in the table makes such claims, we view these dinners as virtually indistinguishable.

We do, however, view as significant the difference in method used by the manufacturer to demonstrate nutritional adequacy. With only one exception—Hill's Science Diet—the products in table 12 were formulated to meet AAFCO nutrient profiles. Hill's verifies nutritional adequacy through animal feeding tests, a method we consider more reliable. But is better testing worth paying nearly three times more for a Science Diet product as for Alpo? This, too, you must decide for yourself.

In judging prices, you must be careful to check the package weights. These cannot be judged by appearance. We checked the weights and prices of large-size bags of dog kibble at a Wegmans supermarket in August 2008. Such bags used to be a uniform forty pounds. No more. Most now weigh less; the lowest was thirty-two pounds. The prices were equally irregular; they ranged from a low of $12 per bag to more than $30. The most expensive was an Iams product ($30.99 for forty pounds), but get out your calculator: Purina ONE was more expensive per pound. At $28.99 for thirty-four pounds, it was 85 cents a pound as compared to 78 cents per pound for the Iams. The lowest-priced brand was just 37 cents a pound. A year later, some of the bag sizes were a bit smaller and the prices a bit higher per pound in response to the economic recession, but the principles still held. In Wegmans, the price for the entire bag appears on shelf labels in large print but the price per pound appears in tiny print; that's the one you need to check. Many stores do not provide this information at all and the lack of consistency in shelf labels and bag weights makes it easy for you to pay more than you need to for similar products.

One last example. In 2007, before the sharp rise in food prices drove every company to reduce its package sizes (but keep prices the same or higher), we compared the prices of what looked like identical bags of Iams MiniChunks dry dog food at Walmart ($8.44) and Wegmans ($9.79). This seemed like a big difference, even for Walmart's famously low prices. But then we looked at the weights. The Wegmans bag contained eight pounds; the Walmart held just seven. On a per-pound basis, Walmart saved us one cent per pound: $1.21 as opposed to $1.22.

We cannot distinguish these products by nutritional value; all are formulated to meet AAFCO nutrient standards (although we give points to the companies that use animal feeding tests to verify nutritional adequacy). Among mainstream products, price is unlikely to tell you much about the cost of the basic food ingredients. Instead, price signifies a marketing strategy, one aimed at appealing to your idea about what you think you should be spending on food for your dog or cat. We discuss the price issue further in the next chapter where we examine the premium price charged for certain "alternative" pet foods.

MARKET SEGMENTATION: BY LIFESTYLE

Active animals require more calories than sedentary animals and getting more calories into them can be accomplished in two ways: feed them more calorically concentrated food, or feed them more food in general. Dick Van Patten's Natural Balance Ultra Active Dog Formula takes the first approach. Its label says it has 27 percent more protein and 16 percent more fat. More than what? This, alas, the label does not say.

In contrast, the primary concern about food for indoor animals, especially dogs, is the amount of waste they excrete—their poop production. Royal Canin's dry food for indoor adult dogs advertises "lower levels of highly digestible proteins [which] help to limit the amount and odor of stools in dogs living exclusively indoors." Indoor animals need relatively fewer calories, but this "indoor" food is not a diet product. It is a product formulated to leave as little digestive residue as possible. We discuss the poop problem in the context of premium foods in the following chapter.

MARKET SEGMENTATION: BY BREED

The more market segments you have, the more customers you appeal to, and the marketers at Royal Canin (Mars) are masters of this strategy. For both dogs and cats, they offer products for specific weights, ages, breeds, and health status. Breeds? We must confess that we had no idea that nutrient requirements might vary in any meaningful way from one breed of dog to another.

Royal Canin's marketing implies that all breeds have *unique* nutritional needs. For each of the breeds targeted by Royal Canin, its marketers say: "the special physiology of [fill in the name of the breed], such as [fill in the special characteristics], make it a *very unusual breed that needs special attention, especially in terms of its nutrition*" [our emphasis].

Consider the Yorkshire Terrier. Does its characteristic trusty nature require special attention to the nutritional quality of its diet? Royal Canin does not say but instead explains other differences:

> One special difference between the Yorkshire Terrier and other canine breeds is that it does not have an undercoat. A single hair sprouts from each hair follicle, whereas in other breeds there are usually 3 to 5 hairs. This makes the Yorkshire Terrier more susceptible than other small dog breeds to adverse environmental factors such as extremes of temperature and urban pollution. . . . Coat quality can be directly related to diet and a specially formulated food may help to prevent brittle, dry, greasy or dull hair and itchy skin.

Especially a specially formulated food made by Royal Canin, no doubt.

An examination of the ingredient lists for products targeting each breed does demonstrate some distinctions. We consider the differences subtle, but Royal Canin sees them as grounds for marketing campaigns. For all breeds, the first five ingredients include chicken meal, brown rice, and various grain or soy meals. The calories vary from about 3,800 per kilogram (Labrador retriever) to 4,200 (shih tzu), a difference of about 10 percent. The protein varies from a low of 24 percent (bulldog, German shepherd, shih tzu) to a high of 30 percent (Labrador retriever), and the fat varies from 13 percent (Labrador retriever) to 20 percent (boxer, bulldog, poodle, shih tzu). All percentages generously exceed nutritional requirements. The fiber varies from 2 percent (boxer) to 5.9 percent (poodle).

Some of these differences make just enough sense to be plausible. For example, the diet for the Labrador retriever, said to have a "predisposition to excess weight," is lowest in fat and calories (but the amount of food given to the dog also determines caloric intake). Fiber is an important determinant of poop volume, and it is understandable why owners would want as little as possible from a big dog like a boxer. Poop from a toy poodle is a lot easier to manage.

The ingredient lists of these products include a large number of additives—omega-3 fats, antioxidant nutrients (vitamins A, C, and E), extracts of green tea, taurine, and dietary supplements such as chondroitin sulfate and glucosamine, most of them coming well after the salt on the ingredient list. It is difficult to know how these supplements (which we discuss in chapters 17 and 18) might affect "special nutritional needs." The predisposition of Yorkshire terriers to cataracts might be countered by vitamin A and other antioxidants, but the essential ones are present in all pet food vitamin mixes. We cannot guess the special purposes of the extracts of green tea, rosemary, and marigolds that are among the last of dozens of ingredients listed for these products. The only good reason we can think of for adding taurine to dog food is marketing. Dogs, as we repeatedly point out, make their own taurine.

Royal Canin explains the rationale for the supplements in the boxer diet, for example: "The Boxer is a highly energetic dog that is always on the move, requiring a diet that supports its active lifestyle. . . . The addition of glucosamine (780 mg/kg) and chondroitin (220 mg/kg) may contribute to the health of the Boxer's joints, which are under constant pressure." Yes, but joints in *all* dogs are under constant pressure and, as we discuss in chapter 18, the evidence for the effectiveness of these supplements is not always as strong as one might wish.

A final difference is in the shape and size of the kibble. In 2008, Royal Canin explained why it extruded wave-shaped kibbles for boxers:

> It's easy to see that a Boxer's jaw has a distinct shape. This unique morphology is called "brachycephalic." A specific kibble shape has been carefully selected in order to make grasping easier. The texture, density and size of the kibble have been designed to fit the Boxer's unique facial characteristics, leading to slower ingestion and increased digestibility. These benefits may help to prevent bloat and help diminish stool quantity.

This is brilliant marketing. The explanation for kibble shape seems rational and scientific. Royal Canin maintains that the company has "never allowed our approach to be diluted by marketing gimmicks. Our nutritional innovation is sincere, authentic and built on studies published in the most reputable and scrupulous scientific journals." What studies? The brochures for each breed provide long lists of studies that establish breed characteristics and review the data for use of supplements, but we cannot find a single study that compares the effects of one breed-specific diet to another or, for that matter, to a nonbreed-specific diet. If the company has such studies, it is keeping them well hidden. Although scientists do find genetic differences among breeds of dogs, we have not seen evidence that breeds differ in their response to diets in any way that can be attributed to "unique nutritional needs." But for truly clever marketing, nothing beats "premium," as we next explain.

Products at a Premium

PET PRODUCT TRADE shows display dozens of foods and treats produced by large and small manufacturers who advertise their products as natural, organic, free of undesirable ingredients, human-grade, holistic, and premium, not to mention superholistic and superpremium. The companies making these products market them as better—of higher quality—than conventional pet foods. They design the foods to address concerns of pet owners about where the ingredients come from, how they were produced, and their effects on the health of pets and the environment. Food marketers lump consumers who share such concerns into the category of LOHAS—Lifestyles of health and sustainability.

In turn, the makers of conventional pet foods lump products aimed at LOHAS owners into the category of "alternative." They view this category as a small but interesting niche market. As a group, alternative pet foods accounted for less than 10 percent of total pet food sales in 2007. But sales of these foods are growing so rapidly that many small companies are encouraged to get into this business, and all of the large pet food companies are snapping up these smaller companies or starting alternative lines of their own. This trend closely reflects similar trends in sales of foods for humans.

Among the alternatives, the largest and fastest growing categories are natural and organic. In 2005, organic pet foods accounted for just $30 million in sales, but that was 46 percent higher than the year before. According to *Nutrition Business Journal*, sales of the natural and organic pet food category "skyrocketed" after the 2007 recalls, as owners sought safer foods to feed their pets. Together, the alternative categories brought in more than a billion dollars in sales in 2007, up sharply from previous years.

The makers of alternative pet foods claim that their products offer substantial improvements in the quality of ingredients offered to cats and dogs, so substantial that they are worth premium prices. Are they? Let's go shopping.

THE "NATURAL" CLAIM

You might think that the word "natural" on a pet food means that every one of its ingredients comes straight from an animal or plant and has not been processed in any way other than cooking. Not quite. AAFCO has an official definition:

> **Natural:** A feed or ingredient derived solely from plant, animal, or mined sources, either in its unprocessed state or having been subject to physical processing, heat processing, rendering, purification, extraction, hydrolysis, enzymolysis, or fermentation, but not having been produced by or subject to a chemically synthetic process and not containing any additives or processing aids that are chemically synthetic except in amounts as may occur unavoidably in good manufacturing processes.

Got that? You can render or extrude an ingredient to mush but you can call it natural if it hasn't been processed with anything synthetic—except when you have to use something synthetic. AAFCO says companies can use the term as long as they do so in a way that is not misleading. If the word "natural" appears on the label, *every* ingredient in the product must meet the definition. Oops. This will not be easy. For a complete-and-balanced product, AAFCO warns that "it is very difficult to have all ingredients meet the feed term definition of "natural," particularly for vitamin, mineral, and other trace nutrients." Indeed. We can't quite understand what the problem might be with minerals—they come from earth and rocks, after all—but as we learned during the 2007 recalls, vitamins, amino acids, and taurine are typically synthesized chemically and unnaturally in Asian pharmaceutical factories.

Because synthetic vitamins cost a good deal less than those extracted from food sources, even the most expensive pet foods use commercial vitamin, mineral, and amino acid mixes. AAFCO knows this and leaves a loophole; it allows companies to label their pet foods as "natural with added vitamins, minerals, and amino acids." It also lets labels say things like "cat food with natural added flavor." Here, the label does not claim that the cat food is natural, just that the flavor ingredient is.

AAFCO is able to make such exceptions because federal labeling laws do not define what natural means for human foods. The FDA and USDA (which regulates meat and poultry) loosely define "natural" as meaning minimally processed with no artificial additives, using statements that are truthful and not misleading. In 2009, the USDA announced that it was working on a definition. In the meantime, manufacturers of human foods can define for themselves what they mean by the term. That is why the makers of high fructose corn syrup can say it is a natural sugar because the enzymes that convert starch to glucose and glucose to fructose occur in nature. The mere fact that AAFCO developed a definition, however ambiguous, means that "natural" on pet foods has a more precise meaning than it does on human foods.

Some pet food companies call themselves natural—Natural Balance and Natural Life, for example—and you can buy any number of cat and dog foods labeled "naturally healthy," "all natural," or "natural nutrition." These products generally contain ingredients other than meat or poultry by-products, and use vitamin E instead of chemical preservatives (BHA, BHT, ethoxyquin). Otherwise, their ingredient lists look much the same as those of any other product.

That is why we were interested in a new Hill's Science Diet product—Nature's Best—handed out as samples by hawkers outside Manhattan's Pennsylvania Station one late afternoon in June 2008. Penn Station is a frequent site for product giveaways, and customers crowded around the boxes to pick up the free packages along with a brochure and a $3 coupon for later purchases. Nature's Best ("complete, natural, and clinically proven") does something we hadn't seen before; it cites the sources of its ingredients. The back of the box said that the chickens and eggs come from USDA-inspected facilities, and the rest of the ingredients—soybeans and soy oil, grains, flaxseed, vegetables (carrots, peas, broccoli), and fruits (apples, cranberries)—are grown by farmers in North America. But the bag inside the box was a lamb and brown rice dinner for which no sources were listed. Nor were sources listed on the box or bag for the vitamins, taurine, and citric acid. Natural, the brochure says, means "natural, wholesome ingredients like premium chicken and premium lamb. . . . Simply put, it has all the ingredients you want and none that you don't . . . no artificial additives or preservatives, no fillers, no corn." So that's how Hill's defines "natural."

In part to fill the definition gap, Natural Pet Nutrition, the maker of Pet Promise foods, developed a certification system for its qualified ingredient suppliers. These must guarantee that meat and poultry ingredients consist only of liver, heart, meat, and "frames" (leftover bones and meat scraps); that they come only from animals fed vegetarian diets, reared without antibiotics or hormones, and raised on U.S. family farms using humane animal husbandry practices; and that they are minimally processed without any artificial or synthetic ingredients. Nestlé Purina PetCare, which owns Natural Pet Nutrition, must have thought these standards would give Pet Promise an edge in the alternative niche market. As far as we know, the parent company had no intention of applying such standards to the rest of the Purina PetCare portfolio. Indeed, Nestlé discontinued Pet Promise in January 2010. In the absence of a consistent definition, "natural" still means whatever the manufacturer says it does.

THE "ORGANIC" CLAIM

As late as 2009, federal organic rules for human foods did not apply to pet foods. The AAFCO *Official Publication* lists a definition of organic feed, but does not explain how it might apply:

> **Organic (process):** A formula feed or a specific ingredient within a formula feed that has been produced and handled in compli-

ance with the requirements of the USDA National Organic Program.

Until the National Organic Program (NOP) gets around to establishing rules for organic pet foods, they remain in a regulatory limbo.

In the odd way in which the U.S. government sometimes does things, it put the USDA—not the FDA—in charge of the NOP. The NOP functions through the National Organic Standards Board (NOSB), which sets organic rules (or standards) for food production and labeling, and recommends them for NOP approval. When the NOSB issued standards for organic certification of human foods in 2002, it did not include pet foods. The NOSB was baffled by how organic standards might apply to such products. Organic standards for livestock production do not apply easily to pet foods for at least three reasons: livestock standards restrict the feeding of mammalian tissues to other mammals (this is allowed in pet foods); they do not permit a "made with" claim on the label (a frequent claim on pet food labels); and they exclude some feed additives and processing aids that are allowed in pet food production. The NOSB explained: "We have not addressed the labeling of pet food within this final rule because of the extensive consultation that will be required between the USDA, the NOSB, and the pet food industry before any standards on this category could be considered."

In 2005, the NOSB appointed a Pet Food Task Force to work all this out. The Task Force submitted its recommendations in April 2006. Quite sensibly, it suggested that the rules for organic certification of human foods apply to pet foods. To be certified as organic, plant ingredients in pet foods would have to be grown without pesticides, artificial fertilizers, genetic modification, irradiation, or sewage sludge fertilizers. Animal ingredients would have to come from animals raised on organic feed, not treated with antibiotics or hormones, and given access to the outdoors, among other provisions.

As the NOSB understated, "These requirements will present challenges for pet food manufacturers, especially sourcing non-genetically engineered ingredients in the non-organic fraction of the products." It was not kidding. More than 90 percent of soybeans and 60 percent of the corn grown in the United States in 2009 were derived from genetically modified varieties and 90 percent of finished beef cattle in the United States were implanted with hormones to promote lean meat production.

Developing new organic regulations occurs at glacial speed. In due course, the NOSB finally dealt with the task force report and settled on standards for organic pet foods. It said production of pet food ingredients should follow the rules for organic livestock feed. In contrast, label claims should follow the organic rules for human food. It allowed one exception: pet foods could be labeled organic even if their vitamin, mineral, and other approved nutrient ingredients were not produced according to organic standards. The NOSB sent these recommendations to the NOP in November 2008, where they still languished as this book went to press.

This unsettled situation leaves AAFCO with the unenviable job of trying to explain how pet foods made with organic ingredients should be labeled. As it interprets the situation in its labeling guide, AAFCO says that until the NOP institutes organic standards for labeling of pet food (numbers added for clarity):

[1] The NOP will not allow pet foods to display the USDA organic seal, and pet foods may not imply or represent that they are produced or handled to the USDA NOP standards.

[2] The NOP has indicated that labeling terms such as "100 percent organic," "organic," or "made with organic ingredients" on pet food products may be truthful statements and do not imply that the product was produced in accordance with the USDA NOP standards, nor that the producer is certified under the NOP standards.

[3] AAFCO recommends that the formulation criteria for labeling of human food products be used for labeling pet foods with organic claims.

What is one to make of this? The first statement sounds to us as though pet foods are not allowed to claim they are organic. But the second statement implies that pet foods may use terms that describe the organic content of the food but are not necessarily Certified Organic. Stores certainly carry plenty of pet foods claiming to be organic. To pick one example, Blue Buffalo has a line of foods called Blue Organics. The bag is illustrated with a truck labeled Blue Organic Farms and with the statement "made with organic chicken, brown rice, and carrots." A look at the ingredient list reveals the first three ingredients to be organic—organic deboned chicken, organic brown rice, and organic oatmeal. This product must be USDA certified organic, right? No, it is not.

For an explanation, we must look again at the AAFCO statements. We interpret them as saying that the NOP has decided not to make a fuss about organic claims on pet foods even though it knows perfectly well that not all of the ingredients meet organic production standards. AAFCO recommends that pet food companies do the best they can to follow the standards for human foods. If they do so, they will stay out of trouble. Some states—California, for example—have passed laws that make this interpretation explicit.

So let's take a look at the NOP's rules for labeling human foods as organic. These, as you see in table 13, are rather complicated.

Table 13

CATEGORIES OF USDA-CERTIFIED ORGANIC FOODS

LABEL STATEMENT	USDA ORGANIC REQUIREMENTS*
100% organic	Must contain 100% organic ingredients. Can display the Certified Organic seal on the front of the package.
Organic	Must contain 95–99% organic ingredients. Can display the Certified Organic seal on the front of the package.
Made with organic ingredients	Must contain 70–94% organic ingredients. Can list up to three organic ingredients on the package front. Cannot display the organic seal anywhere on the package.
Less than 70% organic	Can list organic ingredients on the information panel. Cannot use the word "organic" on the front of the package. Cannot display the organic seal anywhere on the package.

* These USDA categories, established in 2002, are explained further by the National Organic Program at www.ams.usda.gov/nop.

By these guidelines, products that display the USDA organic seal must contain at least 95 percent organic ingredients. We bought a package of certified organic Party Animal Organic Dog Food ("made with the finest organic ingredients!") in which every ingredient—except the vitamins and minerals—is organic, even the guar gum thickener. But just a glance at other "organic" pet foods on the market suggests that this is rarely the case, and that the organic rules apply to pet foods only casually.

The organic rules can be casually applied in part because the regulatory agency is the USDA, not the FDA, and the USDA allows more leeway in marketing. Pet food companies, for example, may use the word "organic" in their name, even when it is obvious that their products are not organic. Timber Wolf Organics, the maker of "carnivore specific herbal pet foods the way nature intended," is allowed to call itself organic even though we bought one of its dry dog foods and observed that it did not contain a single organic ingredient, not even one.

Newman's Own Organics, in contrast, seems to be doing its best to comply with standards, at least for some of its products. Its foods usually contain some organic ingredients, but the amounts vary. We bought a can of its Chicken Formula for dogs, which listed organic chicken as the first ingredient, but that was the only one. The other ingredients were salmon, whitefish, brown rice, flaxseed, oat bran, kelp, and the usual vitamins and minerals, none of them organic. The label said "made with organic chicken," which tells you it must make up at least 70 percent of the dry ingredients if it is following the NOP rules (which it is not required to do). We found a higher-end Newman's dog food labeled "made with organic grains and vegetables." Although nonorganic chicken was the first ingredient, ten of the next thirteen ingredients were organic. The company appears to be trying hard to expand its repertoire of organic ingredients, but even the foods with the most organic ingredients do not display a certified organic seal. By NOP rules, the ingredients would have to be at least 95 percent organic to do so.

But we have no trouble finding pet foods labeled certified organic. Party Animal dog foods, for example, display a certification seal from OCIA, the Organic Crop Improvement Association in Lincoln, Nebraska. PetGuard Organics Adult Dog Food ("made with more than 95 percent organic ingredients") is certified by OneCert, also of Lincoln, Nebraska, and displays the USDA certified organic seal. We guess that it is ignoring the nonorganic vitamins and minerals.

Another certifying agency, Quality Assurance International (QAI), has more stringent standards. It certifies pet foods as organic. But because the vitamin and mineral mixes are not included in the organic standards, it does not allow companies to display the USDA seal. It allows treats and food supplements to display the seal as long as they do not contain synthetic vitamins and amino acids. Buddy Biscuits Sweet Potato Madness treats display the USDA seal as certified by ODAFF (Oklahoma Department of Agriculture, Food, and Forestry), which must not be concerned about the nonorganic ingredients, calcium sulfate and vitamin E.

Organix [Castor & Pollux Pet Works] Feline Formula displays the USDA organic seal and lists all of its ingredients as organic, except chicken broth and the vitamins and minerals. Does chicken broth not count? You have to go to the website to identify the certifier, in this case, Oregon Tilth. The lack of federal regulation allows such inconsistencies. In late June 2009, we bought a package of Natural Planet ORGANICS (in capital letters on the package) cat formula made with organic free-range chicken. The front of the package said "certified organic by Oregon Tilth" but we could not find an organic seal. Organic chicken is listed as the first ingredient but nonorganic chicken meal came second. We have to assume that Oregon Tilth was certifying the separate ingredients, not the product itself.

We think following the organic rules as best they can is nowhere near good enough. If pet foods are marketed as organic, they ought to be certified organic, and should have to follow the rules—all of them—for labeling, organic certification, and display of the organic seal. If organic products are going to command higher prices, their organic claims have to be credible. We hope the NOP acts quickly on this matter.

THE "WE DON'T USE IT" CLAIMS

We got a kick out of the catchy slogan used by Pet Promise: "Let byproducts be bygones." In 2009, the label of a can of Pet Promise "Bison & Brown Rice Formula" dog food still promised:

- NO animal byproducts
- NO added growth hormones
- NO antibiotic-fed protein sources
- NO rendered meats or fats
- NO factory farm meat or poultry
- NO artificial colors, flavors or preservatives

The Pet Promise website assures customers: "We know our ranch of origin for all of our meat and poultry," and "natural meat, free-range chicken, or ocean-caught fish [is] always the #1 ingredient." The website contrasts these points with a matching set of bullet points explaining that other brands contain all those presumably evil things, and "If a pet food doesn't make this PROMISE OF PURITY, it's probably because it can't."

Hormones, antibiotics, and factory farming refer to the way most meat and poultry is produced in America. The animals and birds are raised in large confined animal feeding operations (CAFOs) or factory farms. These farms raise tens of thousands of cattle or hundreds of thousands of chickens in close quarters and often treat them with antibiotics to promote growth or prevent infections. Beef cattle are implanted with hormones to promote growth. The hazards of CAFOs to animal and human health, to the environment, and to the communities in which these places operate, have been well documented. Better production methods are highly valued by many pet owners and alternative pet foods offer choices that support such value systems.

Production concerns, and those about animal by-products, constitute explicit critiques of the other commercial pet foods. Hence: alternative. Dave Carter, one of the founders of Pet Promise, explained how the company got started. Carter was executive director of the National Bison Association, a trade group for bison ranchers. Pet Promise, he said, was founded as an outlet for hearts, livers, and other organs from slaughtered bison that nobody wanted to eat and would otherwise go to waste. He and his partners founded Pet Promise's parent company, Natural Pet Nutrition, in large part to improve the income of bison ranchers.

In 2004, they sold their company to Nestlé Purina PetCare, but you would never have known that from viewing the Pet Promise website. To learn who owned it, you had to go to the Nestlé website to discover that Pet

Promise was a key component of the corporation's sustainable agriculture initiatives. Pet Promise, Nestlé Purina explained, "provides a stable, profitable market for hearts, livers, trim meat, and poultry frames—all portions of the animals that the ranchers have had difficulty in selling . . . [Pet Promise works] with independent ranchers who are restoring once-endangered herds of American bison." Back on the Pet Promise site, the company explained that it was devoted to "Changing the way farm animals are raised and companion animals are fed. . . . Can pet food save the earth? We think so."

We think supporting bison ranchers is a terrific idea, and we greatly favored the values represented by former Pet Promise products. Nevertheless, we are amused by the no by-products claim. The company did not consider hearts, livers, trim meat, and poultry frames to be by-products, because it did not have to. AAFCO definitions permit specific meats and organs to be listed as themselves—bison, bison liver—as long as: "If it bears a name descriptive of its kind, it must correspond thereto." Otherwise, the AAFCO definitions leave plenty of room for creative interpretation: "**By-product:** secondary products produced in addition to the principal product."

Others prefer less creative interpretations, apparently. In 2009, Hill's Pet Nutrition complained that one of its competitors, Blue Buffalo, was advertising its products with a "no animal by-products" claim when in fact they contained fish and meat meals. Because meat meals contain parts of animals humans would not ordinarily eat, Hill's argued that the advertisements were misleading and got the case referred to the Federal Trade Commission.

Whether you consider bison, bison livers, and fish and meat meals to be by-products or not is a matter of semantics. As noted earlier, we view practically all ingredients in pet foods as by-products of human food production. If they weren't, we would be competing with our pets for food. And this would be some competition. On the basis of calorie requirements alone, the 172 million dogs and cats in America need to eat as much food as 42 million people, a population larger than that of Canada in 2009. It's a good thing these animals are eating by-products. But "let byproducts be bygones" was such good marketing, and Pet Promise products were so attractive to consumers interested in alternative pet foods, that we could easily understand why Nestlé Purina PetCare wanted to add this company to its portfolio. We were disappointed when the company was discontinued.

THE "HUMAN-GRADE" CLAIM

We bought a package of Back to Basics Super Premium Food for Dogs with a list of bullet points similar to those of Pet Promise. "100 percent human-grade ingredients" tops the list for both dog and cat foods, and the company's website displays the seal shown in figure 7.

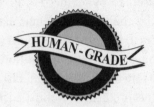

Figure 7
Back to Basics' human-grade seal. AAFCO has not issued a definition of "human-grade."

Source: Beowulf Natural Feeds at www.beowulfs.com.

Products made with human-grade ingredients constitute another growing segment of the alternative pet food category. At Pet Expo in 2008 we were offered any number of foods and treats said to be human-grade, implying that they were good enough for us to eat. The Back to Basics statements and seal are rare, however. We do not see too many of these kinds of claims on package labels, mainly because AAFCO has no official definition of the terms "human-grade" or "human quality." Without an approved AAFCO definition, an ingredient or term is not supposed to be used (recall our discussion of Old Boots in chapter 7). AAFCO says that use of "human-grade" is false and misleading and constitutes misbranding unless every ingredient in the product—and every processing method—meets the standards of the FDA and USDA for producing, processing, and transporting foods suitable for consumption by humans, and that every ingredient producer is licensed to perform those tasks.

AAFCO's unease about the term does not stop pet food makers from using it, particularly because the legal situation seems to be on their side.

In 2007, a case against The Honest Kitchen pet food company led the Ohio courts to rule that it had a constitutional right to truthful commercial free speech and could use "human-grade" on its labels. The Honest Kitchen says "all ingredients are guaranteed 100 percent Human Food Grade" and that it "has been the only pet food manufacturer in the United States to have proven to the Federal FDA that every ingredient it uses in its products are [*sic*] suitable for human consumption." If Back to Basics had also proven this to the FDA by mid-2008, it was not saying so on its website. Instead, it said: "BACK TO BASICS chicken is specially processed from USDA inspected facilities which produce the same chicken we eat at our tables. It is the highest quality chicken available, costing 40 percent more than the second best chicken available."

Although only a few companies are claiming human grade on their food labels, a great many use the term freely in their in-store materials and websites. Eagle Pack says: "Our ingredients are sourced from human grade suppliers. Chicken Meal is produced from chickens passed by the USDA; meals are antibiotic free with no added hormones. Fruits and veggies are all human grade." Newman's Own Organics even provides a Q and A on the topic:

Q: Does Newman's Own Organics use human grade materials? Why isn't that written on the bag?
A: Newman's Own Organics organic pet food uses human grade and fit for human consumption ingredients such as natural chicken and organic grains. The AAFCO Board . . . actually prohibits the printing of "Human Grade" on pet food packaging.

THE "HOLISTIC" CLAIM

We are not sure what holistic means exactly, and even less sure what it means when applied to pet foods. Companies that use the term rarely bother to define it. Consider Bench & Field's Holistic Natural Canine Formula with "quality protein sources for superior nutrition & palatability, including certified Free Range chicken grown by Amish farmers," Artemis Pet Food's Holistic Approach to Cat Food, Azmira's Holistic Animal Care (As Nature Intended), or Burns Feline Maintenance for Cats ("developed by a holistic veterinarian . . . the holistic approach to health and nutrition"). The ingredient lists of these products are no help at all. They look just like any other pet food, but without by-products. The first five ingredients of the Burns cat food, for example, are brown rice, chicken meal, peas, ocean fish meal, and maize (corn).

From reading these labels, we imagine that holistic pet foods are supposed to encompass everything that is good about food in its most natural state. Heidi Hill, who owns Holistic Hound, an alternative pet products store in Berkeley, California, told us that holistic should refer to the totality of the physical, mental, and emotional state of the animal—the whole pet. But by this definition, she says, holistic pet food is an oxymoron because it only addresses the physical aspect of the animal. Something more is needed, perhaps like the definition that appeared in an advertisement for Solid Gold Health Products for Pets, a company that claims ownership of the entire concept:

> In 1985, we introduced the first holistic dog/cat food into the U.S. . . . They had no idea what holistic meant. It doesn't mean natural and it doesn't mean organic. It is a philosophy of life. It means the whole body works together—mind, body and spirit. It saddens us that other dog food companies incorrectly throw around the word holistic just because Solid Gold uses it. It saddens us that they try to fool the public by trying to copy our philosophy.

We were interested to check the first five ingredients in this company's Hund-n-Flocken Adult Dog (Lamb): lamb, lamb meal, brown rice, cracked pearled barley, and millet. These are fairly common ingredients in many dog foods—meals, but no by-products. As far as we can tell, "holistic" in practice must mean "no by-products."

THE "PREMIUM" CLAIM

The meaning of premium, according to people who have been in this business a long time, used to be easy to understand. The term referred to products that you could not buy at supermarkets but had to get from pet stores, breeders, or veterinarians. These days, the meaning has changed. When we ask pet food makers to define "premium," we love the answers we get:

- It means nothing, it's about marketing.
- You can charge more for the food.
- The animals won't make as much poop.

Without an AAFCO definition—AAFCO has yet to develop one—premium is a marketing term. You are supposed to think that the product is better than your average run-of-the-mill pet food and worth the higher price—sometimes *much* higher price—that is inevitably attached to it. As usual, we like to check the first five ingredients, but we have a hard time telling the difference between premium and non-premium pet foods. Sometimes the premium ingredient lists begin with meat, but the next several are usually grains of one type or another. We bought a can of Precept Premium Nutrition dog food, for example, that began with chicken meal, but then came ground rice, ground wheat, ground corn, and chicken fat. As for superpremium: Walmart's Maxximum Nutrition Super Premium dog food lists the first five ingredients as lamb, chicken meal, ground sorghum, brewer's rice, and ground barley. Worth a premium price? That is for you to decide.

We are not alone in our skepticism. In 2005, researchers at the University of Georgia's College of Veterinary Medicine recruited dog owners to feed three premium dry pet foods in random order and judge their effects on the dogs' body condition. The products were from Purina ONE (Nestlé Purina PetCare), Eukanuba (Procter & Gamble's Iams), and Science Diet (Hill's Pet Nutrition), but the owners were given the foods in plain white bags and were not told which was which. When blinded to the product name, owners perceived no significant difference in the dogs' response to the diets. The researchers were forced to conclude that "factors other than the diets themselves play a role in how owners perceive the performance of dog foods." So premium is about brand recognition more than discernable quality (think Coke vs. Pepsi). As a marketing strategy, it works well. Among dog owners responding to a survey in 2007, 42 percent said they had purchased a premium food during the past year, and one-third said premium products were their most frequent choice. We looked for research studies comparing the responses of pets to premium and grocery brand foods, but found none. No pet food company wants to do a study like this.

THE "POOP" CLAIM

We think the real meaning of premium is low poop. Cat boxes and kitty litter have solved the poop problem for cats that live indoors, but the poop issue is a critical one for the owners of dogs living in apartments or places where the animals do not have free access to the outdoors. Left to their own devices, dogs typically defecate five or six times a day. Even the most diligent dog-walking owner will have a hard time keeping up with that kind of schedule. This puts a "premium" on anything that keeps the volume and urgency of poop to a minimum. The poop problem explains why the PETCO store in Union Square, Manhattan, posted this sign throughout its dog food section:

SUPREME NUTRITION

More Nutrition / Feed Less: Only the highest quality ingredients are used in Premium Pet Foods, so they are more nutritious and digestible than Supermarket Brands. It takes less food to meet the nutritional needs of your pet.

Better Value / Spend Less: Rich in energy, Premium Pet Food packs more protein and energy per mouthful than Supermarket Brands. It takes less food to feed your pet, so you get more for your money.

Easier Clean Up / Less Waste: Feeding smaller amounts of highly digestible Premium Pet Food means lower stool volume and easier backyard cleanup.

In case this message is too subtle to understand, the sign provides photographs of two bags: a small "stool volume for premium pet food," and a bag twice as large of "stool volume for supermarket brand food."

Nutro (owned by Mars) makes the issue even more explicit. It provideed a graphic illustration of the pounds of stool produced by dogs eating one hundred pounds of food of different brands, which we reproduce in figure 8. Nutro does not give details about how this study was accomplished, but we are glad we were not the ones doing it.

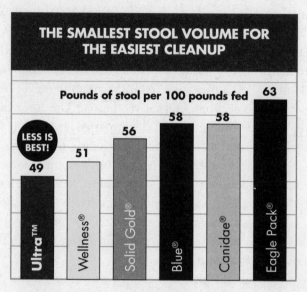

FIGURE 8
Nutro Ultra-Holistic Nutrition explained why its dog foods are premium quality on its website in 2008.

Source: www.ultraholistic.com/stool/shtml/

Meat produces less residue than grains, so you would expect premium foods making "low poop" claims to have relatively more meat, chicken, or fish, but relatively less corn, rice, wheat, barley, soybeans, or beet pulp, all of which are sources of poop-making fiber. The benefit of marketing lower poop to owners is well established. Prior to the mid-1980s, dry dog foods were higher in fiber. As Americans began working longer hours and staying away from home for longer periods of time, dog owners began looking for foods that would reduce fecal volume. The older styles of pet foods are said to have produced an average of 400 grams or nearly a pound of wet feces for each 400 grams of dry food consumed (feces mostly consist of bacteria, some undigested fiber, and water). In contrast, today's premium brands can produce as little as 85 grams, and the consistency will be harder and less messy to clean up.

THE COST OF PREMIUM ALTERNATIVES

Issues related to food production methods—how animals and plant crops are raised—and to the quality of the ingredients fed to pets are important to many people (including us). Alternative pet foods offer choices designed to address those values, but at a cost. In May 2008, we went to Whiskers Holistic Pet Care, a store in our Manhattan neighborhood that caters to pet owners seeking alternative choices. The store carries only a few products made by Big Pet Food companies. Instead, it specializes in products labeled natural, organic, holistic, premium, and superpremium, and containing no by-products or other components perceived as undesirable. We bought a can of every alternative chicken dinner for dogs we could find, and did some price comparisons. Later, since none of the labels claimed that the ingredients were human grade, we went to the companies' websites and checked to see if they were making that claim. Table 14 shows what we found.

During that week, the lowest price for a conventional chicken dinner for dogs was 44 cents for Ol'Roy at Walmart (table 12). The mark-up for alternative pet foods ranges from three- to nearly sevenfold. Within the alternative products themselves, the prices ranged more than twofold, from $1.39 to $2.99. We could not discern any clear trend within this range. The ingredients are quite similar: chicken appears first, chicken broth or water comes second, and various chicken, fish, and vegetable ingredients follow. Perhaps the quality of the ingredients varies, but we cannot know that without comparing the company's actual practices to its promises. Within the alternative category, we think the price has more to do with marketing than anything else. Ordinarily, our first choice would be an organic product because we believe that organic production methods are better for the environment, but through 2009 at least, the standards for organic pet foods were full of loopholes. If we wanted an alternative pet food, we'd pick the cheapest we could find unless we were sure that a more expensive one would more closely reflect our values.

Table 14

COMPARATIVE PRICES OF "ALTERNATIVE" CHICKEN DINNERS, ~13-OUNCE CANS, MAY 2008[a]

PRODUCT	LABEL CLAIMS	PRICE, $	FIRST FIVE INGREDIENTS
Eagle Pack Holistic Select	Holistic (human grade[b])	1.39	Chicken, chicken broth, ocean fish, oat bran, carrots
Evangers's Super Premium	Natural, superpremium; no preservatives, artificial color, or added salt (human grade[b])	1.69	Chicken, chicken broth, carrots, peas, apples
PetGuard Organics	Organic, holistic, super-premium	1.89	Organic chicken, chicken broth, organic brown rice, organic oats, organic carrots
Wellness (Old Mother Hubbard)	No by-products, wheat, corn, white rice, or artificial flavors, preservatives, or colors (human grade[b])	1.99	Chicken, chicken broth, chicken liver, ocean whitefish, ground barley
Pet Promise (Nestlé Purina PetCare)	Natural; no by-products, hormones, antibiotics, rendered meats or fats, factory-farmed meat or poultry, artificial colors, flavors, or preservatives	2.15	Chicken, chicken broth, chicken liver, brown rice, potatoes
Newman's Own Organics	Organic	2.49	Organic chicken, water, ocean whitefish, brown rice, organic turkey
California Natural (Natura Pet Products)	Natural	2.59	Chicken, chicken broth, brown rice, natural flavor, ground flaxseed
Natural Balance (Dick Van Patten)	Natural, ultrapremium	2.99	Chicken, chicken broth, chicken liver, carrots, oat bran

a. Products differ in can size (range: 12.7 to 13.2 ounces) and name (Chicken and Brown Rice Formula, Chunky Chicken Dinner, etc.). All meet AAFCO dog nutrient profiles for adult canines or for all life stages. All were purchased at the same time at Whiskers Holistic Pet Care, Manhattan, except for the Pet Promise, obtained at another store during the same week. b. Claim given on company website.

Nancy Kerns, who edits the excellent publication *Whole Dog Journal*, and whose work we greatly admire, has more specific recommendations for choosing high-quality pet foods. These, she says, should contain:

- Superior sources of protein: whole, fresh meats or single-source meat meals (chicken rather than poultry)
- Whole-meat sources as one of the first two ingredients
- Whole, unprocessed grains, vegetables, and other foods
- Organic ingredients
- A minimum of food fragments such as brewer's rice or wheat bran
- No meat or poultry by-products (mainly because they are poorly handled)
- No generic fats or proteins, or artificial preservatives, colors, or sweeteners
- No propylene glycol moisturizer

We concur with most of these recommendations, particularly the last two, but are not convinced that the others make that much of a difference. Canning and processing into kibble are great levelers and we are hard-pressed to argue that anyone should pay more for products that we find virtually indistinguishable.

SPECIAL
PRODUCTS for
TARGET MARKETS

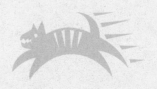

For Young and Old

PET FOOD COMPANIES market special products for puppies and kittens and for senior animals. Do young and old cats and dogs need anything special in their food? Many brands targeted to young, growing animals contain supplements of the omega-3 fatty acid DHA. Many products aimed at older animals are supplemented with antioxidants. But during the time we were working on this book, not many owners were buying products for young animals—fewer than 10 percent of dog owners and 5 percent of cat owners. Foods for older animals were selling a bit better, as they were purchased by 15 percent of dog owners and 14 percent of cat owners. Should you help fill the market gap by buying special foods for your young or old pets? Let's take a look.

MARKET SEGMENT: PUPPIES AND KITTENS

Puppies and kittens require more protein, calories, and other nutrients than adult animals in order to support their rapid growth. They can get extra nutrients from foods that are more concentrated, but they also eat more food relative to their body weights than do adults. The National Research Council (NRC) says newborn puppies require twice as many calories per pound of body weight as adults do. By the time animals reach half their adult weights, the proportion falls to about 1.6.

AAFCO nutrient profiles usually call for amounts that are higher than those recommended by the NRC, and these higher levels are reflected in the composition of pet foods targeted to young animals. Such foods provide more protein and fat than products aimed at adults. Nutro Max Cat Kitten dry food, for example, is for kittens as well as pregnant or nursing cats (these also need to eat more than nonpregnant adults). It lists a guaranteed analysis of 34 percent protein and 19 percent fat, compared to 30 percent protein and 15 percent fat in the adult formulas. This is a higher-protein, higher-fat product, with plenty of of calories.

The feeding guidelines on pet foods targeted to puppies and kittens take the calorie and growth needs of the animals into consideration. We think the feeding directions are worth following carefully. Giving too much food to young animals, especially to large-breed puppies, encourages them to grow too quickly and can cause problems with their bones.

But we remain unconvinced that special formulas are needed to support the growth of kittens and puppies. They may be great for marketing purposes, but foods that meet the AAFCO profiles for *all life stages* also meet the needs of puppies and kittens. That is the point of such complete-and-balanced products. But the *all life stages* profiles present a marketing challenge. If complete-and-balanced pet foods for all life stages meet the needs of growing animals, why would anyone want to pay more for special foods for them? The answer to a marketer's prayer: DHA.

DHA-Supplemented Formulas

Let's hear applause for the omega-3 fatty acid DHA. On the basis of research performed on rats and humans, DHA appears to be essential for proper development of the brain, vision, and other critically important functions. It is now routinely added to human infant formulas. We and other animals, including dogs and cats, make our own DHA from a precursor, alpha-linolenic acid (ALA). Leafy greens and vegetable seed oils—flaxseed, canola, and soy, for example—are good sources of ALA. But the best sources of omega-3 fatty acids are fatty fish that ate small algae when they were young, and the meat and eggs of chickens fed on ALA-rich seeds. Eating vegetables and seeds provides ALA, but the conversion of ALA to DHA occurs slowly in the animal body and there is some speculation that the amounts of DHA formed from ALA may not reach optimal levels.

How much is optimal? Because only small amounts of DHA seem to be required, it is difficult to do studies to define how much is best. Studies of dogs and cats, for example, would have to be done on a large number of animals over a long period of time and would be difficult and expensive to perform. Instead, the amounts needed by dogs and cats are extrapolated from human studies and from the few studies done on small groups of dogs. Both types find DHA to accumulate in neural tissues during fetal development and to be linked to improved performance on certain tests of vision and behavior in young infants and puppies. These short-term test results look impressive but the long-term benefits of the early improvements have yet to be documented.

In one typical study in humans—not coincidentally funded by Martek Biosciences, a manufacturer of DHA—investigators gave preschool children doses of either 400 milligrams DHA per day or a placebo. As would be expected, the children who received DHA supplements had higher levels of this fatty acid in their blood. Higher blood levels seem good, but do they make any real difference? The children supplemented with DHA did not perform any better on four tests of mental acuity than children who were given the placebo. Nevertheless, Martek claimed the study constituted "an extension of the evidence of the beneficial effects of DHA supplementation seen during pregnancy and infancy." The inconclusive nature of such research is not viewed as an impediment to adding DHA to infant formulas—and to charge more for such formulas. Pet food makers are now using the same strategy for products aimed at puppies and kittens.

Pet food companies say they have research to back up the benefits of adding DHA. In one published study, investigators raised puppies on diets supplemented with omega-3 fats. They observed the same kind of improvements in visual acuity as those observed in human infants, but did not say or predict whether the supplemented puppies would see better as adults.

At this point, we must deal with another frustrating barrier erected by this industry. The details of many DHA research studies were not available for our review. They were conducted by pet food companies that consider the methods and results of their investigations to be proprietary. On its website, for example, Iams describes a study in which its scientists gave DHA supplements to pregnant dogs. The company says the supplemented dogs produced puppies that were "more trainable" than those born to unsupplemented mothers; they were able to work their way more effectively through mazes. What were the doses of DHA? Did the puppies born to unsupplemented mothers have any DHA in their diets at all? If not, they might have been suffering from nutrient deficiencies to begin with. The significance of this study cannot be evaluated without having access to its methods and data.

Iams notes on its website that details of the study are on file. We wrote the company and asked to see them. We soon received a response from Iams Pet Care Team Member, Mary Lou:

> Thanks for your message about DHA and its effects on a puppy's trainability. We've found feeding pregnant bitches and young puppies food rich in DHA results in a smarter more trainable puppy. I'd be happy to send you some printed information via postal mail if you write back with your complete name and postal mailing address. It will arrive about three weeks after I receive your information. . . . Best wishes to you and all of your four-legged friends for many more happy and healthy years together.

Three weeks seemed like a long time to wait in this era of instant access to online research reports, but we are patient. Team member Mary Lou did get back to us within the promised time, but why bother? The mailing consisted of precisely the same one-page summary of the study that we had seen on the website. The reluctance of Iams (which is owned by Procter & Gamble) to share the details of its research does nothing to instill confidence in its DHA label claims.

The 2006 NRC pet food committee noted the lack of convincing research on which to base a recommended allowance for omega-3 fatty acids. Nevertheless, the committee suggested that adult dogs need about 880 mg/kg of omega-3s in their food each day, and even more—1,300 mg/kg—for puppies and for pregnant and lactating dogs. This seems high to us. Although poultry fat and poultry by-product meals contribute omega-3s to the diet, the suggested allowances are so large that they can only be attained by adding DHA-rich fish meal or fish oils to the formulas.

In contrast, the NRC recommended much lower omega-3 allowances for cats. Although the NRC cited no research as a basis for the allowance, it recommended only 100 mg/kg for adult cats, and 300 mg/kg for kittens and pregnant and lactating queens. Given the lack of research on which to base such figures, we have no idea why the NRC proposed such different allowances for dogs and cats. Our uneasy suspicion is that the difference simply reflects the differing ways in which the members of the cat and dog subcommittees interpret the science.

It is possible that omega-3 fatty acids in general, and DHA in particular, may be especially useful for puppies, kittens, or children, but we would like to see more research on long-term benefits before setting recommended allowances. We particularly want to know whether consuming omega-3 fats in infancy makes infants, puppies, or kittens more visually acute, smarter, or healthier as adults.

Others would like to know these sorts of things as well. When the FDA agreed to allow DHA to be added to infant formulas, it did so in response to a petition from Martek Biosciences. Without research one way or the other, the FDA had no grounds for denying the petition, but still had reservations, as the agency explains in a Q and A on its website:

> The scientific evidence is mixed. Some studies in infants suggest that including these fatty acids in infant formulas may have positive effects on visual function and neural development over the short term. Other studies in infants do not confirm these benefits. There are no currently available published reports from clinical studies that address whether any long-term beneficial effects exist.

We think such studies are badly needed. Here's why. The FDA first allowed DHA and other omega-3 fats to be added to human infant formulas only in 2002. Prior to that year, generations of American children—in the millions every year—were raised on infant formulas without added DHA. Somehow, they made it to adulthood. No studies of adults show signs of visual or other deficits linked to the lack of extra omega-3s in infancy. Is DHA more about marketing than health? Without research, we cannot be sure.

MARKET SEGMENT: SENIORS

With the increase in human life expectancy, the effects of diet on aging have become a subject of intense personal and professional interest. Many of the diseases common to aging populations—coronary heart disease, cancers, diabetes, and kidney disease, for example—are influenced by diet. Advances in treatment of these diseases have contributed to longer life expectancy of humans, as have antibiotics, improved sanitation, and other public health measures. Although much less is known about the role of diet in longevity, researchers are especially interested in two types of interventions that might extend the human and animal life span: caloric restriction and antioxidants.

Food Restriction

Caloric restriction as a means to extend life span has a long history. In the 1930s, Dr. Clive McCay and his colleagues at Cornell University conducted now famous studies of diet and longevity in rats. They allowed rats to eat only about 60 percent of their normal ration each day, a near-starvation level. To their surprise, the rats fed restricted diets lived nearly twice as long as rats allowed all the food they wanted. Since then, other investigators have observed the same phenomenon with mice, fish, flies, worms, and yeast.

Studies like these are in progress using primates, but none has yet been done in humans. This level of food restriction would not be easy to attain. We do not enjoy starvation. Even a 20 percent reduction in calorie intake for more than a day or two makes us cranky. We feel hungry and lethargic, obsess about food, and display all kinds of symptoms of psychological distress. The consistency of the results of the animal experiments, however, has induced some intrepid individuals to voluntarily restrict their calorie intake in the hope of delaying the onset of chronic diseases and living longer. This does not sound like much fun to us, but we await the results of their efforts with great interest.

What about cats and dogs? Nestlé Purina PetCare examined the effects of food restriction on twenty-four pairs of Labrador retrievers. The way they did the study was complicated. Researchers fed an unrestricted diet to one member of the pair, but just 75 percent of the normal ration to the other. Fine, but after three years, they changed the protocol. To prevent the dogs on the unrestricted diets from becoming obese, they limited the ration of these "control" dogs, as well. Then they adjusted the calorie intake of the dogs on the restricted diets downward to 75 percent of the amount fed to the less-restricted controls. In effect, *both* members of the pair were fed diets restricted to at least some extent. Nevertheless, by the end of the study, the more restricted dogs weighed 26 percent less than their partners. They also were healthier and lived two years longer—to an average age of thirteen years as compared to eleven.

These are impressive results but we are not sure how they might translate into taking care of a pet at home. The mere thought of living with a constantly hungry dog or cat is not a happy one. The dogs in this experiment were confined to pens and the report gives no information about their comparative behavior or activity levels. One of the first signs of starvation is to become lethargic, which also might not be much fun in a house pet. We cannot recommend that you try severe caloric restriction at home. But we do think the study provides good evidence that pets should not be overfed or allowed to become obese.

Use of Antioxidants

One theory of aging is that it is due to the accumulation of oxygen-induced damage to protein, fats, and DNA. This damage causes age-related diseases. Caloric restriction, according to this theory, reduces or slows oxidative damage. If so, could you take—or give pets—antioxidants to prevent or reverse the damage? Antioxidants are widely distributed in nature, and several essential nutrients such as selenium and vitamins A, C, and E either act as antioxidants or promote their activity. Vitamin E, for example, prevents the oxidation of body fats, and is commonly added to pet foods to prevent fats from going rancid, as are the synthetic antioxidants ethoxyquin, BHT, and BHA. Many other isolated constituents of fruits, vegetables, beans, and grains also have antioxidant activity, among them beta-carotene, flavonoids, and polyphenols. Perhaps these substances could promote longer and healthier lives? Researchers have addressed this very question in humans as well as in pets.

Antioxidants in human foods. Epidemiology provides much evidence that eating fruits and vegetables delays the onset of chronic diseases and the deterioration of function that occurs with aging. Much effort has gone into trying to figure out which specific components of these foods might be protective. Because fruits and vegetables are rich sources of substances that act as antioxidants, researchers have focused on single nutrients that might be responsible for these benefits. Unfortunately, the results of research on single antioxidant nutrients have been deeply disappointing. By now, several studies have shown that supplements of vitamin A, beta-carotene, or vitamin E have no effect on the risk of cardiovascular disease or cancer. Worse, they might actually increase the risk. Research on the effects of antioxidants on Alzheimer's disease or macular degeneration also does not show consistent benefits. To date, antioxidants do not appear to reverse problems of aging or to increase longevity in humans.

Antioxidants in pet foods. The lack of evidence for benefits of antioxidant supplements in humans has not stopped pet food companies from trying the same kinds of experiments in pets. If a company could find some research evidence for the health benefits of antioxidants, it could add antioxidants to its foods and market them as promoting health and longevity.

As in people, the brains of aging dogs develop plaques and deposit proteins that are characteristic of dementia and Alzheimer's disease. This makes dogs good candidates for the study of aging. Many beagles, for example, begin to lose cognitive ability when they are about eight years old. After age twelve, their brains sometimes decline to the point of dementia. In a study sponsored by the National Institute of Aging in partnership with Hill's Pet Nutrition, a mixture of antioxidant substances—and "environmental enrichment" (translation: play)—improved the ability of dogs to learn how to recognize where their food was hidden. Playing with the dogs alone improved their learning ability, but the combination of antioxidants in the food and keeping them actively engaged worked best.

Although Hill's uses these results to market an antioxidant-enriched food for older dogs, we cannot tell whether this study provides evidence for the claim. The investigators did not disclose the composition of the diet they used; apparently, this information is proprietary to Hills. The treatment mixture contained several antioxidant substances—vitamin E, carnitine, lipoic acid, and ascorbic acid—as well as very small amounts of spinach flakes and by-products (skin, pulp, seeds) of tomatoes, grapes, carrots, and citrus fruits. It is difficult to know which of these components might be responsible for the reported effects. Most troubling, the "control" dogs, the ones that were not fed antioxidants or given behavioral stimulation, were older—by an average of seven months—than the dogs given the most effective treatment. This difference may be equivalent to two or three years in humans and could account for the difference in results all on its own.

Nestlé Purina PetCare did a similar study using cats. When investigators fed cats a diet supplemented with an antioxidant mix, the animals lived a year longer than cats fed unsupplemented food. The mix consisted of beta-carotene, extra vitamin E, a mixture of linoleic (omega-6) and linolenic (omega-3) fatty acids, and dried whole chicory root (as a promoter of the growth of "friendly" intestinal bacteria). The investigators did not disclose the composition of the diet, nor did they report the amounts of the supplement ingredients. They did note that the cats fed the supplemented diet ate substantially less than those fed the unsupplemented diet. Could eating less be the real reason the supplemented group lived longer? The report does not say.

All the major pet food companies that conduct research seem to be doing such studies. Researchers at Mars Petcare report stronger responses to immunizations in kittens and dogs fed a diet supplemented with an antioxidant cocktail of vitamins C and E and lutein, with some taurine tossed into the mix. Once again, details of the study are not available. The Mars investigators reported their results only in a short abstract in a professional journal and as a summary in the company's publication, the *Waltham Focus* (now *Veterinary Focus*).

Given the limited number of dogs (usually twelve or fewer) used in these studies, the lack of information about the composition of the diets, and the commercial sponsorship of the research, we cannot help but be skeptical about the claims for benefits of antioxidants in pet foods. The NRC notes that vitamin and mineral antioxidants are demonstrably beneficial as sources of essential nutrients, and for preventing fat oxidation. But it also questions the benefits of supplemental antioxidant nutrients for aging cats and dogs. If human studies suggest harm from excessive intake of antioxidants, shouldn't we expect similar results in animals? Indeed, vitamin C supplementation has been reported to slow the running time of racing greyhounds, and a group at Cornell advises against using vitamin C to treat bone disease in growing, large-breed dogs (recall: dogs make their own vitamin C).

On the other hand, we also find the evidence for harm of antioxidant intake to be as limited and preliminary as the evidence for benefits. Even so, enough studies are around to cast doubt on the wisdom of feeding excessive amounts of antioxidants to people or to pets. Until more research is available on the safety of antioxidant supplements, we recommend sticking to levels that are adequate to meet nutritional requirements and to keep fats from going rancid.

14

For Special Health Problems

 THE FOOD LABEL in chapter 10 lists "five ways Whiskas food benefits your cat." Whiskas, says the label:

- Is 100 percent complete and balanced
- Helps to clean teeth
- Has everything needed for a healthy skin and a shiny coat
- Is easy to digest
- Helps your cat live a long, healthy life

Some of these promises—teeth, skin and coat, long life—are health claims and AAFCO has pages of model rules governing their wording. From the standpoint of federal regulations administered by the FDA, three kinds of health claims are allowed on the labels of human foods and supplements: nutrient content, disease, and structure-function. Nutrient content claims deal with such matters as the benefits of added nutrients and low fat. Disease claims are statements like "reduces the risk of heart disease." Structure-function claims refer to benefits for a body part or activity such as "supports a healthy immune system" or "helps maintain healthy bones."

Health claims are governed by Acts of Congress, none

of which say a word about pet food. Prior to 1990, when Congress passed the Nutrition Labeling and Education Act (NLEA), the FDA did not permit food manufacturers to claim that their products could prevent, mitigate, treat, or cure a particular disease. Such claims, the FDA said, would be the same as those made for drugs, and drug claims must be supported by clinical trials that prove safety and efficacy. No food manufacturer wanted to go through something like that to prove that a breakfast cereal might help lower cholesterol.

The NLEA put the nutrition facts label on the packages of foods for humans. Food manufacturers complained to Congress that the new labeling requirement forced them to disclose what was wrong with their products (too much saturated fat, salt, sugars), and that they should be allowed to say what was good in them. Congress agreed and ordered the FDA to review the science behind certain disease claims and to approve the ones substantiated by a reasonable amount of science. Eventually, the FDA approved a few claims, but said such statements had to be accompanied by a disclaimer. You can see the results of this decision on boxes of breakfast cereal labeled "helps prevent the risk of heart disease," with the disclaimer in very small print: "when eaten along with a diet low in saturated fat and cholesterol."

Even with a disclaimer, such claims were quickly shown to increase sales. They turned out to be such effective marketing tools that all companies wanted to use them. Whenever the FDA refused to approve a claim that did not have much science behind it, petitioners took the FDA to court. Health claims, food companies argued, were an expression of free speech protected by the First Amendment. Although you might think it unlikely that the founding fathers introduced the First Amendment to protect the right of food marketers to make health claims, the courts have consistently ruled in the companies' favor. The FDA gave up fighting unsubstantiated health claims and now permits food labels to display "qualified" health claims minimally backed up by science.

The NLEA and its legal interpretations apply only to human foods. Nevertheless, the FDA "incorporated the philosophy of the . . . [NLEA] in its policies to permit meaningful 'health' information on the labels of some animal food products." Pet food companies understand this philosophy to mean that the FDA allows them to say that their products help prevent or treat hip problems, skin allergies, or the risk of heart disease in dogs and cats as long as they can come up with a study or two to support the claims.

You might think that the Whiskas' statement, "has everything needed for a healthy skin and a shiny coat," requires at least some scientific substantiation, but it does not. It is a structure-function claim governed by the Dietary Supplement Health and Education Act (DSHEA) of 1994. This act, which we discuss further in chapter 17, required the FDA to permit claims that foods "help," "maintain," and "support" body structures or functions. The purpose of this act was to allow dietary supplements greater leeway in making health claims. Unless they are outrageous, structure-function claims can be left to the discretion of manufacturers. The supplement industry likes this arrangement. So do pet food companies.

Because neither the NLEA nor DSHEA have anything to say about pet foods, health claims are open to interpretation. In theory, the NLEA forbids health claims on pet food labels; if they appear, they are subject to the FDA's "regulatory enforcement." Also in theory, DSHEA means that supplements permitted in the human food supply are unapproved food additives when added to pet food. But in practice, the FDA has better things to do than to worry about health claims on pet food labels. It looks the other way as long as the labels more or less follow rules that apply to human foods or supplements. As the FDA puts the matter, pet food health claims are subject to the agency's "discretionary enforcement." The FDA is unlikely to invoke regulatory discretion and take action against pet food labels unless the labels say something that might cause overt harm.

The result is that products in the pet food aisles of supermarkets look just like products in any other area of the supermarket. They abound with claims that the products support overall pet health as well as healthy teeth, skin, fur, joints, and immune systems. Without specific federal guidance about claims on pet food labels, AAFCO says only that states may require documentation of a scientific basis for health claims and that structure-function claims must be based on ingredients with approved definitions for use in pet foods. And, says AAFCO, if a claim is based on a particular nutrient, that nutrient must be listed in the guaranteed analysis.

AAFCO model regulations do deal with one health claim: tartar control and bad breath. The Whiskas label is an example of how this works. The label says the product "helps to clean teeth." This wording is permitted because it does not imply that the food does anything more than control dental plaque through abrasion. It also does not imply that the product helps prevent or treat gum disease, cavities, or loss of teeth. If it did, it would be making a disease claim that requires scientific substantiation. AAFCO makes one exception for claims about breath odor. Its model regulations permit the labels of products containing chlorophyll or approved flavoring ingredients to claim that these ingredients control breath odor.

How this murky regulatory situation came about is something we discuss in detail in appendix 3, in which we review the history of the current oversight system. The effect of all this is that pet foods—as well as pet supplements—are allowed to be marketed with claims that their ingredients prevent or reduce risks for a host of common health problems. Like the makers of foods for humans, pet food makers sometimes add nutrients or other substances to their foods for the express purpose of making health claims. Such foods are referred to as "nutraceuticals." We review the evidence for the effectiveness and safety of the most common nutraceutical substances added to pet foods in chapter 18. In this chapter, we discuss some of the health problems for which pet food companies typically make health claims.

PRESCRIPTION DIETS

The FDA particularly ignores disease claims on veterinary prescription diets. These are products sold or marketed by pet food companies and veterinarians to treat specific disease conditions that affect almost any organ of a cat or dog's body. Hill's Prescription Diets, for example, are advertised as "therapeutic nutrition for dogs [or cats] with specific diseases." In prescription diets, food is medicine. One, for example, is a cat food (g/d Feline) advertised as a "nutritional aid in managing heart disease and heart failure." It also "is formulated to be helpful in older cats." To achieve this help, the formula reduces the amounts of sodium and phosphorus and adds extra taurine. Table 15 compares the composition of these nutrients in this Prescription Diet to a Hill's Science Diet product that is also designed for older cats—Minced Savory Chicken Entrée Mature Adult 7+—and to the amounts suggested by AAFCO nutrient profiles.

Table 15

AAFCO PROFILES COMPARED TO AMOUNTS OF THREE NUTRIENTS IN HILL'S PRESCRIPTION AND SCIENCE DIETS FOR CATS, % DRY INGREDIENTS

NUTRIENT	AAFCO NUTRIENT PROFILE	HILL'S PRESCRIPTION DIET*	HILL'S SCIENCE DIET*
Phosphorus	0.5	0.52	0.69
Sodium	0.2	0.32	0.49
Taurine	0.2	0.44	0.45

* Both products are canned cat food.

Phosphorus, sodium, and taurine are present in small amounts in these foods, less than 1 percent each. The Prescription Diet contains more phosphorus and sodium than is required by the AAFCO profile, but 17 percent less of each than the Science Diet. Both Hill's diets contain more than twice the amount of taurine required by AAFCO profiles. Is the Prescription Diet substantially better than the Science Diet for the health of older cats with heart disease? Hill's website does not cite research that might help answer that question.

The question of effectiveness is a critical one because Prescription Diet products are only sold through veterinarians (see chapter 24). In February 2008, we received a letter from a reader of *The Bark* whose dog, Jasper, had kidney disease and was put on a Prescription Diet but didn't like it much:

Jasper . . . hates the prescription kibble . . . but the vet (whom we really like) thinks we're nuts to contemplate anything other than a strict kibble regime. . . . The pet food industry makes me feel it's a heresy to even consider using anything other than prescription kibble. . . . I'd like to know what percentage of pet food companies' profits comes from special prescription diets, and why the basic facts about the composition of these diets don't seem to add up.

We would like to know these things too. Jasper's human thinks home cooking would be better for him but was discouraged from doing so by the dog's veterinarian. Veterinarians do not like home cooking, and we have no trouble understanding why they prefer to prescribe diet products and discourage alternatives. Prescription diets give them something plausible to recommend to owners of animals with chronic diseases, and companies market the products to veterinarians for precisely that purpose. Most pet owners given prescriptions for diets are likely to feel better when they know they are doing something special for their animals. Some of these foods may be sufficiently distinct from other commercial products to make a difference to a pet's health. They also are likely to do less harm than prescription drugs.

As is so often the case with pet foods, it is difficult to know just how much good prescription diets actually do. Mr. Big, the half-Havanese, half–shih tzu dog that belongs to some Canadian cousins of ours, often threw up after eating his once-a-day portion of dry food. His veterinarian prescribed a canned Medi-Cal Gastro Formula made in Guelph, Ontario, "available exclusively from your veterinarian." Our cousins were instructed to feed Mr. Big small portions of this wet food three times a day. This took care of the problem, but at considerable expense. The veterinary formula cost five times as much as a standard pet food. The ingredient list of this product included no by-products but otherwise looked much like that of any other premium pet food. We wondered whether the improvement occurred as a result of the formula, or simply because Mr. Big was eating smaller portions of wet, rather than dry, food, three times a day instead of once. This would be impossible to know without doing some experimenting, something our cousins preferred not to do with their now healthy dog.

In all fairness, some prescriptions are demonstrably effective. Hill's, for example, traces its origins to Dr. Mark Morris, a New Jersey veterinarian who developed a diet to treat chronic kidney failure in dogs. The modern equivalent of his diet is Hill's k/d Prescription, a low-protein, low-phosphorus, low-sodium formula with added omega-3 fatty acids. This bland formula is similar to the one used to manage kidney disease in humans. Although dogs also may find it bland, peer-reviewed research indicates that the diet prolongs the life of dogs with kidney disease. This research is sponsored by Hill's and, as is all too typical, the published report does not include complete information about dietary composition.

Veterinarians, of course, receive a percentage of the profits on any foods they sell, and it is no surprise that they want to keep control over the use of prescription products. Irate customers, however, have filed suits to make these foods more accessible. The pharmacy board of at least one state—Ohio—ruled that consumers have the right to buy therapeutic pet foods without a veterinarian's prescription. Ohio law, says the board, considers therapeutic pet food to be equivalent to products like Tylenol that can be sold over the counter. We are willing to grant that therapeutic pet foods do some good for some pets. We would feel more confident about this company's claims, and health claims in general, if the methods and results of the research were more freely available.

With that said, let's take a look at some of the conditions prescription pet foods are designed to address. We review the evidence for these kinds of claims in chapter 18.

ALLERGIES

Most pet owners we talk to say they have heard that allergies in pets are increasing. We are unable to corroborate that rumor because of the lack of surveys of the health of cats and dogs over time. But we have no trouble thinking of factors in a pet's environment that might contribute to allergies: air pollution, household dust, household cleaners, insufficient exercise and time outdoors, and, of course, diet. Pets are exposed to plenty of chemicals in their environments that could induce allergic reactions.

But the basic components of pet foods have not changed substantially in decades. We have seen many pet food labels from the 1950s or 1960s with ingredient lists that look much like the ones we see today. The Rivets dog food label shown in figure 9 is a typical example. The one major difference between ingredients then and now is that today's pet foods contain a complete complement of vitamins and minerals; these, however, are highly unlikely to cause allergic reactions. For one thing, they are essential to life. For another, they are not proteins. True allergies are a reaction—an overreaction, really—of the immune system to foreign proteins. But because animals can react badly to other components of the diet as well, all food-related problems are lumped into the category "adverse food reactions."

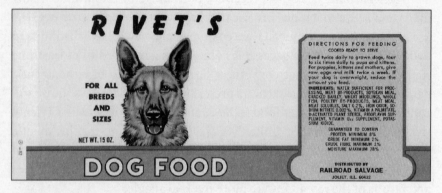

FIGURE 9
The ingredients in mid-twentieth-century dog foods look much like those in use today. On this list, soybeans, wheat, and fish are among the top eight foods responsible for food allergies. Identifying the dates of older pet food labels is not easy, but this one is likely to be from the mid-1960s. Vitamin B$_{12}$ was discovered in 1948 but not added to animal feed until the mid-1950s. Railroad Salvage was in business in Joliet, Illinois, from 1953 to 1974. Postal zip codes began in 1963. The label does not conform to AAFCO models that came into use in the late 1960s. Authors' collection.

Pet foods claiming to be hypoallergenic (note: a disease claim) interest us, as we wonder what especially allergenic substances have been eliminated and what has been added as a replacement. Although any food containing a protein can be allergenic, just eight foods account for 90 percent of human food allergies: milk, eggs, peanuts, tree nuts, fish, shellfish, soy, and wheat. Pets also can develop adverse reactions to some of these foods. Companies marketing hypoallergenic pet foods tend to eliminate the usual suspects but it is not at all clear that those particular foods are the ones that cause problems.

Food allergies are hard to deal with mainly because there is no easy way to figure out their cause. Like people, animals can be allergic to anything they eat and pet foods contain a large number of ingredients. Skin tests are often unreliable, and challenge tests—feeding a potential allergen and waiting to see what happens—can be tricky and not always safe. This leaves elimination trials in which you must remove everything from the diet except one or two foods unlikely to cause reactions, and reintroduce new foods one at a time until something bad happens. Elimination diets for pets used to start out with lamb and rice. Because those ingredients were unusual in pet foods, animals were thought unlikely to be allergic to them (allergies usually—but not always—require more than one exposure, and the more frequent the exposure, the greater the risk). Now, those ingredients are also common, which doesn't leave many feeding options. Elimination trials can take months to do, and are no fun at all for the pet or its human.

Once the source of the allergy is discovered, treatment requires strict avoidance of the offending food, and forever. This also is not much fun. One alternative is to try products advertised as helpful for animals with allergies. California Natural, for example, says its pet foods provide "all the nutrients they need to stay healthy and strong, without enduring allergic reactions that can make its life miserable." The company says it eliminates by-products and artificial flavors and fillers and uses limited sources of protein and carbohydrate in its products. We are not aware of evidence that by-products, artificial flavors, or thickeners cause more allergic reactions than any other ingredients, but a product like this might work if you and your pet are lucky. In theory, diets containing hydrolyzed (predigested) proteins ought to work, but in practice they apparently do not. Because so many questions about allergies in either humans or pets do not yet have answers, prevention is difficult and you have to play this one by ear. We recommend switching products until you find one that works better.

DENTAL HEALTH

Claims that dry pet foods can "clean teeth" have appeared on product labels for decades, but only recently have labels displayed more explicit claims about tooth and gum care. The FDA considers claims that a food

can treat or prevent gum disease or control plaque and tartar to be disease claims requiring scientific substantiation. Officially, the FDA does
not allow them. Unofficially, such claims fall into the grey area of FDA
"regulatory discretion," meaning that the agency does not consider
them a threat to public health and is not going to bother doing much
about them. AAFCO has issued guidelines for the wording of "structure-
function" claims that raise no regulatory problems. These say that the
products help reduce tartar formation through mechanical action and
help control breath odor with chlorophyll. Hence: Greenies toothbrush-
shaped chew:

> An independent, third-party dental test showed that using
> Greenies dental chews once a day resulted in a 69 percent reduc-
> tion in tartar and a 10.5 percent reduction in plaque (vs. dogs
> who ate the same dry dog food diet minus the Greenies dental
> chew). Isn't a good healthy smile reason enough to start feeding
> your pet Greenies?

The Greenies site (the company is now owned by Mars) does not cite
the third-party researchers or provide references to published data from
the independent study. This makes us wonder how the study was conducted and whether any other chew or dry food might have the same
benefit. This is not an unreasonable wonder. Our review of available
evidence for the benefits of such products concludes that the results are
not particularly specific. Any chewing of foods with "enhanced textural
characteristics" (translation: the foods don't crumble easily) does the job
quite well. This matters, because dogs eating the wrong-sized Greenies
have sometimes choked on them. If you feed your dog such products, you
must follow the size advice carefully.

To deal with the marketing problem raised by nonspecificity, an
organization of the American Veterinary Dental College, the Veterinary Oral Health Center, developed a protocol for companies to use to
demonstrate that pet foods control plaque and tartar. Companies that
follow the protocol get to display a special logo. The initial fee for the
logo is $10,000 and $2,000 annually thereafter, but the fee is reduced for
products marketed through veterinarians. Some companies must think

the seal is worth the investment. In July 2009, the organization's website listed twenty-two products that bear its seal.

GLYCEMIC CONTROL

Merrick products offer "5-star entrées for dogs"—"Grammy's Pot Pie and Cowboy Cookout," for example—with gold stickers on their labels saying "Low Glycemic," as certified by the Glycemic Research Institute. For those in the know, this is a claim that the food will not cause high blood sugar in the dog, a usual symptom of diabetes. Glycemic refers to the ability of the carbohydrates—starches and sugars—in foods to cause a spike in an animal's blood sugar and insulin levels. Scientists measure the glycemic level by feeding an animal a defined amount of a specific food, and measuring the rise in blood sugar over time. Foods ranked "high glycemic" usually contain sugars or starches that are quickly digested to sugars; these are absorbed quickly. Animals digest and absorb low-glycemic foods more slowly, which is better for metabolism.

We would expect *all* complete-and-balanced pet foods to be "low glycemic," even the ones based on corn, rice, barley, or any other grain. Pet foods hardly ever contain sugars. They do contain starches, some of which are digested to sugars and quickly absorbed. But pet foods also contain proteins and fat; these are digested more slowly and slow down the absorption of sugars. That is why ice cream (high in sugars, but also high in fat) has a much lower glycemic index than a Coke (just sugars), even though ice cream is higher in calories for its weight. It is also why scientists find that complete-and-balanced diets made with cassava, brewer's rice, corn, sorghum, peas, or lentils do not raise the blood sugar or insulin levels of cats by much. Merrick uses Low Glycemic as a marketing tool but its ingredients look much like those of other premium pet food brands.

HAIRBALL CONTROL

Cats do lick themselves as part of their grooming rituals, and their raspy tongues pick up hair. Cats swallow the hair and get rid of it by coughing it up, a habit that owners find annoying and disgusting, if not alarming.

Sometimes the hair is too thick to cough out and it obstructs the intestine. At that point, it becomes more than a nuisance and requires veterinary intervention. Wouldn't it be nice if pet food could prevent hairball coughing? Yes, it would, and pet food companies are happy to oblige. They take two approaches: add fiber to increase the amount of poop and the speed with which poop passes through the intestine, or add petrolatum (Vaseline or some other lubricant) to ease the hairball through the digestive tract. About one-fourth of cat owners use such formulas.

Purina ONE Advanced Nutrition Hairball Formula is one such product. According to Purina, its product is better than those of its competitors, Iams Hairball Care and Hill's Science Diet Hairball Formula, on the grounds that its "natural fiber blend helps minimize hairballs and promotes healthy digestion." This is a bit confusing because Purina ONE guarantees 5 percent fiber whereas the other two guarantee 8.5 and 10 percent, respectively. The ingredients do not look all that different. All three contain some kind of corn meal or corn gluten meal and two other sources of plant fiber: brewer's rice and soy flour (Purina ONE), dried beet pulp and powdered cellulose (Iams), and brewer's rice and powdered cellulose (Hill's). Purina ONE substitutes soy fiber for cellulose fiber. Does this make it control hairballs better? You decide.

HIP AND JOINT HEALTH

Hip problems and other forms of arthritis are common problems in certain breeds of dogs and it would be terrific if diets could prevent them. Typically, products aimed at preventing joint problems contain "chondroprotectives," chemicals normally found in cartilage. The two most common are chondroitin sulfate and glucosamine. Because these chemicals are not nutrients, they are regulated as dietary supplements in human food and are also considered as supplements in pet foods. We discuss them along with other supplements in chapters 17 and 18.

KIDNEY DISEASE

Cats evolved from desert animals that do not drink much water, produce concentrated urine, and are susceptible to kidney disease. Cat

owners rightfully worry about how commercial pet foods might affect
their animals' kidneys. Pet food companies make special foods aimed
at minimizing the risk of kidney disease. For some reason, the FDA has
taken a special interest in label claims for prevention of feline lower urinary tract disease (FLUTD), a problem that the agency says occurs in less
than 1 percent of cats in America. As we have seen, the FDA considers
such claims to be disease claims requiring some level of scientific proof.
But "in an effort to get some meaningful health-related information to
the consumer," the FDA does not bother to do anything about statements that a food reduces (acidifies) urine pH, which is a disease claim,
or "helps maintain urinary tract health" or "promotes healthy kidney
function," which are structure-function claims.

The acidity of urine matters because alkaline (higher pH) urine
predisposes dogs and cats to kidney stone formation. Grain-based,
carbohydrate-rich diets neutralize the acidity of urine and make it more
alkaline. This favors the crystallization of struvite (magnesium ammonium phosphate) kidney stones. Struvite crystals impair kidney function
through mechanical blockage, and can lead to infections and metabolic
imbalances. The relationship of alkalinity to kidney stone formation is
not simple, however. Acidic urine favors the formation of calcium stones.
When the struvite problem was discovered in the mid-1980s, pet food
companies began to reformulate their foods to make them more acidify-
ing. The result was that fewer cats were brought to veterinary clinics with
struvite crystals, but more came in with calcium oxalate stones.

Some foods designed to address kidney disease use a different approach; they are low in magnesium, one of the minerals involved in struvite formation. The FDA says that if a label says "low in magnesium," the
food must contain less than 25 mg of magnesium per 100 calories. This
is a magnesium level well below the amount that forms stones. In both
dogs and cats, the risk of any kind of stone formation can be reduced by
feeding low-magnesium foods but also making sure the animal drinks
enough water.

But getting pets to drink water raises another set of problems. Water
is easier to get into dogs; they drink water anyway. But cats don't. Some
commercial dry kibbles add salt to stimulate cats to drink water. But if
you want to get water into cats, it is easier to feed them wet pet foods that

are mostly water to begin with. Cats and dogs are protected against struvite if they eat grain-based diets that are not too alkaline, are low in magnesium, and provide some moisture. Commercial foods do these things,
which is one reason why the prevalence of cat struvite has declined.

SKIN AND COAT PRODUCTS

Pet food labels promise "healthy skin" and "glossy coat." And why not?
Any complete-and-balanced pet food contains all the nutrients needed—
and then some—to support these characteristics. Not that anyone other
than a company lawyer or the FDA can tell the difference, but skin and
coat claims must be worded carefully. As long as companies stick to
statements like "promotes healthy skin and coat" (a structure-function
claim), they are on safe ground. If they claim to be able to prevent dry,
flaky, or itchy skin or to restore shine to coats, they are making disease
claims that supposedly are not allowed. Once again, the FDA exercises
regulatory discretion and doesn't bother enforcing the distinctions since
it no doubt has more important things to do than to split proverbial hairs
over the wording of coat claims.

As you can see from these examples, health claims on pet food labels
are not regulated stringently, if at all, meaning that companies have a
great deal of leeway in advertising the health benefits of their products.
Like health claims on products for human consumption, it is best not to
take them too literally. If your pet has a condition that might be related to
food, the special foods might be worth a try. If one doesn't work, try another. But it is now time to discuss health claims where diet demonstrably
makes a difference: those that promise that the foods will help a dog or
cat lose weight.

For Weight Loss

The label of Lick Your Chops D'Lite Low Calorie Formula for cats says: "Calorie Content (Calculated): 910 kcal/kg, 142 kcal/can (5.5 oz)." This product is aimed at owners of obese cats. Obesity is just as much a problem for pets as it is for people. U.S. government health agencies estimate that nearly one-third of American adults are overweight and another third are obese, using body mass index (BMI) as a criterion. No equivalent surveys or criteria exist for pets so it is anyone's guess how many are overweight and we are not surprised that estimates range widely, from 20 percent to 60 percent.

As in people, obesity in pets is the result of eating too many calories for the number needed. Excess calories, no matter where they come from, are stored as fat. Although extra fat is good to have when food supplies are limited, it is not so good in situations where pets are kept indoors and fed frequently. The consequences of obesity in dogs and cats are similar to those in humans. Heart disease, diabetes, hip and joint problems, urinary tract disorders, respiratory problems, and reproductive disorders occur more frequently in obese animals. And, as we discussed in chapter 13, thinner animals live longer.

Veterinarians do not use an obesity index similar to the BMI, but some consider dogs and cats to be overweight if their body weight is more than 15 percent above optimal body weight, and obese if they are 30 percent above the optimum. Optimal weights are not well defined, however, so this classification is not particularly useful. In practice, veterinarians use scoring systems that evaluate the way cats and dogs look and feel. Nestlé Purina PetCare and Mars's Waltham Center for Pet Nutrition offer such scoring systems—with photographs—on their websites. So does Hill's. Everyone tells us that pets are getting fatter, but we are unable to find reliable studies reporting the weights of dogs or cats over time and have to take the trend on faith.

Several studies have examined the causes of obesity in dogs. Because owners are responsible for what pets eat, researchers looked at the characteristics of owners of overweight dogs. One study, by Nestlé Purina, found that among the owners of dogs judged by veterinarians to be overweight, half viewed their dog's weight as ideal. A German study compared the owners of obese dogs to owners of normal-weight dogs. The owners of obese dogs, it said, were more likely to treat their pets as fellow humans, and to sleep and eat with them. They also were more likely to feed the dog from the table, to give it frequent treats, and to view exercise as less important. Among owners of overweight dogs, 24 percent were overweight themselves as compared to just 8 percent of owners of normal-weight dogs.

Studies of cat owners yield similar results. Owners of normal-weight cats tend to reward their animals with extra play time, while owners of overweight cats use extra food as rewards. One large study looked at the characteristics of overweight cats, rather than owners. The overweight cats were more likely to be male, neutered, middle-aged, living in an apartment, kept indoors, and consuming dry cat foods.

These studies form the basis for typical explanations of obesity in pets. Dogs and cats increase in weight with age, especially if they are neutered. Pets kept indoors get less exercise. The use of dry dog and cat foods has increased in recent years. Dry foods are more concentrated in calories per weight of food than canned foods (which are mostly water). Dry foods are designed to be highly palatable and highly digestible so they will be low-residue and produce smaller feces; fewer calories in them are wasted. The use of treats also has increased. All of these trends make it easier to feed pets more calories than they need.

CALORIES IN PET FOODS: "METABOLIZABLE ENERGY"

A word about calories: they are a measure of the amount of energy (heat, for example) in food. They are produced through the metabolism of food fats, proteins, and carbohydrates (starches and sugars). The Whiskas dry cat food discussed in chapters 7 and 10 contains several calorie sources: the carbohydrate and protein in ground yellow corn, wheat flour, and rice; the protein and fats in chicken by-product and corn gluten meals; and the fat in animal fat. Digestion breaks these down to sugars, amino acids, and fatty acids, which are absorbed and used to construct the pet's body parts or to produce energy.

When you see "Calorie Content" on food labels, it really means "Kilocalorie (kcal) Content." In common (but not chemical) usage, calories and kilocalories mean exactly the same thing and can be used interchangeably, as we do here. "Calorie Content (Calculated)" means that the maker of Lick Your Chops, Healthy Pet Foods, Inc., did not actually measure the calories. Instead, the company estimated the calories from the nutrient composition, as is now common practice. This product lists the calories as kcal/kg (kilocalories per kilogram) of food, but also for the total amount of food in the can, which in this case is 142 kcal, quite a bit less than an average cat might need in a day. This product is meant to be lower in calories; it is a diet food.

But if you are curious about the number of calories in most pet foods, good luck. You will not see calories listed on the labels of most products. Calories do not appear in the guaranteed analysis. AAFCO model regulations merely say that calories listed on food labels "shall be separate and distinct from the Guaranteed Analysis and shall appear under the heading Calorie Content." Its models only require pet food companies to disclose calories when the label says the product is light, "lite," or low-calorie, or reduced in calories. For regular products, calorie labeling is voluntary. How come? We suspect that most pet food companies would rather that you did not know how extremely caloric the average pet food really is.

Some pet food companies list calories anyway, even though they don't have to. Merrick's Cowboy Cookout with Beef, Sweet Potatoes, Carrots, Green Beans, and Granny Smith Apples voluntarily provides "Calorie

Contents: 1,046 kcal/kg (calculated)—A 13.2 oz can provides 394 kcal of Metabolizable Energy (calculated)."

Metabolizable Energy? Unlike the calories on the labels of human foods, this is the term used to describe calories for dogs and cats. It refers to the *usable* calories in food—the ones left after the calories excreted in feces and urine are subtracted out from the total. "Calories" for humans means that too. For foods that humans eat, nutritionists say that a gram of fat provides 9 usable calories, and a gram of protein or carbohydrate provides 4 usable calories. The 9,4,4 values really refer to metabolizable energy but we do not use that term in human nutrition. We use "calories" instead. Even for pet foods, we think "metabolizable energy" is unnecessarily confusing, and is another reason why pet food labels should more closely resemble those on human foods.

Part of the confusion is due to the fact that the human values are slightly higher than those used for pet foods; human food is considered to be more digestible than pet food. We have our doubts about whether pet food really is less digestible than human food; we think of food for people, pets, and farm animals as highly interconnected and much the same. But by convention, metabolizable energy values used in AAFCO calculations of the energy content of pet foods are lower: 8.5 calories per gram for fat, 3.5 for a gram of protein, and 3.5 for a gram of "nitrogen-free extract," meaning carbohydrates (yet another point of confusion).

Carbohydrates do not contain nitrogen and are estimated by difference. You add up the grams of protein, fat, fiber, ash, and moisture, and subtract them all from 100; what remains is carbohydrate. Fine, but we see little real difference between calories in human nutrition and metabolizable energy in pet nutrition. The values are close enough to be treated similarly. Throughout this book we use the more familiar term calories to indicate and to substitute for both the more formal kilocalories and the animal feed-specific metabolizable energy.

PET WEIGHT LOSS PRODUCTS

Products designed to help dogs and cats lose weight work exactly the same way dieting does for humans: they provide fewer calories. With so many dogs and cats now overweight, weight management products present a growth opportunity for pet food companies. At a pet trade show, we picked up a flyer for Hill's Science Diet that describes the "weight management opportunity gap"—the gap between the 35 percent of pets that veterinarians judge obese, and the mere 9 percent of pet foods designed for weight control ("with only a 9 percent share, the Weight Management category has the potential to triple in size"). Hill's markets its foods directly to veterinarians, and it advises them to:

- Capitalize on a continuously growing weight management category that was worth $350 million in 2006.
- Help your customers' pets GET FIT with the real light and STAY HEALTHY with our clinically proven antioxidants.
- [Use our products as] tools you need to drive your business forward.
- Build loyalty and educate consumers by leveraging your position as the expert in pet care.

You may think your veterinarian's job is to take care of your pet's health but, as we discuss in chapter 24, selling pet foods constitutes a piece of their income and diet pet foods can be a big income booster. Hill's also sells products directly to consumers. In an Agway store that sells pet food, we picked up a shelf card in the Hill's section that compares the company's diet products to those of its competitors. According to this comparison, which we reproduce in table 16, Hill's diet products are the only ones that contain fewer calories than the AAFCO standard.

The FDA rules that apply to "lite" labels on human foods do not apply to pet foods. AAFCO model regulations say that if pet food labels use "lite" or similar terms, they must display the calorie content. For dogs, dry foods may contain no more than 3,100 kcal/kg or 87 per ounce, and wet foods no more than 900 kcal/kg or 25 per ounce. Wet foods make better diet products because they are much lower in calories per volume of food. The standards for diet foods permit slightly more calories for cats: 3,250 kcal/kg for dry foods (91 per ounce) and 950 kcal/kg for wet foods (27 per ounce).

Table 16

CALORIES IN DIET DRY DOG FOOD COMPARED TO
AAFCO STANDARD FOR DIET PRODUCTS*

PRODUCT	CALORIES PER KILOGRAM FOOD
AAFCO standard for light (diet) dog foods	3,100
Hill's Science Diet Light Adult (Hill's Pet Nutrition)	2,997
Pro Plan Weight Management Formula (Nestlé Purina PetCare)	3,342
Iams Weight Control (Procter & Gamble)	3,853
Eukanuba Adult Reduced Fat (Procter & Gamble)	3,875

* Shelf card, Hill's Pet Nutrition, 2005, collected at Agway, Ithaca, NY, 2008. A kilogram is 2.2 pounds.

How much of a reduction over nondiet products do these figures represent? As with much else in pet foods, the comparison is not easy, in this case because calories on regular pet foods labels are rarely listed. Hill's, however, helpfully provides calorie information on its Science Diet website in the usual kcal/kg of metabolizable energy, but also in kcal/cup. Even more helpfully, it gives the ounces of food per cup. From this information, the figures can easily be translated to calories per ounce. We give the figures in table 17 along with the AAFCO diet standards for some chicken-based diet foods for adult animals.

If these figures are correct and representative (and as far as we can tell, they are), regular wet pet foods already come close to meeting AAFCO standards for the calories allowed in diet foods. This is why pets can maintain weight so much more easily when they eat canned foods rather than kibble (canned foods are more expensive, of course). The calories in regular dry foods, however, are roughly 20 percent higher than those in the "lite" dry foods.

PUTTING PETS ON DIETS

The body weight of a cat or dog (or human) is the result of the balance between the calories it eats and those it uses in physical activity. You can-

Table 17

COMPARISON OF THE CALORIES IN HILL'S
ADULT REGULAR FOODS TO AAFCO "LITE"
STANDARDS, CALORIES PER OUNCE*

TYPE OF FOOD	HILL'S DOG FOODS		HILL'S CAT FOODS	
	REGULAR	AAFCO "LITE" STANDARD	REGULAR	AAFCO "LITE" STANDARD
	CALORIES PER OUNCE			
Wet	27	25	31	27
Dry	105	87	115	91

* Calculated from information given at www.hillspet.com.

not really measure either one without using special equipment. If you don't have that equipment handy, the only way to know whether your pet is eating the right amount of calories is to monitor its weight. If your pet is losing weight, you are not giving it enough to eat. If it is gaining weight, you are giving it too much. So far, so good. But the hard part is to know what "right amount" means. For this, you need to know two things: the number of calories in your pet's food, and the number your pet needs. Neither is obvious.

Problem #1: Calories in Pet Foods

What if the food label does not disclose the calories? Finding out how many calories a food contains is no task for the faint of heart. You can make a very close estimate from the guaranteed analysis, as we explain in appendix 4. Without calorie labels, you must have both a calculator and no math anxiety. Even with these things, you need the skills of a detective. Here, for example, is how we determined how many calories are in an Iams Weight Control dry food for cats labeled as "10 percent less fat." The product gives no information about calories on the package label. This is because AAFCO considers "10 percent less fat" to be in a different category than "lite." "Less fat" merely requires an explanation of "less than what," in this case, the Iams Original with Chicken.

We began by going to the Iams website. There we discovered that the product contains 3,545 calories per kilogram of food, or 99 calories per ounce. That seemed reasonable for a diet product until we saw further information that the product contained 319.2 calories per eight-ounce cup. This just seemed weird. Calories are hard enough to measure to the nearest 10, let alone to the first decimal place. And when we divided that overly precise 319.2 by the usual eight ounces per cup, we came up with 40 calories per ounce, which is much lower than 99.

Something did not compute. Perhaps the ounces of food per cup were wrong? We bought the product, measured out a cup of kibble, and weighed it on a kitchen scale—4.5 ounces. That gave 70 per ounce, still much lower than 99. At that point, we wrote the company and asked for the ounces of food per cup. We received a prompt answer: 3.3 ounces, a weight that gives 99 calories per ounce but is still lower than the amount we measured. So which number is correct? And why doesn't Iams just say how many calories the product provides? Some companies, such as Natural Balance, do give this information. If you read the small print on its website, you see that its diet product contains 385 calories in a 120-gram cup (4.3 ounces), for about 90 calories per ounce. The point of all this? It's hard to know how much to feed your pet if you can't count the calories.

Problem #2: The Calories Pets Need

We like to think of the calorie needs of cats in "mouse units." Working cats and those free to hunt can obtain some or all of their calories from the mice they catch. At some point, scientists measured the calorie content of mice; each provides about 30 calories. An average cat needs eight or nine mouse units per day, or 240 to 270 calories. For owners who like to serve natural, raw food to their cats, Gina Spadafori and Paul Pion provide a handy recipe in their book, *Cats for Dummies*.

Take one small mouse from the freezer.
Thaw.
Put in a blender and hit "frappé."
Serve at body temperature on a clean plate.

Do this nine times a day, and you will have one well-fed cat. Like people, larger animals require more calories than smaller ones. Active animals need more calories than sedentary ones. Mouse-chasing outdoor cats require more mouse units than indoor ones. As always, the calorie needs of puppies or kittens are higher for their weight than those of adults because the animals are growing. Pregnant and lactating animals also need more calories for their weight.

The National Research Council (NRC) has developed tables of calorie needs for dogs or cats of different weights, activity levels, and stages of life. These can be difficult to use, mostly because they are based on a complicated formula that accounts for the fact that smaller animals need more calories for their size than larger animals (they have a proportionally larger surface area which increases the rate of heat loss). Using the formulas, which differ for dogs and cats, requires a fancy calculator that does exponential functions. We give the formulas in the notes.

On the basis of such formulas, the NRC estimates that an active adult dog weighing thirty pounds needs about 920 calories per day; an inactive dog of the same size needs only 670 calories (see table 18). A sedentary adult cat weighing 4 kg (about nine pounds) needs about 250 calories per day (table 19). Larger dogs and cats will need more, but not exactly in direct proportion. Some breeds need more calories than others; active terriers may need nearly 30 percent more energy at the same body weight than other breeds. In comparison, most pet owners need on the order of 1,800 to 2,500 calories per day, depending on how much they weigh and how active they are.

Activity levels make a big difference to calorie needs. An Alaskan sled dog needs a lot more food than an apartment-dwelling city dog taken out once a day for a walk. We visited the colony of working Alaskan huskies at Denali National Park and took a good look at their diet. They eat dog kibble, but one specially formulated to be high in fat (guaranteed analysis 37 percent) and, therefore, calories. During their summer holidays, these thirty to fifty pound dogs eat "only" a pound a day of this food or about 1,850 calories, an amount appropriate for an average human female. Once they go to work, the food gets serious. When transporting rangers and supplies throughout the park at distances of 10 to 100 miles a day, the dogs get twice that amount—along with frequent treats of scoops of restaurant-grade, frozen lard (115 calories per tablespoon). In appendix 5, we give a shopping list for the impressive quantities of food needed to supply a team of dogs running a 1,000-mile race such as the Yukon Quest.

If you are not sure how many calories your pet is supposed to eat, weigh it and follow the feeding directions on the food label as best you can. But be sure to account for the additional calories in treats or tidbits that you might give your pet.

Table 18

ENERGY NEEDS OF DOGS, CALORIES PER DAY*

WEIGHT IN POUNDS	YOUNG ADULT, ACTIVE	ADULTS, ACTIVE	SENIOR, ACTIVE	ACTIVE TERRIERS	INACTIVE ADULT
15	590	550	440	760	400
20	730	680	550	940	500
25	870	800	650		590
30	990	920	740		670

* Values rounded off to the nearest 10 calories. Calculated from formula given in National Research Council, *Nutrient Requirements of Dogs and Cats* (Washington, DC: National Academies Press, 2006), 359.

Table 19

ENERGY NEEDS OF CATS, CALORIES PER DAY*

WEIGHT IN POUNDS	LEAN, DOMESTIC CAT
6	190
9	250
12	310
15	360

* Values rounded off to the nearest 10 calories. Calculated from formula given in National Research Council, *Nutrient Requirements of Dogs and Cats* (Washington, DC: National Academies Press, 2006), 366.

Problem #3: Practical Advice

Diet pet foods typically instruct owners to feed smaller portions as a way to reduce calories, even when the foods do not claim to be low in fat or calories. This is excellent advice. For example, the label of Purina

ONE Healthy Weight Formula for dogs says that the product contains 25 percent less fat and 15 percent fewer calories than Purina ONE Total Nutrition Lamb & Rice Formula. For a weight loss of 25 percent, you are to reduce the portion size by 25 percent. A dog weighing twenty-one to thirty-five pounds usually gets 2.5 cups a day, but you must reduce the feed to 2.0 cups a day to achieve a 25 percent weight loss. The moral: smaller portions have fewer calories. This is a good lesson to remember.

PET FOOD POLITICS: CALORIE LABELS

It makes no sense to us that calories are not required to be stated on pet food labels. In early 2008, the AAFCO pet food committee agreed to look into the matter but like most such committees, this one will be doing a thorough study that could take years. The American Veterinary Medical Association and the American Academy of Veterinary Nutrition are in favor of calorie labeling, but the Pet Food Institute (PFI), which represents manufacturers, strongly opposes it on the grounds that information about calories is unnecessary and will not help prevent obesity in pets.

We are baffled by the PFI's stance, since it seems so consumer unfriendly. Owners are totally responsible for the food intake of their pets, but figuring out how much food a dog or a cat might need—as we have explained—can be a challenge. Dogs and cats vary in their calorie needs. Some regulate their body weight well and will not become overweight even when given continuous access to food: others are gluttons and will happily eat everything in sight. The feeding directions on pet foods offer general guidelines but cannot account for a particular animal's activity pattern or disposition.

Will calorie labeling eliminate obesity in pets? Not on its own, but it certainly could help, especially if accompanied by information about the calorie needs of dogs and cats of various sizes, ages, conditions, and activity levels. Our conclusion: calorie labeling is a useful part of the nutrition facts labels on human foods, and would help pet owners take better care of their cats and dogs. We cannot think of a single reason not to do it.

The
PET FOOD
EXTRAS

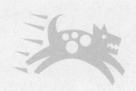

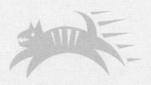

Snacks, Treats, Chews, and Bottled Waters

PET SUPPLY STORES are filled with products intended to supplement complete-and-balanced diets for dogs and cats: snacks, treats, chews, and various kinds of dietary supplements. Food supplements must meet the minimal federal labeling standards, but AAFCO exempts them from having to provide certain other kinds of information. They must provide the same guaranteed analysis and ingredient lists that are required for complete foods. But because they are meant to be extras, they do not need to display a statement of nutritional adequacy.

SNACKS

We consider snacks to be commercial food supplements that make no claim to be complete and balanced, but instead are meant to boost the nutritional value or palatability of a pet's diet. Some commercial foods labeled 100 percent or 95 percent meat fall into this category. These foods are not complete and balanced. They lack nutrients that can only be provided by other foods, ingredients, or supplements.

The Canadian Wysong Corporation, for example, produces Turkey Au Jus (*"nourriture pour chiens et chats"*) labeled 95 percent poultry, excluding water. The short ingredient list—just turkey, water, turkey liver, animal plasma, and guar gum—tells you that this product is unlikely to be formulated to meet AAFCO nutrient profiles. The feeding directions make this explicit: "Use as a supplement to and top dressing for dry Wysong Diets in conjunction with the Wysong Optimal Health Program, which includes fresh food supplementation." As you might suspect, this program suggests that you include other Wysong diet and supplement products to complete the pet's diet.

Any food that provides calories is a snack, but this definition blurs distinctions between commercial food supplements, table foods, and treats. Tobi, a mixed-breed dog who belonged to some friends of ours, loved to eat raw carrots. We consider carrots to be a snack and a good one at that; carrots don't have many calories but are high in nutritional value. Treats, in contrast, are almost always high in calories.

TREATS

Treats are a lively part of the pet food business. Pets love them and so do owners and trainers. We love them too, but view them as kitty and doggie junk food. They are extras. They add calories that few pets need. But treats are fun. They also are happily profitable for the companies that make them.

In February 2008, we were given *Bark* press credentials to attend Pet Expo in San Diego, a huge exhibition of pet products open only to the trade. Treats dominated the thousands of food products on exhibit. We saw—and enjoyed tasting—treats in every imaginable shape and size, many of them said to be made from human-grade ingredients. We nibbled on cheese-flavored, bone-shaped biscuits and cookies that looked just like Oreos; meat-flavored treats that looked like vegetables; and real meats and vegetables dried and ready to feed. International treat makers from Brazil, China, and New Zealand were well represented, and we particularly appreciated the dried treats made from Australian kangaroos.

The reason exhibitors show their products at Pet Expo is to encourage retailers to stock them. Treat sellers have a good chance of finding buyers because treats are serious moneymakers. In 2007, they accounted for nearly $2.4 billion in sales, or about 14 percent of total pet food revenues. As might be expected from the joy with which dogs respond to treats, those designed for dogs greatly outnumber those for cats. Dogs also eat more food than cats. That explains why the PetSmart store in Ithaca, New York, devotes more than two hundred feet of linear shelf space to dog treats, but just twenty-eight feet to cat treats.

Many small companies are trying to get into the treat business. And why not? Many pet owners buy them. According to the American Pet Products Association, 88 percent of owners gave treats to their dogs and 68 percent gave them to cats in 2008. The market concentration for these products is still relatively low so small companies still have a chance to make some money on them. The ten leading treat brands accounted for less than 60 percent of total sales in 2006. Milk Bone (Del Monte) holds the largest market share followed by some private label brands and Beggin' Strips (Nestlé Purina). And treats are easy to make. They are not required to meet any nutrition standards at all. Best of all, they are handsomely profitable. Treat sellers at Pet Expo were offering markups of 50 percent or more to wholesale buyers.

As Revenue Generators

On our return from Pet Expo, we wanted to see the kinds of treats offered by pet stores, so we headed off to our local PetSmart. As mentioned earlier, this PetSmart devotes more than 200 feet of precious shelf space to treats, and the treat aisle is close to the front of the store. We had our choice of many options. We bought the smallest sizes available of several regular treats (not the ones advertised for special health purposes), and took a look at their labels. Because the packages come in a huge range of sizes, we converted their prices to price per pound. Table 20 summarizes our observations.

Our first impression: treats are expensive, sometimes shockingly expensive. Because the packages vary so much in size, it is difficult to relate the price to what you are actually getting and you must pay close attention to the package weight. In this small sample, the prices ranged from a bit more than $4 for a pound of Del Monte's Milk Bone biscuits to nearly $37 per pound for Mark and Chappell's Green Ums. The ingredient lists

Table 20

SELECTED EXAMPLES OF REGULAR COMMERCIAL TREATS AVAILABLE FOR ADULT ANIMALS AT THE ITHACA, NY, PETSMART STORE, JULY 2008*

PRODUCT (MAKER)	PRICE PER POUND	FIRST FIVE INGREDIENTS	FEEDING INSTRUCTIONS	CALORIES PER PIECE
Milk Bone Original (Del Monte)	$4.04	Wheat flour, beef meal and beef bone meal, **sugar,** cooked bone marrow, dried digest of poultry by-products	None	10
Milk Bone Filet Mignon Flavor (Del Monte)	$9.97	Beef, chicken, soy grits, **sugar,** corn starch	None	Not given
Pup-Peroni Ribs (Del Monte)	$10.26	Beef, soy grits, beef by-products, **sugar,** maltodextrin	None	Not given
Beggin' Strips (Nestlé Purina)	$11.28	Ground wheat, corn gluten meal, wheat flour, ground yellow corn, water	Feed as a treat	Not given
Feline Greenies Salmon Flavor (Mars)	$15.94	Chicken meal, brewer's rice, wheat, corn gluten meal, poultry fat	6 to 8 pieces per serving	2
Green Um (Mark & Chappell)	$36.67	Wheat flower [*sic*], sunflower oil, **sugar,** rice flour, wheat bran	2 to 3 per day for dogs up to 22 lbs	Not given

* Smallest package. Most treats cost about $5.50 per package, but their sizes varied from 2.0 oz to 15 oz. Sugar is indicated in bold (our emphasis).

were no help in understanding the pricing strategies. To us, the first five ingredients look like those in any other pet food, except that treats have more binders and sugars—just what your pet does not need. Ordinary pet food is more nutritious and often sells for less than $1 per pound. No wonder so many companies want to get into the treat business.

As Junk Foods

Several of the treats in the table add vitamins and minerals. At what levels? The labels do not say. The lowest cost Milk Bone seems to be a wheat flour cookie with small amounts of meat ingredients added for flavor. Its protein guarantee is 12 percent, which is low for a dry food (the Whiskas example in chapter 7 guarantees 31 percent protein), and it has no added nutrients. This and other dog treats often list sugars or syrups as one of the top five ingredients. Dogs, like people, have a sweet tooth, and they like sweet snacks. Cats, however, seem indifferent to sugars and we wonder whether the sugars are added to appeal to owners' tastes. Overall, our impression is that treats provide minimal nutritional value for the calories they provide. Hence: junk foods.

As Calorie Sources

To know how treats fit into the calorie needs of your pet, you need to know how many calories each treat contains and how many calories your dog or cat needs. But package labels are no help at all. Treat packages hardly ever state calorie values on their labels. Even if you knew how many calories a treat provided, you would still need to know how its calories compared to your pet's daily needs. As we discussed in chapter 15, a twenty-pound adult dog needs about 680 calories per day. The low-cost Milk Bone treats are small and contain just 10 calories each. But give your dog ten of them and they add up to 15 percent of its daily calorie needs. As with portion sizes for humans, larger treats have more calories.

Our educated guess: each gram of treat provides 3 to 4 calories, depending on how much fat it contains. This means that treats run 80 to 110 calories per ounce—let's call them 100 calories per ounce, an average.

To figure out the calories, multiply the treat weight in grams times 3 or 4. Or you can:

- Look up the weight of the package in ounces.
- Multiply ounces times 100 calories per ounce to get the approximate number of calories in the package.
- Count the number of treats in the package.
- Divide calories per package by the number of treats to get calories per treat.

A treat weighing 14 grams, as does each of the Pup-Peronis we bought, is likely to be about 50 calories. That is why the lack of feeding directions on treat packages is a problem. You must substract treat calories from those your pet needs each day.

But the job of treat sellers is to encourage you to feed more treats to your pet, and as many as possible. Treat makers know perfectly well that calories are an issue. Blue Dog Bakery makes 100 calorie packs (in peanut butter and bacon and cheese flavors, no less) just like the ones sold by Frito-Lay and Kellogg for humans. Pup-Peroni (Del Monte) makes 50-calorie packs. Those calories count.

So do the calories in bakery products. We love visiting pet bakeries. There, lined up on shelves, are colorful and delicious-looking treats shaped like pretzels, donuts, sweet rolls, cookies, French and Italian pastries, cupcakes, and birthday cakes. These are fun and so appealing that it is easy to forget their calories, particularly since calories are not labeled. We have a flier from the Barking Dog pet bakery in Oklahoma City. It makes "human grade" dog treats marketed for their health benefits. A Cinnamon Apple treat (red apple, white flour, egg whites, vegetable oil) is said to have these "health benefits: metabolism, sugar leveling, anti-bacterial, boosts estrogen, anti-viral." This seems like a lot to ask of any food, let alone a treat, but this kind of marketing distracts you from calorie counting.

As Medicines

In advertising the purported health benefits of its treats, Barking Dog Bakery is participating in a hot new trend. Pet food makers consider snacks and treats to be convenient delivery systems for supplements aimed at preventing or treating all kinds of pet diseases. The Dogswell company, for example, produces Happy Hips (with chondroitin sulfate and glucosamine), Vitality (flaxseed and vitamins), Breathies (mint and parsley), Mellow Mut (chamomile and lavender), and Happy Heart (taurine, turmeric, and flaxseed).

We see labels on many treats stating that they have medicinal uses or help support some structure or function of the body. As we explain in the next chapter, you would never know from seeing these labels that such statements are neither backed up by much science nor AAFCO-approved. We are particularly intrigued by frozen yogurt products marketed as healthy pet treats because they are loaded with probiotic friendly bacteria. Alas, freezing destroys many if not most probiotic bacteria.

We found an Authority hip and joint treat listing a guaranteed analysis of 550 ppm (550 mg/kg) of glucosamine plus chondroitin sulfate. The label suggests giving a twenty-pound dog one of these treats a day. One treat weighs 4.4 grams, meaning that it would supply a mere 2.4 mg of these compounds. We discuss whether glucosamine and chondroitin sulfate really promote joint health in chapter 18, but in this situation the science is irrelevant. This dose is too small to do much good.

The toothbrush-shaped Greenies treat ("Cleans teeth! Freshens breath!") claims: "helps clean teeth down to the gum line." How it does this is beyond us. The first five ingredients are gelatin, wheat protein isolate, glycerin, soy protein isolate, and sodium caseinate; these are gummy rather than abrasive. We bought the petite size for dogs weighing fifteen to twenty-five pounds. Each Greenie weighed 17 grams and we guess it contains at least 50 calories. The feeding guide comes with a caveat: "ATTENTION: As with any edible product, monitor your dog to ensure the treat is adequately chewed. Gulping any item can be harmful or even fatal to a dog." Follow this advice!

We cannot resist mentioning Green Um Treats for Dogs, manufactured for Mark & Chappell in Slovenia, of all places. This is a "Health Management Treat" that "helps keep your lawn green." "Formulated by animal nutritionists," this product is supposed to control lawn burn from dog urination. The active ingredient is the amino acid methionine, which is a urine acidifier, at least in cats. Why methionine would keep lawns from urine burns is beyond us, even at guaranteed analysis of 2.5 percent. At nearly $37 per pound, it is an expensive treatment, especially for lawns.

CHEWS

At Pet Expo, we saw no end of treats advertised as whole grain or wheat-free, or all-natural, organic, kosher, no preservatives, no added sugar, no animal by-products, vegetarian, or vegan. Owners of pet food stores tell us they get "buy my product" requests from the sellers of such treats all the time, particularly from the makers of chews. The owner of a neighborhood store in San Francisco forwarded one such request to us from the marketing director of a company called Himalayan Dog Chew:

> Five years ago as a Peace Corps Volunteer in Nepal I took in an abandoned puppy off the streets. . . . I had to improvise with locally available products. I discovered that a hard, cheese-like product consumed by the Nepali people was the perfect answer to my problem. It is made by boiling yak and cow milk with lime juice which separates the curds. The curds are then packed tightly into sticks and dried for days. The result is a long-lasting chew treat that dogs just can't seem to get enough of.

On its website, the company adds: "We are satisfied that the product we are offering to the North American consumer is safe and will fill the void for an edible treat that can keep the attention of even the most powerfully neurotic canine jaws." Chews are great for keeping dogs happily occupied and for keeping their teeth clean (if the ingredients are abrasive), and we like the idea of giving those powerfully neurotic jaws something benign to chew on.

At Pet Expo, we saw dozens of displays of knotted rawhide chews and pigs' ears. These, which are meant to be chewed, not eaten, were mostly made in Brazil but many of them came from China. AAFCO does not require natural treats, those made from the hide, hooves, or ears of animals, to follow feed labeling requirements. Unless these products claim to have some nutritional value, AAFCO considers them to be toys, not foods. AAFCO specifies, however, that standard labels are required on chews made from more nutritious parts of animals: tracheas, lungs, livers, hearts, and pizzles (the euphemism AAFCO uses for penises). You will no doubt be pleased to know that AAFCO's pet food committee recommended exempting pizzles from labeling requirements, even though it requires full labels on other dried meat, fish, and poultry products.

Natural chews are by-products of the meat processing and leather tanning industries. Depending on how far they have to travel, they arrive at the chew factory frozen or fresh. The factory thaws them if necessary, and cooks and dries them before packaging. These processes ought to kill pathogens. Rawhide chews twisted into bone and other shapes require special handling. The hides have to be treated by cooking or tanning before they are cut, trimmed, and dried.

Whole Dog Journal's Nancy Kerns warns against chews made from wood, plastic, or any other material that might splinter. She recommends oversized, intact, rolled rawhide made from a single sheet, even though these are more expensive. And, she says, not even the best may be safe for every dog. Her advice: supervise.

On a visit to the Bravo! raw-food factory in Connecticut, we saw slabs of sliced venison liver drying on racks in a walk-in oven. These are broken into fragments and packaged. As far as we can tell, the company takes any part of an animal it can find and turns it into an edible, chewable treat. The company's labels state the single ingredient—buffalo livers, turkey hearts, chicken breasts—with a guaranteed analysis. The protein content is 60–70 percent. Sometimes the fat goes as high as 15 percent. These too will have calories.

As with people, we think junk foods have a place in pet diets, but a small one. Treats and chews are fine for dogs and cats as long as they are real foods. Others are more for the pleasure of owners than the pets. Pets should be just as happy—and better off nutritionally—if given real food. Calories add up quickly and it's harder to maintain a pet's weight if you give it frequent treats. The same rule applies to dogs and cats as it does to humans: the more times a day you feed your pet—and the more you feed it—the more calories it is likely to take in.

BOTTLED WATER

At a time when bottled waters have become a flashpoint for concerns about environmental pollution, for the failure of city governments to protect the safety of municipal water supplies, and for their breathtakingly inflated cost, we have doubts about the wisdom of bottled waters made especially for dogs and cats. But we have learned never to underestimate the creativity of pet food marketers. Bottled water is liquid gold. Its main ingredient costs practically nothing (it comes out of a tap), the tiny amounts of added nutrients are a trivial expense, and the markup can be enormous. The marketing must be working. The American Pet Products Association estimated that 5 percent of dog owners and 6 percent of cat owner bought flavor-enhanced water for their pets sometime in 2008.

Still, we were surprised to see so many bottled waters at Pet Expo in 2008, and even more surprised to see such candid explanations for their existence. Fortifido Fortified Water (Cott Beverages), for example, displayed a peanut-butter flavored, calcium-fortified water ("for healthy bones") with this explanation: "Today's dog owners spare no expense to make sure their pet is happy and healthy. . . . Consumers who purchase Fortifido spend $3.45 more on other items in the store vs. consumers who do not purchase Fortifido." Hero Enhanced Dog Water (Century Foods International) displayed an Exercise Recovery water, "triply purified by reverse osmosis," and fortified with electrolytes, amino acids, and vitamins: "Dog owners are passionate about their pets and respond well to products that are healthy for their dogs . . . many lavish their dogs with luxuries unheard of in the past." Dog-Wa (Hitchen' Spot) is a concentrate of leafy greens to be added to your dog's water—at a markup of 48 percent to the retailer. So consider these products as liquid dietary supplements targeted to an upscale, treat-loving audience.

The targeting is interesting to observe. The European company Special Waters displayed Water Cat, a "True and healthy alternative to tap water." The company's products "contain natural spring water, and only use organic/natural active ingredients." Organic water? According to the label, a liter contains less than a combined total of 90 mg of added calcium, magnesium, sodium, and potassium, an amount too small to make much of a difference in a cat's diet. These may be dietary supplements, but they are weak ones. Some of the targeting is aimed at convenience: Wetbone waters come in a resealable and leak-resistant pouch.

Yes, bottled water is convenient and some pets don't like the taste of chlorinated water. One of the first entrepreneurs to go into the bottled pet water business developed her product to overcome the disgusting (to owners) tendency of dogs to drink anything they can find: "toilets, puddles, gutters." But an Australian developer of a sports drink for dogs explained the true genesis of his products. His visits to supermarkets made it clear that "The fastest growing markets were bottled water for humans and high-value pet treats. . . . Bottled water for dogs . . . I just had to follow through with it." *Advertising Age* considers the fortified pet water category to be "hot." Fortified waters for humans earned $1.46 billion in sales in 2006, more than a tenfold increase in just the five years since 2001. Of Fortifido, *Advertising Age* explains: "For those who would snicker at the idea of a major beverage company moving into the pet category . . . it was not a hasty decision. The product-development phase took nearly 18 months, and the company poured $80,000 into research." This, for *water*.

If you like the products and don't care about the environmental and financial costs, we see no reason not to buy them. But fortified pet waters are about marketing, not health. If you need portable water for your pet, bring some tap water along in a reusable nontoxic plastic container and take advantage of another product we saw displayed at Pet Expo: Wow-Bow's Acqua BōL, a "folding water bowl for dogs that's stylish, reusable, and the size of a credit card!" We disagree with writers who say "tap water is just as harmful for your pet as it is for you" and insist that you use bottled water. If your cat or dog turns up its nose at chlorinated water, you can easily get rid of the chlorine smell. Just leave an open container of water out overnight and most of the chlorine will be gone by morning.

Many bottled waters are meant as delivery systems for nutritional or herbal supplements. We look at these products in the next two chapters.

Dietary Supplements

DIETARY SUPPLEMENTS ARE a relatively small, but growing segment of the pet food marketplace. They include nutrients or other substances taken or given, usually as pills, to promote health or prevent disease. More than half of American humans take some type of a dietary supplement, at least occasionally. The most common supplements are vitamins and minerals, but people also choose supplements from among hundreds of antioxidants, enzymes, gland extracts, herbals, and plant extracts in order to improve one or another aspect of health. Supplements are marketed to pet owners for the same health reasons. If supplements are good for humans, aren't they also good for dogs and cats? You might think so but remarkably little research has evaluated the benefits (or risks) of supplements for either humans or pets, leaving many questions about their effectiveness and safety unanswered.

The lack of evidence for benefits does not stop anyone from either selling supplements or taking them. Supplements are highly profitable. The sellers of both human and pet supplements want to market their products. Because the pet supplement market is still in its infancy, pet supplement makers are especially eager to increase sales.

Supplement manufacturers need distribution channels. Pet Naturals of Vermont ("helping pets live healthier lives") explains why pet supply stores should sell its supplement products. For example:

- Category growth. The Natural Pet Health and Nutrition category is growing at a remarkable 20% per year. Now your opportunity to carry a phenomenally profitable pet nutrition and health line is here.
- Highest margins per linear foot. Dedicating just 24″ of shelf space to Pet Naturals can generate $3000 in profits a year!

The profitability of supplements drives their marketing. It is one thing to sell bone meal and potassium salts to people who feed raw foods or home-cooked diets to their pets. These supplements provide minerals that have been demonstrated to be essential for a pet's health. But it is quite a different challenge to market supplements that *might* do some good but are less demonstrably beneficial. Health claims address the selling problem, and supplements are marketed with claims that cover the entire range of health problems likely to beset humans and pets. Keeping these claims honest presents especially difficult challenges for regulatory agencies.

OVERSIGHT OF SUPPLEMENTS: HUMANS

Because supplements are not foods, they are not regulated as foods. But they also are not drugs. If they were, they would have to undergo testing to prove that they were safe and more effective than placebos in producing the claimed benefits. The supplement industry has long argued that its products are safer than drugs and should be exempt from having to prove safety or efficacy. Categorized neither as foods nor drugs, supplements fall into a regulatory grey area that over the years has embroiled the FDA and the supplement industry in endless controversy.

As we noted earlier (chapter 14), claims that dietary supplements could prevent or treat disease have been allowed only since 1994 when the supplement industry successfully lobbied Congress to pass the Dietary Supplement Health and Education Act (DSHEA, pronounced d'shay).

This act effectively deregulated dietary supplements. Supplement companies no longer had to prove products effective or safe before marketing them. Instead, they could use a new kind of health claim called "structure-function." Companies could claim—without much in the way of scientific proof—that products supported or promoted a particular structure or function of the body. Such claims permitted statements like "enhances immune function" or "promotes heart health." The act, however, continued to block companies from making statements that the FDA considered drug claims, such as "prevents colds" or "reduces the risk of heart disease."

For anyone other than a company lawyer or FDA regulator, "promotes heart health" and "reduces heart disease risk" sound much alike, and that was just what supplement marketers wanted. The supplement industry grew rapidly in the years immediately following DSHEA. Sales of herbs and botanicals increased nearly 70 percent between 1994 and 1997, and sales of supplements such as glucosamine and fish oils grew 60 percent during those years.

One additional provision of DSHEA directed then president Bill Clinton to appoint a Commission on Dietary Supplement Labels to evaluate how DSHEA was working in practice. The president appointed one of us (Nesheim) to serve as chair of the commission, which issued its final report in 1997. The report recommended a series of actions to improve supplement safety, require evidence to substantiate health claims, and convey information about supplements to the public, but few of its recommendations were implemented.

Finally, DSHEA required the National Institutes of Health (NIH) to establish a research program on dietary supplements. As part of this program, the NIH Office of Dietary Supplements maintains a library of research studies on these products. The NIH also began to fund clinical trials of the effectiveness of some of the more widely used supplements. To the dismay of everyone concerned, the results of these trials have been consistently disappointing. In most trials, the groups of people receiving dietary supplements fared no better than those given a placebo, and they sometimes did worse. Perhaps as a result of the lack of evidence for benefits, sales of herbal supplements declined in the early 2000s, and only increased slightly beginning in 2007.

OVERSIGHT OF SUPPLEMENTS: PETS

DSHEA does not apply to pet foods or, by extension, to pet supplements. As we have explained, pet foods are regulated as animal feed under guidelines set by FDA and AAFCO; these apply to supplements, but awkwardly. AAFCO does not develop model regulations for supplements specifically, but its model food regulations do specify that nonessential nutrients such as extra vitamins, omega-3 fatty acids, omega-6 fatty acids, and taurine (for dogs) can be marketed "for the purpose of having an effect on the structure or function of the body."

The AAFCO models say that if a product label claims a health benefit for a nonessential nutrient, the amount of that nutrient must be listed in the guaranteed analysis with an asterisk: "*Not recognized as an essential nutrient by the AAFCO [dog or cat] food nutrient profile." Supplement makers have their own interpretation of this rule. They say it applies to *any* substance in their products that has no nutritional value. Such substances are useful for marketing purposes when they can be used as a basis for structure-function claims.

Here comes the awkward part: Under FDA and AAFCO model regulations, nonnutritive substances in pet supplements or treats are considered unapproved—and, therefore, forbidden—food ingredients unless they have been previously approved as additives to animal feed. This "unapproved" category includes many of the supposedly active ingredients in pet supplements for which marketers make health claims. If companies adhered to the FDA and AAFCO guidelines, they could not make health claims for unapproved additives. But they do. And they get away with this because the FDA says it follows the philosophy of the laws governing human supplements in allowing "meaningful health related information on pet food labels." The bottom line is that health claims on pet supplements are illegal but the FDA allows them. A situation like this is not only awkward, but unstable. The FDA could (and, we think, should) change its policy at any time.

We have reason to be concerned about this situation. In January 2002, for example, AAFCO announced a "uniform enforcement event" to help states remove unapproved and potentially harmful feed and pet food ingredients from the market. AAFCO and the FDA announced that they planned to enforce rules against unsafe, unapproved ingredients distributed through all channels of commerce, including catalogs and the Internet. In the absence of more specific information, supplement makers speculated that AAFCO state regulators would begin removing natural remedies from the market and that the regulators would especially be going after glucosamine supplements.

The reaction? Consternation. The American Veterinary Medical Association (AVMA) wrote AAFCO stressing the importance of glucosamine products for treating joint problems in companion animals. Susan Wynn, an officer of the Veterinary Botanical Medicine Association and the American Academy of Veterinary Nutrition, and an advisor to the National Animal Supplement Council (NASC), quickly put up a website:

> It is time to start a letter writing campaign, the likes of which we have never had before. Preventing this drastic action is likely to take an act of Congress, just like the Dietary Supplement Health Education Act (DSHEA) in 1994 . . . to replicate that success for our animals, we will need tens of thousands of letters. At least. This will be a political fight, and you need to inform your federal legislators as well as your state feed control official of your opinion on this matter. . . . Send your letters and petitions to ALL of the people suggested below.

NASC, which had just been formed by twenty-five supplement companies the year before (and in 2009 listed more than a hundred members), counterproposed that industry and regulators work together to bring unapproved ingredients in compliance with federal and state laws. It designed a program of industry self-regulation, "Compliance Plus," to deal with labeling, manufacturing practices, oversight, and reporting.

These pressures and countermeasures worked. In August, the president of AAFCO, John Breitsman, assured veterinarians that the rumors of a crackdown on supplements and targeting of glucosamine were unfounded. Yes, AAFCO wanted to conduct the enforcement event in the spring but because of a "misinformation campaign directed at consumers" had decided to postpone it. AAFCO's goal, he said, was to increase consumer awareness of the hazards of harmful supplements, limit their availability, establish uniform regulations, and create a level playing field for the industry. Perhaps, but nothing further has come of this.

Since then, the emphasis has shifted from regulation to self-regulation. NASC reports that its members are working to obtain legislation that will allow pet supplements to follow the same rules as those for human supplements. In the interim, it offers a seal of approval to companies that comply with criteria involving process and quality controls, a reporting system for adverse reactions to supplements, and some labeling disclosures. The seal does not require companies to offer proof that their products are safe and effective. Even so, we see few supplement products bearing the NASC seal.

The "threat" of regulation of health claims on pet foods has not gone completely dormant, however. In June 2008, the AVMA executive board, "in the interest of public safety . . . recommends the FDA require all pet food products with implied or explicit health claims [to] include a prominent statement on the label indicating that these claims have not been evaluated by the FDA." This kind of statement is required on human supplement labels, and this proposal would make the labels of pet supplements look more like those for human supplements. At the time of this writing, the FDA had not acted on the recommendation.

Without national legislation, pet supplements are in regulatory limbo. The FDA considers them to be "unapproved drugs of low regulatory priority." Our guess is that as long as unapproved feed supplements are not noticeably making pets, farm animals, or humans sick, the FDA will ignore them. We understand that the limbo is awkward for supplement companies but we think it is worse for pets and their owners. Pet stores sell a huge array of unregulated supplements, hardly any of them (other than vitamins and minerals) known to be safe or effective, and none under independent oversight.

One question worth asking is whether pet supplements really contain what their labels claim. Apparently, some do not. Tests by an independent laboratory, Consumer Lab, showed that four of six pet supplements did not contain the promised amount of chondroitin; one contained only 17 percent of the stated amount. Of eighty-seven chondroitin brands tested by NASC, 28 percent failed to meet label claims. Perhaps chondroitin supplements are particularly subject to manufacturing errors. One investigation of taurine and carnitine supplements concluded that nearly all contained within 10 percent of the amounts stated on the labels. Even so, these particular supplements dissolved so poorly that they were likely to be excreted unabsorbed and intact. In the absence of regulation, NASC certification seems like a reasonable first step.

With this background, let's take a look at some of the supplement products we found on store shelves in mid-2008.

THE PET SUPPLEMENT MARKETPLACE

Reliable data on the use of pet supplements are hard to come by. In 2004, a telephone survey found nearly 10 percent of 1,100 pet owners to be giving dietary supplements to their pets. Most gave vitamins and minerals, but many also used chondroprotective agents (glucosamine and chondroitin sulfate), and omega-3 fatty acids. The American Pet Products Association (APPA) reported in 2009 that 10 percent of dog owners said they gave vitamin supplements to their dogs, and about 2 percent said they gave them to cats. The NASC considers these figures as underestimates because the APPA survey mostly asked about vitamins. It guessed that about 20 percent of pet owners use supplements. In 2008, the National Research Council (NRC) estimated that up to one-third of dogs and cats in the United States are fed a dietary supplement, so the proportion could be increasing. Sales certainly are increasing, reaching $1.4 billion in the United States in 2008.

We went to the Whiskers pet food store in Manhattan, which specializes in alternative health products, and took a look at what the store carried in the way of supplements. Table 21 presents a few selected examples.

Supplements are marketed with a remarkable range of structure-function claims and, in the case of "alleviates pain associated with exercise," an occasional drug claim. The Nupro product listed in the table makes several such claims, more than might be expected of just one supplement. We hardly know what to make of the ingredients in these products. Some of them are vitamins with well-established functions in the body. But pets consuming foods labeled as complete and balanced should not need vitamin supplements. Such foods are already supplemented with vitamins at levels that meet AAFCO nutrient profiles and exceed

Table 21

SELECTED EXAMPLES OF DIETARY SUPPLEMENTS
FOR DOGS AND CATS, 2008

PRODUCT (MANUFACTURER)	HEALTH CLAIMS	LEADING INGREDIENTS IN GUARANTEED ANALYSIS OR INGREDIENT LIST
Wellness WellTabs Dog Formula High-Potency Multi Vitamin & Mineral Supplement (Old Mother Hubbard)	Maintains optimal levels of key nutrients; prevents borderline deficiencies	Vitamin A, vitamin D, vitamin E, menadione (vitamin K), ascorbic acid (vitamin C)
Nupro Dog Supplement (Nutri-Pet Research)	Supports a healthy immune system; helps maintain a full healthy coat which may minimize itchy dry skin; maintains healthy cardiovascular function; promotes healthy digestion; supports allergy protection; nutritive support for healthy bones, teeth, and muscle function	Protein, fat, fiber, moisture, Norwegian kelp, flaxseed, nutritional yeast culture, desiccated liver, proprietary blend of amino acids and enzymes
Canine Slim Results (U.S. Animal Nutritionals of Vermont)	Weight loss in overweight dogs; contains Phase 2 pet starch neutralizer, a clinically tested weight loss ingredient	*Phaseolus vulgaris*
Ark Naturals Joint Rescue for Dogs and Cats (NASC seal)	Supports cartilage and joint function; alleviates pain associated with exercise	Glucosamine sulfate, Boswellin extract, curcumin extract, chondroitin sulfate, yucca extract

(continued on next page)

PRODUCT (MANUFACTURER)	HEALTH CLAIMS	LEADING INGREDIENTS IN GUARANTEED ANALYSIS OR INGREDIENT LIST
Heart Discovery for Dogs and Cats (U.S. Animal Nutritionals of Vermont)	Heart support formula	Carnitine, taurine, dimethylglycine, alpha tocopheryl (vitamin E), eicosapentaenoic acid (EPA)
Kidney and Heart High Concentration Emulsified Glandular (Doctor's Best for Your Pet/Doctor's Mutual Service Company)	Safe alternative to toxic drugs	Adrenal extract, kidney extract, heart extract
Kidney Strength for Cats (U.S. Animal Nutritionals of Vermont)	Supports and maintains proper kidney function and mineral balance	EPA, DHA, astragalus root powder, lecithin, rehmannia root extract
Liquid Hepato (Rx Vitamins for Pets)	Supports normal liver function, hypoallergenic	Milk thistle extract, lecithin, vitamin B_1, vitamin B_2, vitamin B_6
Digestive Enzymes Feline Formula (Dr. Goodpet)	For general health and digestive support with *Lactobacillus acidophilus*	Beetroot fiber, protease, amylase, lipase, cellulose

NRC recommendations. In any case, pets do not need pet-specific vitamin and mineral supplements. As we explain in chapter 21, pets can be given human multivitamin/multimineral supplements cut to fractions proportional to the weight of the animal.

Taurine is an essential amino acid for cats and is always added to complete-and-balanced cat foods; it is not required by dogs except under rare circumstances. Carnitine and lecithin are compounds synthesized by the body and also should not need to be supplemented. Neither should protease, amylase, and lipase; these are normal digestive enzymes. *Phaseolus vulgaris* is a common green bean. Kelp is seaweed. Yeast is yeast. All have some value as food, although the amounts in supplements are usually quite small. Beet root fiber and cellulose are indigestible fibrous substances; they bind the ingredients in the supplements together. If they do anything special at all, it is to increase stool volume. Glands from cows—adrenals, kidneys, and hearts—contain many different substances and it is not easy to know what any of them might do when eaten by cats or dogs. The same is true of extracts of plants such as astragalus, milk thistle, cumin, and yucca.

We had never heard of Boswellin or rehmannia extracts and had to look them up. Boswellin is a plant extract claimed to relieve symptoms of arthritis. Rehmannia is a plant used in Chinese traditional medicine, presumably to improve kidney function. We were unable to find any supporting documentation for the use of these botanicals or, for that matter, any of the others. Most such substances are not feed ingredients defined by AAFCO, nor are they on the FDA's list of substances generally recognized as safe (GRAS). Despite claims that the value of these ingredients is proven, virtually no scientific evidence supports the claimed benefits, with only a few exceptions. For these exceptions—carnitine, the chondroprotectives, omega-3 fatty acids, and probiotics—some research exists. This research is well worth review, and we do that in the next chapter.

Do Supplements Work?

WITH FEW EXCEPTIONS, the lack of research on ingredients in dietary supplements means that it is not possible to say whether they produce greater benefits than placebos. Pets, as far as we know, are not susceptible to placebo effects. Placebos work on *owners*. Owners want to do something to help their pets. Giving supplements to pets makes owners feel better.

We doubt that most pet supplements do harm, but we can't find much research on that point either. The ingredient lists of supplements make the products seem as if they do wonderful things for health. But do they? In most cases, we just don't know. According to a committee of the National Research Council (NRC), few data are available to establish the safety of dietary supplements for pets. The committee examined evidence for the use of evening primrose oil, garlic, and lutein, for example, but could not find enough information to establish safety limits for these supplements. All the committee could do was to estimate safe levels from the amounts that had been previously used in animal feeds with no apparent ill effects. Just as we have done, the NRC committee concluded that the regulation of animal dietary supplements is in disarray.

We can make some guesses about whether pet supplements do any good based on the few that have some research behind them—carnitine, the chondroprotectives, the omega-3s, and probiotics. In examining this research, it becomes easier to understand why even the most basic questions about dietary supplements in either pets or humans are so difficult to answer.

CARNITINE

Carnitine is a body chemical that transports fatty acids to cells to be "burned" for energy; it also removes toxins from cells. Because carnitine is made in the body, it is not considered a dietary requirement for humans except for early preterm infants or individuals with rare genetic defects in metabolism. Nevertheless, carnitine frequently appears on the ingredient lists of supplements claimed to prevent or treat heart disease and obesity, and to boost athletic performance. These ideas derive from carnitine's transport and detoxification functions and are based on the notion that even though you make your own, more might be better. Researchers have examined this possibility. The results? Some of their studies suggest benefits, but others do not, thereby leaving much opportunity for speculation.

Do carnitine supplements do anything good for pets? The NRC finds "no evidence that dogs in a normal domestic environment require carnitine supplementation nor is there any indication that carnitine is required in the diet for cats." As is the case with humans, however, some dogs have a rare genetic defect that interferes with carnitine synthesis. Such dogs might develop heart problems that resolve when they are given supplemental carnitine. But this says nothing about whether carnitine does anything for normal dogs. A combination of carnitine and lipoic acid has been reported to improve the performance of aging beagles on some choice tests and both chemicals are included in a patented supplement marketed to delay human aging. This study, unsurprisingly, was sponsored by the company marketing the product.

On the basis of its role in fat transport, carnitine shows up in weight-control supplements and diet foods for cats. When investigators gave carnitine supplements to cats on reducing diets, the cats receiving the supplements lost weight a bit faster than cats given placebos. A 2008 review of these and other studies of carnitine concluded that supplements appear to produce some weight-loss benefits. But, the investigators said, the research cannot be independently evaluated: "Unfortunately most of these studies are described only in abstracts, industry publications, and patent applications which makes it difficult to review experimental methods and analysis." We are not the only ones complaining about not having access to research; the authors of this review are scientists from the pet food industry. Even the editor of the trade magazine *Petfood Industry* observes that "there are many questions about the safety and efficacy of functional ingredients in pet food that need to be answered . . . however, much of the science is proprietary and unpublished."

The inability of independent scholars to evaluate pet food research is a pervasive problem in this field but the problem is particularly acute when interpreting supplement studies. Without knowing how the studies were conducted—the composition of the diets, the dose of supplement, the number of animals, the length of time involved, and other such details—it is not possible to determine whether carnitine really has an effect. Cats on reduced-calorie diets lose weight anyway, and eating less still remains the most useful weight-loss strategy in animals as well as in people. Our assessment of the benefits of carnitine: doubtful.

THE CHONDROPROTECTIVES: CHONDROITIN SULFATE AND GLUCOSAMINE

Because these compounds are structural components of cartilage, it seems reasonable to think that eating them might prevent or treat arthritis of the hip or other joints in aging dogs as well as humans. With age, some of the cartilage in joints thins or erodes away and allows bones to rub up against each other. This hurts. Perhaps 20 percent of dogs experience this kind of arthritis, and large breeds are more susceptible than small breeds. Older cats are also affected. As in people, being overweight increases the risk of developing hip and joint problems, and losing weight improves mobility.

Everyone agrees that it would be helpful to prevent cartilage losses. Several clinical trials in humans have examined the effects of glucosamine and chondroitin sulfate, singly and in combination, on pain and loss of mobility associated with arthritis of the knee. These studies included a control group taking a placebo, not least because pain and mobility are highly subjective and would be expected to be just the kind of condition to respond to placebos. Alas, a federal review of such studies concluded that chondroprotectives are no better than placebos in relieving pain and improving physical function. Within some of the clinical trials, however, small subgroups of individuals responded well to the treatment. Analysis of these cases showed that in these particular individuals, symptoms improved no matter what they were taking: the chondroprotective or the placebo. Our interpretation: joint pain is highly subject to placebo effects.

Pets do not respond to placebos: owners do. So studies in dogs also must include a placebo control. In the largest placebo-controlled study to date, one using fifty-eight dogs, neither owners nor veterinarians could see any difference in whether the disease got better or worse in dogs given chondroitin sulfate, a mussel extract (with anti-inflammatory properties), or a placebo. But again, a small group of owners in all three groups—including those whose dogs had been given the placebo—reported that their dogs were doing much better. This study also demonstrates the power of placebo effects to produce observable benefits.

Investigators conducted a systematic review of sixteen clinical trials of drug and chondroprotective treatments for arthritis in dogs. They concluded that the strongest demonstrable benefits of treatment were mostly limited to anti-inflammatory drugs like aspirin, ibuprofen, or naproxen. About glucosamine and chondroitin sulfate, the reviewers concluded that no conclusions or recommendations could be drawn because the results of clinical trials were too limited to interpret. The uninspiring conclusion: more research is needed.

Despite the lack of evidence for the benefits of chondroprotectives, the results of these studies have been widely interpreted as holding out a glimmer of hope to sufferers from joint pain. On this basis, many owners believe that chondroprotectives are important for their pets' health. Pet food makers tell us that chondroitin sulfate and glucosamine *must* be on ingredient lists in order to get anyone to buy their products, and many pet foods and treats contain them. Some products promote the sources of chondroprotectives as "natural." Natural, in this case, usually means poultry and meat by-product meals; these meals contain the cartilage that remains when meat is removed from chicken breasts and the ends of animal bones. Cartilage naturally contains chondroprotectives. Trachea chews are another "natural" source.

Do natural meals contain enough chondroprotectives to do any good? Purina ONE Lamb and Rice Formula, for example, guarantees 400 mg of glucosamine per kilogram of diet (from natural sources, lamb and poultry by-product meal). At recommended feeding levels, this would provide about 6.5 mg of glucosamine per kilogram of a dog's body weight. But most of the disappointing studies investigating the potential benefits of chondroprotectives used doses three to four times higher: 20 mg to 25 mg/kg body weight. If the higher doses do not work, lower doses are also unlikely to work. Supplements contain higher doses. The Ark Naturals joint supplement (table 21) is said to contain 500 mg of glucosamine and 50 mg of chondroitin sulfate per chewable tablet. If nothing else, it could be a better placebo.

Our view is that the evidence for the benefit of chondroprotectives is minimal for anything beyond a placebo effect. But placebo effects are enough to encourage people to believe that the supplements might work for their pet. Chondroprotectives are normal components of diets containing poultry or meat by-products and, therefore, unlikely to cause harm. Supplements can make owners—and veterinarians—feel better because at least they are doing something. Chondroprotectives make manufacturers feel *much* better because health claims help sell supplements as well as supplemented pet foods and treats.

OMEGA-3 FATS

Neither humans nor pets can make omega-3 fats: we must eat them. In talking about pets' needs for omega-3 fats, we need to consider three types, each with its own mind-numbing abbreviation: ALA (alpha-linolenic acid) from plants, and EPA (eicosapentaenoic acid) and DHA (docosahexaenoic acid) from fish and fish oils. As we mentioned earlier, pets and people can convert ALA to EPA, and EPA to DHA, but slowly. DHA is the one for which most health claims get made. It is said to do good things for an astonishing array of health conditions, among them

Alzheimer's disease, asthma, cancer, depression, diabetes, heart disease, and stroke. In theory, if omega-3s are good for people, they could also be good for cats and dogs.

But as is typical, the evidence that links omega-3 fats to protection against such diseases is limited and subject to interpretation. Omega-3s first came to public attention when Danish investigators observed low rates of heart disease among indigenous Greenlanders eating diets high in fish fats rich in EPA and DHA. Since those initial observations, numerous studies have examined the effects of eating fatty fish and fish oils on a variety of health conditions. Systematic reviews of such studies give mixed results.

Because humans cannot make their own omega-3 fats, ALA is considered a nutritional requirement. Dogs and cats cannot make their own omega-3 fats either, but AAFCO profiles do not include them as required nutrients. This is because no definitive experimental studies have confirmed them as requirements. This omission is not as surprising as it may seem; the studies would be difficult to do. The amount of omega-3s needed in people—and by extrapolation, in cats and dogs—is so small that the fatty acids would need to be completely eliminated from the diet for a long time before symptoms of deficiency would appear. Instead of trying to perform such difficult and expensive research, experts find it easier to assume that cats and dogs need omega-3s and establish recommended allowances based on whatever evidence is available from human and animal studies. The NRC did just that when it recommended allowances for ALA as well as for EPA and DHA in its 2006 publication. AAFCO generally goes along with the NRC's recommendations and we expect AAFCO to establish profiles for omega-3s at some point.

Much of the evidence for benefits of omega-3s in pets is by analogy to human studies. These, for example, suggest that consuming omega-3s from fish or fish oil may reduce the risk of death from heart attacks. On this basis, the American Heart Association says people who have experienced a heart attack should eat fish twice a week. In 2006, the Institute of Medicine, a think tank of health professionals, appointed a committee to review the evidence linking fish consumption to health. One of us (Nesheim) chaired that committee. The committee concluded that the human evidence was insufficient to say much about the benefits of fish or fish oil for any condition other than heart disease. Eating fish appears beneficial for heart health, but eating fish *oils* less so. The committee cautioned against assuming that the benefits of fish rich in omega-3s could be achieved just as well by taking fish oil supplements containing omega-3 fatty acids.

The research in dogs is much less extensive than that in humans. One study found consumption of fish oil omega-3s to be helpful to dogs with surgically induced kidney insufficiency. In contrast, safflower oil, which mostly has omega-6 fatty acids, seemed to worsen the kidney problems. Investigators have used fish oils to treat heart arrhythmias and congestive heart failure in dogs, with some evidence of benefit. In chapter 13, we reviewed the uncertain evidence linking omega-3s to learning ability in young animals.

As for arthritis: scientists at Hill's Pet Nutrition report that dogs fed EPA-supplemented diets have fewer symptoms and less pain than dogs fed the same diet without the added EPA. But because the investigators did not provide details about the composition of the diets or of the supplement, it is impossible to know whether the study really did what it claimed. Nevertheless, Hill's uses this study as the basis for marketing a Prescription Diet product for joint disease.

Veterinarians sometimes recommend supplements of omega-3 fats for skin disorders in dogs and cats. In general, diets high in fats of any type seem to improve coat quality. For example, one study compared the effects of omega-6 fatty acids (from sunflower seeds) to a mixture of omega-6 and omega-3 fatty acids (from flaxseed). Both diets led to observed improvements in the dogs' hair and skin. But both groups of dogs were fed more fat than usual, and the investigators could not distinguish the effects of omega-3s from that of the higher fat content.

One other complicating factor is that although fish are a good source of omega-3s, some are also sources of methylmercury, a neurotoxin that accumulates in the fish food chain. Large, predatory fish that have eaten other fish for most of their lives—albacore tuna, for example—accumulate levels of methylmercury that sometimes exceed safety standards. Concerns about the neurotoxic effects of methylmercury on the developing fetus have induced federal agencies to advise pregnant women to limit or avoid eating albacore tuna and other large predatory fish.

In 2008, the Environmental Working Group (EWG) released a study of toxins in the blood and urine of cats and dogs in an animal hospital in Virginia. The EWG investigators found blood levels of methylmercury in cats to be 6 times higher than in dogs, and 4.4 times higher than in the average human in the United States. They attributed this finding to the large amounts of tuna that cats eat. We do not know whether the EWG results are typical of cats in the United States (or just hospitalized cats) or whether the high levels have any clinical significance. We cannot tell, for example, whether high levels of methylmercury induce neurological impairments in kittens. But why take chances? It is always a good idea to vary food intake and to rotate fish-based foods with other kinds. Most pet food manufacturers offer any number of nonfish foods for cats that can easily be substituted for tuna.

So are omega-3 supplements useful? Omega-3 fats and omega-6 fats are needed in the diets of pets, but in small amounts. Commercial complete-and-balanced pet foods are supposed to provide both in adequate amounts. We are not convinced by current evidence that supplemental amounts are needed. Could omega-3 fats be harmful? That too seems unlikely. Overall, as we discuss in chapter 21, if you are cooking for your pet and use a wide variety of relatively unprocessed foods, you should not need supplements except maybe bone meal, some calcium and potassium salts, taurine for cats, and a daily multivitamin for insurance.

PROBIOTICS

Probiotics means the opposite of antibiotics—living bacteria, but friendly ones. The theory is that if you eat probiotic bacteria, they will replace unfriendly bacteria in your intestinal tract, improve your immune response, and help prevent the diarrhea that sometimes comes with antibiotic treatment. Bacteria have to eat too, and that introduces another term—prebiotics—meaning foods that stimulate the growth of probiotic bacteria. Your digestive tract cannot extract nutrients from the fiber in fruits, vegetables, and whole grains, but bacteria can digest (ferment) some fiber carbohydrates in the large intestine. A supplement like Dr. Goodpet's (table 21) adds beet and cellulose fibers to feed those bacteria.

The best source of probiotics in the human diet is yogurt, traditionally made from milk fermented with friendly *Lactobacillus bulgaricus* and *Streptococcus thermophilus*. Because these bacteria are rather delicate and are easily killed by food processing and stomach acid, supplement makers prefer to use the hardier *Lactobacillus acidophilus*. In yogurt, such bacteria digest lactose, which makes dairy products more tolerable for people who are unable to use this sugar.

Probiotic bacteria are good candidates for supplements for other reasons. They survive digestion, multiply in the intestinal tract, and alter the composition of fecal bacteria. Feeding probiotic bacteria to infants with diarrhea reduces the severity of their symptoms, and helps to prevent allergic reactions to milk or other food proteins. Feeding probiotic bacteria to adults with antibiotic-induced diarrhea also relieves symptoms and may enhance immunity. In 2004, a group of scientists reviewed research examining the effects of yogurt on health. Probiotics, they said, showed "promising health benefits," suggesting that foods or supplements might alleviate symptoms of constipation, inflammatory bowel disease, colon cancer, stomach ulcers, and allergies. This review, initiated and paid for by the National Yogurt Association, concluded that "Patients with any of these conditions could possibly benefit from the consumption of yogurt." Subsequent reviews, also sponsored by companies with a vested interest, have come to similar conclusions: probiotics show promise. Promise, we must point out, is not the same as effectiveness, but it is all a supplement seller needs for marketing purposes.

As for prebiotics: although most indigestible food carbohydrates (fiber) encourage bacterial growth in the large intestine, not all kinds promote the growth of beneficial strains. Fiber composed of long chains of fructose sugar seems especially beneficial. So does the carbohydrate in soybeans. These observations have encouraged researchers to feed fructose fiber to dogs in the hope that it would stimulate the growth of friendly bacteria. The results of the one test of this hypothesis, however, were disappointing. In a study sponsored by Iams, investigators at Texas A&M fed dogs a diet supplemented with fructose carbohydrates and looked for probiotic bacteria in their feces. They did not find many.

Because the physiology of humans and pets is so similar, it seems reasonable to suppose that probiotics might prove beneficial to pets, and investigators at pet food companies (or sponsored by them) have taken an active interest in this area. Researchers at Mars's Waltham Centre in Great Britain, for example, demonstrated that probiotic bacteria survive digestion, multiply in the colon, alter the balance of fecal flora, and improve some cellular and biochemical components of the immune system. The immune effects suggested that probiotics might help prevent food allergies in pets.

One study sponsored by Nestlé Purina examined the effects of probiotics on dogs that developed diarrhea when they ate certain foods. The dogs were placed on diets that eliminated those foods but also included either probiotics or a placebo. As you might expect, the elimination diet improved symptoms in all of the dogs. The probiotics, however, did not make much difference. Despite the lack of evidence for demonstrable benefits, pet food makers are increasingly adding probiotics to their foods, supplement makers are increasingly marketing probiotic products, and veterinary researchers are increasingly interested in this area.

Let's deal with food first. Because cooking kills bacteria, probiotics do not survive canning. The heat generated by extrusion means that living probiotic bacteria must be added to dry foods after kibble is formed. To make the experimental dry diets, the Waltham manufacturers froze and dried the bacteria, and then sprayed them on the finished kibble. According to Waltham, 60–70 percent of the bacteria survive manufacturing and storage, but Waltham does not say for how long. Survival depends on reducing the moisture in the kibble to 2 percent before spraying on the probiotics, and sealing the finished kibble in aluminum foil. We wonder about the survival of bacteria in "probiotic" kibbles we see in stores; these typically guarantee 10 percent moisture and are packaged in ordinary paper.

We suspect that probiotic bacteria must be alive to do any good, and we doubt that many survive in pet foods stored for long periods of time. What happens to them when they are eaten? Viability has been studied extensively in yogurt, an excellent growth medium for bacteria. Commercial yogurts typically display a "Live & Active** Cultures" seal. The double asterisks refer to a statement that the product meets criteria for living bacteria set by the National Yogurt Association, a trade group for this industry. That standard is 100 million living bacteria per gram of yogurt at the time of manufacture. Think about this number the next time you eat a six-ounce container of yogurt. If you eat the whole thing, you will have consumed 18 *billion* live bacteria. Frozen yogurt only has to have 10 million bacteria per gram at the time it was made to qualify for the seal—a 90 percent reduction and low in bacterial terms.

Although the Yogurt Association does not test products at the retail level, *Consumer Reports* does and reported a few years ago that most of the yogurts it examined had more than the required number of live and active bacteria—15 billion to 155 billion per serving. Supplements, which have a much less favorable environment for keeping bacteria alive, widely varied in the content of living bacteria, from 20 million to 70 billion per dose.

It is unfortunate that *Consumer Reports* did not test dry probiotic pet foods, because it would be interesting to do so. Tests of probiotic supplements suggest that if they contained bacteria in the first place, the bacteria did not last long. Scott Weese, a veterinarian at the University of Guelph, analyzed the microbial content of eight veterinary and five human probiotic supplements. Only two of thirteen products contained the number of live bacteria claimed on their labels. Most products contained very low levels of living organisms. His conclusion: "Most commercial veterinary probiotic preparations are not accurately represented by label claims. Quality control appears to be poor."

High and low are relative terms and what seems high to one manufacturer may seem low to another. In 2008, Eagle Pack Holistic Select Hairball Relief cat food, for example, reinforced doubts about the probiotic dose of other products: "We added L. acidophilus like the cultures in yogurt. Unless a brand guarantees the effective levels on their bag they are most likely ineffective." A year later, its website said, "Research supporting the effectiveness of our Hairball Relief formula is on file with the FDA. Our research was more scientific than that performed by any other brand. We outperformed the leading brand 6 to 1." How did Eagle Pack do the study? The website does not say. Eagle Pack claims a live probiotic count of 240 million CFU [colony forming units] per pound of food. Other brands, as shown in table 22, claim 20 million to 283 million per pound. But even the highest amounts in pet food are just a few percent of the *minimum* counts allowed in yogurt for human consumption (45,400 million per pound of food), as shown in table 22.

Table 22

COMPARISON OF THE PROBIOTIC CONTENT OF COMMERCIAL DOG FOODS TO HUMAN YOGURT STANDARDS, JULY 2009

SOURCE	MILLIONS OF LIVE PROBIOTIC BACTERIA PER POUND OF FOOD
National Yogurt Association standard for "Live & Active Cultures"*	45,400
Nutro Ultra Holistic Adult for Dogs	283
Edge Pack Dog Food (guaranteed analysis)	240
Canidae for Dogs	100
Evo Ancestral Dog Food (guaranteed analysis)	90
Wellness Complete Health for Dogs	20

* The human food standard is 100 million per gram (a pound is 454 grams).

It is possible, of course, that lower counts still might do some good in dogs and cats. In human clinical trials of probiotic effects, the doses were 10 to 100 *billion* bacteria per day. The Waltham clinical trials in dogs and cats used doses of 0.2 to 1.0 billion per day, at least 100 times lower. Dogs and cats are not 100 times smaller than most humans, and we question whether the amounts of live probiotic bacteria added to dry foods or given as supplements can be high enough to be meaningful. If you want to try probiotics as a way to improve your pet's digestion, immune function, and resistance to allergies, you might be better off feeding them a tablespoon or two of plain, ordinary yogurt. Just make sure the yogurt is unsweetened. And don't expect frozen yogurt to contain as many living bacteria.

ALTERNATIVES to COMMERCIAL PET FEEDING

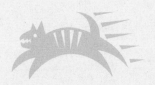

19

Unconventional Diets

AT THIS POINT we turn to a new market segment: the small percentage of owners who distrust commercial products and want to feed their pets according to their own "unconventional" (non-mainstream) dietary principles and values. People do not eat food just for fuel. We choose foods for reasons of culture, religion, identity, and any number of belief and value systems. If you are someone who holds strong opinions about your own diet, the question of what to feed your dog or cat is not simply a matter of nutrients. It gets into much more personal issues.

From the standpoint of veterinarians, unconventional diets—kosher, vegetarian, "ancestral," raw-food, and home-cooked—pose challenges, especially to those accustomed only to dealing with commercial complete-and-balanced products. Some of the challenges are nutritional. Diets that restrict one or another food group can be lacking in certain nutrients and cause deficiency symptoms. To deal with such challenges, veterinarians are advised to:

- Ask clients about their knowledge, beliefs, concerns, and expectations about dietary practices.

- Take a thorough dietary history of the pet (foods consumed, frequency, amounts).
- Ask clients about their pets' treats, supplements, table foods, and access to other foods.
- Ask clients whether they are ready and willing to make dietary changes for their pet.
- Take such factors into consideration when giving dietary advice or advising dietary changes.

This is excellent advice for any veterinarian-client discussion about dietary practices, unconventional or not (and we also note its value for doctor-human dietary interactions, as well).

Although the proportion of pet owners who feed their pets non-mainstream diets is small, a small percentage of the nearly $17 billion in dog and cat food sales represents a substantial market. The potential growth of this market makes it worthwhile for small companies to start manufacturing non-mainstream commercial products and for large companies to be interested in them. With that introduction, let's take a look at some of the more popular of the unconventional diets used to feed pets and the nutritional challenges, if any, that they pose.

KOSHER PET FOODS

The label on a can of Evanger's "Super Premium Holistic Pheasant Dinner for Cats" is labeled "Endorsed by the Chicago Rabbinical Council KOSHER FOR PASSOVER." Kosher refers to Jewish dietary laws. The Chicago Rabbinical Council certifies that the food is produced according to those laws. These are based on biblical injunctions against eating two kinds of animals, those that do not ruminate and do not have completely cloven hooves (Leviticus 11:26), and young animals cooked in their mother's milk (Deuteronomy 14:21). Thus, they forbid such things as eating pork or mixing meat and dairy foods at the same meal. The Passover celebration requires one additional restriction: Jews are not allowed to have in the house or to consume any foods containing potentially fermentable *chametz*—wheat, wheat starch, wheat gluten, barley, oats, oat fiber, and other grains—precisely the ingredients in many pet foods.

Given the multiple and not always identifiable sources of ingredients in pet foods, it is difficult to imagine how pet foods can conform to Jewish dietary laws at any time, let alone at Passover. Can pet foods be kosher? Is it acceptable to hold Passover seders for dogs and cats, as some do? And must pet owners who observe Jewish dietary laws feed their animals according to such laws? The answers are typically Talmudic: yes, and no.

According to Rabbi Mendel Weinbach, "Your pet certainly does not have to keep kosher but you do! This includes not deriving any benefit from those foods which the Torah has prohibited us to eat and to derive benefit from." He is saying that if you follow the kosher dietary laws, you must adhere to two restrictions. The first is that you must not feed your animals beef and dairy foods cooked together because you are not allowed to derive any benefit from them. Mixing meat and dairy in the same meal would not be kosher. But Rabbi Naftali Silberberg argues, "It is permissible to feed non-Kosher food to your pet. In fact the Torah says (Exodus 22:30): 'you shall not eat flesh of an animal that was torn in the field, to the dog you shall throw it.'" And Rabbi Eliezer Danzinger explains:

> In general, the laws of kosher are for (Jewish) humans, not for animals ... the "meat" that we may not cook with milk, or may not benefit from if it was cooked with milk, is meat from a *kosher* animal. Therefore, if it can be determined that the meat in the pet food comes from a non-kosher animal (such as horse meat), then it is "kosher" for your pet.... Some authorities permit feeding *stray* animals meat and milk mixtures, since you don't derive any apparent benefit. But other authorities forbid this as well, maintaining that by fulfilling your desire to feed a stray, you benefit too.

The second restriction applies to the Passover celebration. You are not permitted to feed pets *chametz* at Passover because "it is forbidden not only to eat, but even to own or gain any benefit from *chametz*." Although some observant Jews forbid consumption of *kitnyos* (legumes) at Passover, pets are exempt from this restriction.

What all this seems to mean is that with the exception of mixing meat and milk and using *chametz* at Passover, pets can be fed just about anything, including pork. Observant owners may not want to, however, and neither may Muslim pet owners who observe Halal dietary laws. But pork is a relatively infrequent ingredient in pet foods, so it should not be difficult to avoid. Pork-containing pet foods usually are called such things as "Pork Blend," "Pork Dog Food," or "Pork Flavor," but it is best to check the ingredient list to be sure.

Pork may not be much of a problem in pet feeding, but certification of kosher status is a huge concern. The Chicago Rabbinical Council, which certified the Evanger's product, is one of hundreds of such certifying groups. These differ—sometimes substantially—in their interpretation of the dietary laws. Some groups favor lenient interpretation, while others do not. The degree of stringency of kosher certification is a subject of much debate within the Jewish religious community and, we suspect, for good reason. One of us (Nesheim) visited a plant that made dry pet foods, including some labeled kosher. According to its manager, the kosher certification process was effortless. A rabbi came by once a year or so and asked if anything had changed in the manufacturing process. That took care of it.

Because application of dietary laws is so much a matter of interpretation, kosher certification of pet foods has little to do with religious observation. Kosher Pets, a company that sells pet foods to owners who observe Jewish dietary laws, says "kosher" means "clean, healthy, and fit." On this basis, no doubt, kosher foods and treats are attractive to many owners, Jewish and not. But pet foods are not certified kosher for Passover because they are especially clean; they are certified kosher because they do not contain *chametz*. Kosher pet foods may be acceptable for feeding cats and dogs, but these products are not kosher for humans. Observant Jews are forbidden to eat pet food (as if they would anyway). They also are forbidden to prepare or serve pet foods using kosher dishes or utensils.

This means, as some commentators make clear, that the principal purpose of kosher certification is marketing: "Kosher or Halal supervision is taken on by a company to expand its market opportunities. It is a business investment that, like any other investment, must be examined critically."

VEGETARIAN AND VEGAN

Among humans, vegetarianism encompasses a variety of dietary practices that have in common a partial or complete reliance on plant foods as the principal source of nutrients. People choose vegetarian diets for reasons of health, philosophy, religion, environmental impact, animal welfare, or just personal preference. The single common feature of all vegetarian diets is the avoidance of red meat—beef, pork, and lamb—but some people who consider themselves vegetarians even waive this restriction at times. The world of vegetarians encompasses people who occasionally eat red meat as well as vegans who never consume products from animals at all. Table 23 summarizes the most common categories of vegetarian diets.

Table 23
FOODS PERMITTED IN VARIOUS CATEGORIES OF VEGETARIAN DIETS

VEGETARIAN DIET CATEGORY	RED MEAT	FISH & POULTRY	MILK & DAIRY	EGGS
Partial	No	Yes	Yes	Yes
Lacto-ovo	No	No	Yes	Yes
Lacto-	No	No	Yes	No
Ovo-	No	No	No	Yes
Vegan	No	No	No	No

When vegetarian diets are adequate in calories and sufficiently varied, they promote excellent health. Vegetarians tend to have lower rates of heart disease, cancer, diabetes, and other such conditions than the general population. The risks of nutrient deficiencies in vegetarians are few; they are occasionally seen among adults and children eating highly restricted diets that do not provide enough foods containing vitamin B_{12} or some other nutrients. Supplements, more varied diets, and, sometimes, more food in general are easy remedies for such problems.

When it comes to pets, however, the idea of vegetarian diets seems counterintuitive. Dogs and cats evolved from a carnivorous past. But owners who practice vegetarian lifestyles often want their pets to do so too, and mainly for reasons of animal welfare.

The Ethics of Pet Vegetarianism: Pro and Con

When asked, people who feed vegetarian diets to their pets say they are doing so for ethical reasons. Eating meat, they say, is unethical. The Vegetarian Society of the United Kingdom, for example, argues that dogs ought to be vegetarian:

> Even with government subsidies, the cost of meat is high in monetary terms. To the cow, sheep, chicken, rabbit, pig, or fish the cost is even higher: they lose their lives . . . spent imprisoned in intensive rearing conditions. Imported meat may come from countries where slaughter methods are extremely cruel. . . . Furthermore, eating meat is a means of prolonging human suffering across the world. While half the world is starving, we continue to rear animals for food, an inefficient means of food production.

Animal rights groups make the choice simple: "If you are concerned about your companion animals' health and about the cruelty of the meat industry, now is the time to stop buying meat-based commercial food." If, they say, you feed your dog a vegan diet, "your companion can have a cruelty-free diet, too!" Never mind that dogs and cats ate meat in the wild. It's the raising of animals for the sole purpose of feeding humans and pets that troubles such groups.

If the animal-rights argument does not seem sufficiently compelling, proponents of pet vegetarian diets also maintain that meatless diets are healthier for pets. Such diets, they say, improve coat condition; reduce the risk of allergies, arthritis, diabetes, cataracts, kidney disease, and other degenerative conditions; and improve vitality. The proof? The benefits are "attested to by glowing accounts from their owners."

Pet food companies are happy to make products targeted to the vegetarian market segment, and they do. Avoderm says its Natural Vegetarian food is "for meat-sensitive dogs." We are not sure whether meat sensitivity refers to allergies or some other problem, but the first five ingredients are rice, soy, barley, canola oil, and avocado meal, which should be fine for dogs that do not have allergic reactions to any of them. Dick Van Patten's Natural Balance vegetarian formula is "true vegan" and contains "no animal or dairy products, which may cause allergies in some sensitive dogs." The calories have to come from some other nutritious ingredients, in this case, grains. The Evolution Diet Pet Food Corporation specializes in vegetarian and vegan foods. Since 1989, says the company's director of health and nutrition, Eric Weisman:

> Evolution Diet has manufactured both Dog and Cat Foods that has [*sic*] no artery clogging animal fat. . . . Animal Fats progressively block and destroy all the arteries in Dog and Cat Heart, Brain, Liver, Immune System, Kidney and virtually all other organs every time they are eaten. . . . [W]e have proven that Dogs, Cats and even Ferrets . . . can live longer and healthier on a Flesh Free—Animal Fat Free Diet with none of the Drugs, Radiation, Nitrates and Carbon Monoxide Gas found in Meat, Poultry and Fish Products.

Testimonials like this, no matter how glowing, do not constitute science. The value of feeding vegetarian diets to carnivorous pets is not, to understate the matter, universally accepted (ask any advocate of raw-food diets, for example). Some critics go so far as to say that imposing vegetarian diets on pets—especially cats—is a *breach* of ethics. The U.S. Humane Society, for example, says "it's unfair and unrealistic to impose humane ethical standards on cats. And forcing a cat to eat a diet that isn't based on meat imperils its health and its life." Are vegetable-based diets good or bad for pets? Fortunately, a few studies have addressed this question.

Do Vegetarian Diets Meet the Nutrient Needs of Pets?

Evanger's Vegetarian Dinner for Canines & Felines is labeled as meeting AAFCO nutrient profiles for all life stages with no preservatives, no artificial color, no salt, and no meat. Its first five ingredients are potatoes, carrots, oat groats, sunflower oil, and peas. Among the lesser ingredients are taurine, vitamin B$_{12}$, and biotin—nutrients that in nature would mainly come from meat sources.

The first question to ask is whether vegetarian diets meet the basic nutritional needs of dogs and cats. Dogs are omnivores and have few nutritional requirements that cannot be met by eating grains and vegetables. Vitamin B$_{12}$ is one exception. It must be obtained from meat. But as long as this vitamin is added to complete-and-balanced vegetarian foods, dogs should be able to meet their nutritional needs from such products. Cats, however, require several nutrients that derive exclusively or mainly from meat: vitamin B$_{12}$, but also taurine, arachidonic acid, and vitamin A. These nutrients also should be added as supplements to vegetarian cat foods.

But are they? In one small study, investigators sent a single sample of two commercial vegan diet products for cats—both labeled as meeting AAFCO nutrient profiles—to be tested for nutrient content. Neither met AAFCO standards for complete-and-balanced products. Both were especially low in some essential nutrients commonly found in meat. Since these deficiencies could easily have been corrected with supplements, it is difficult to know how representative the results might be or whether similar problems might be observed in an analysis of any commercial pet food.

A European study examined the clinical status of eighty-six dogs and eight cats that had been fed vegetarian diets. Compared to AAFCO profiles, the animals were consuming diets below standards for protein and several vitamins and minerals. The dogs, however, displayed no obvious clinical signs of nutritional deficiencies. This finding is not as surprising as it might seem. Nutrient profiles are set high to encompass the needs of animals of all life stages, and intakes well below profile levels can be quite adequate. A few of the cats in the study, however, displayed clinical signs of eye and reproductive disorders, suggesting that cats may be more sensitive to nutrient deficiencies. Other reports also document occasional problems in cats fed vegetarian diets. The moral? If you must feed your pets a vegetarian or vegan diet, be sure to supplement the diet with essential nutrients (we explain how in chapter 21).

Can Dogs and Cats Digest Plant Grains?

The answer to this question is yes, definitely (whether they should is a different question). As the history of pet feeding reveals, oatmeal was commonly fed to dogs. By 1945, the ability of dogs to digest and use starch was well established experimentally, and corn flakes and grain meals were frequent ingredients in pet foods. More recently, researchers tested the ability of dogs to digest flours made from barley, corn, potato, rice, sorghum, and wheat, and found all of them to be almost completely digestible and usable. Their conclusion: "Any of these flours could be used without negative effects on digestion." But because stool weights tended to be higher among dogs fed barley, feeding large amounts of that particular grain "may not be advantageous for dog owners who house their animals indoors for most of the day." These researchers also tried soybean meal, soy flour, and soy concentrate. Dogs could digest soy proteins as well as meat proteins, but produced bulkier feces and more flatulence. The moral: if you keep dogs indoors, you might want to avoid feeding them products based on barley or soy.

What about cats? Investigators have looked at whether cats can digest starches from various sources and whether these starches raise levels of blood sugar and insulin. Indeed, cats can digest the starches in cassava, rice, corn, sorghum, peas, and lentils. Among these carbohydrate sources, only corn stimulated a rise in blood sugar, but not by much. Other investigators have studied the effects of complete-and-balanced vegetarian diets on cats. Cats fared well on them, and displayed normal blood levels of taurine and vitamin B_{12}. These particular researchers especially wanted to know whether grain-based diets would cause the cats to produce alkaline urine, a condition that increases the risk of forming struvite kidney stones. This did not happen in their study, and the researchers concluded that it is quite possible for cats to thrive on well-formulated vegetarian diets.

From this limited evidence, we conclude that dogs and cats can do fine on vegetarian diets if—and only if—the diets are formulated to provide nutrients that are missing or found in low amounts in plant foods. But some commentators think feeding vegetarian diets to pets, especially cats, is flat-out unethical: "If you are going to keep a cat as a pet, the number one ethical concern in terms of diet should always be what is best for the cat . . . and that is a diet that might definitely conflict with one's ethical choices." Even veterinarians who favor vegetarian diets urge some caution. They advise owners of pets fed vegetarian diets ("vegetarian pets") to take them to a veterinarian for frequent health monitoring. They also say "we recommend that people who wish to feed vegetarian diets to their cats be counseled about the potential risks and the need to use a properly formulated recipe or commercial food." Following an adequate dietary formula makes good sense to us, and we provide one for cats and dogs in chapter 21.

"ANCESTRAL" DIETS: MEAT, NOT GRAINS

And now to an opposite view. Ancestral diets are based on the premise that because cats and dogs evolved from meat-eating ancestors, they ought to be eating meat and nothing but. Proponents of ancestral diets say never mind that animals are able to digest grains; they should not be eating them. Companies make products for owners who hold this belief. At our local holistic pet food store, we found a can of Instinct (Nature's Variety) Instinctive Nature, Innovative Nutrition Duck Formula Grain-Free Nutrition for Dogs. This particular complete-and-balanced product is labeled 95 percent duck; its first three ingredients are duck, water, and eggs (of unspecified origin). Flaxseed and peas follow soon after on the ingredient list but the product contains not a drop of rice, wheat, corn, barley, or oats.

The Evo line of Innova brand foods (Natura Pet Products)—"high protein. Low carb. No grain."—also offers a 95 percent duck product: duck, duck broth, and nothing else except flavor and thickening additives and the usual vitamin and mineral mix. A brochure for Evo foods explains the rationale for this product: "An evolutionary diet 10,000 years in the making. The benefits of raw and home-cooked nutrition in a safe and convenient natural food." Evo, it seems, claims the best of both worlds. On the one hand, it is a commercial product that meets AAFCO standards for complete-and-balanced nutrition. On the other, it directly positions itself as an alternative to what it considers unsafe and inconvenient raw-food and home-cooked diets. Evo products, according to their manufacturer, are what pets were designed by evolution to eat:

> Today's companion animals are seemingly much removed from their ancestors in the wild. But after thousands of years of se- lective breeding—achieving an incredible diversity of species— their dietary requirements remain, in many ways, unchanged. Unfortunately, they are only marginally fulfilled by most mod- ern commercial pet foods. Where once wild prey provided en- ergy and nutrients in the form of meat-based protein and fats, grains in modern pet foods have largely taken their place. . . . But "dilution" by carbohydrates means fewer essential nutrients to meet your pet's needs.

At the Ithaca Grain & Pet Supply, we picked up a package of dog kib- ble made by the Canadian pet food company Orijen ("nourish as nature intended"), which uses a similar marketing approach. This label says this food is BARK, "Biologically Appropriate Real-food Kibble," 70 per- cent premium animal ingredients; 30 percent fruits, vegetables, and botanicals; and 0 percent grains. The concept? "By nature all dogs are carnivores—biologically adapted for a diet rich and varied in meats, with smaller amounts of fruits, vegetables, and grasses." The long ingredient list includes two kinds of potato—russet (ingredient #4) and sweet (#7). Are the starches in potatoes really better for dogs than those in corn? We don't see how. From the guaranteed analysis and ingredient list, we assume the kibble is complete and balanced, but the label does not say so in any of six languages (English, German, French, Czech, Japanese, or Korean). It also says nothing about feeding directions or nutritional adequacy. We thought Canadian pet food companies were supposed to comply with AAFCO labeling rules to sell products in the United States, but apparently not all do.

Let's assume that all of these products do meet AAFCO profiles. If so, they are not much different from other commercial products, with or without grains. As we explained in earlier chapters, animals eating wild prey eat *all* of what they catch—intestines, other organs, and bones, as

well as the meat. Meat alone is not sufficient to provide the full complement of needed nutrients and it is especially unbalanced in its ratio of calcium to phosphorus. Diets based mainly on meat must be supplemented
with essential nutrients from other foods. Commercial products do this.

After thousands of years of domestication, "ancestral evolutionary"
diets do not really have much relevance to today's dogs and cats. As is
the case with humans, a wide variety of protein and energy sources can
meet their nutritional needs. Ancestral diets are more about marketing
than health. But these products specifically target pet owners who might
otherwise be feeding raw-food diets or home-cooked table food to their
cats and dogs. Such diets also elicit debates, sometimes angry ones, as we
discuss in the next chapters.

The Raw

THE FIERCEST ARGUMENTS we hear about what to feed dogs and cats concern raw-food diets, and we get more questions about them than about any other topic. This is not surprising. Anthropologists have long maintained that whether foods are eaten raw or cooked is an important marker of cultural identity. Proponents of raw-food diets are adamant that they are best for pet health. Opponents are equally adamant that these foods are dangerous and nutritionally inadequate. Here, for example, are a couple of statements taken from books about pet feeding:

> PRO. "We shall begin to provide our pets with the type of food for which their body was designed. Food that is RAW and WHOLE and in the same form, balance and amount, as they would have received in their natural environment." —Ian Billinghurst, *The BARF Diet*
>
> CON. "Some people believe that feeding your dog raw meat is the best way to go . . . I have researched all aspects of the meat industry, including conditions at many slaughterhouses, and I have decided that I am not willing to risk my dog getting seriously ill from ingesting contaminated raw meat." —Ann Martin, *Foods Pets Die For*

Given the sharp difference of opinion, we were especially pleased at the opportunity to meet and hear Dr. Billinghurst in person at the Pet Food Forum in Chicago in April 2008. Billinghurst is an Australian veterinarian who is often considered the guru of the raw foods movement and the creator of the BARF (Biologically Appropriate Raw Food, or Bones and Raw Food) diet. In 1993, Billinghurst wrote and self-published *Give Your Dog a Bone,* in which he claimed that the ingredients in commercial pet foods reduced the resistance of animals to disease; caused gum disorders, bad breath, and skin problems; and shortened pets' lives. His BARF diet, he said, would not only eliminate these conditions, but also would reduce the risk of arthritis, cancer, and a host of other problems. The book received worldwide attention when it was reviewed favorably in the London *Sunday Telegraph.*

The theory behind the BARF diet is the same as the one behind the ancestral diet: evolution. Because dogs and cats lived exclusively on raw foods in their natural state, they should now eat raw foods. According to Billinghurst, cooking destroys the natural enzymes in food which "contribute to the health of our pets by being part of the anti-aging mechanism." Instead, the principal sources of calories and nutrients should be raw meaty bones, organ meats, fruits, and vegetables. Seasonal fruits and vegetables should constitute 15 percent of the diet of dogs and 5 percent of the diet of cats. The sources of raw meaty bones can be beef, but also chicken backs, wings, necks, and carcasses, and the animals should also be fed liver, kidney, heart, and tripe. It is acceptable to feed ground raw bones to avoid the splinter punctures or broken teeth that dogs sometimes suffer when they chew on whole bones. The diet should be supplemented with garlic, vitamins, antioxidants, minerals, omega-3 fatty acids, and probiotic bacteria.

We addressed some of these claims in chapter 18. Our conclusion: beyond the evident benefit of vitamin and mineral supplements, we are not able to find much scientific support for these ideas. Nevertheless, many pet owners consider the BARF diet to be nothing short of miraculous in eliminating their animals' long-standing health problems. The Internet is full of testimonials from people who attribute their pets' remarkable health to raw-food diets. We even have our own collection of testimonials. A physician friend who knew we were working on this book wrote us this note about her seventeen-year-old dog, Shelly:

For the past few years, as often happens with older dogs, she became a bit smelly with a duller and oilier coat. We lived with that and baths every couple of weeks that seemed to keep us all happy. When she started to suffer various organ failures, I switched her to a raw diet, some I made at home myself . . . and some I bought frozen and fed her from the local pet store. She not only rallied physiologically but after one bath, I never gave her another. She was glossy and clean. Very odd . . . She lasted another summer with good quality that gave us time to say good-bye and prepare for the inevitable.

This is a happy story, but we have to say that we hear similar testimonials from friends who feed their dogs the most ordinary commercial products purchased at Walmart or Grand Union.

In evaluating the risks and benefits of raw diets, we think it useful to concentrate on the nutritional aspects and put aside the ideology. By ideology, we mean the evolutionary rationale, the bits about enzymes and anti-aging, the attitude that cooking is harmful, and the belief that raw foods are superior to commercial foods. Dogs are no longer wolves and cats are no longer desert animals. Enzymes are inactivated by stomach acid and digestion and we are unaware of evidence that enzymes in food protect against the consequences of aging. Cooking makes foods more digestible and some nutrients more available to the body.

Cooking also kills dangerous microbes, and the safety of raw-food diets is a big issue, as we will soon discuss. But from a nutritional standpoint, the BARF diet—as recommended by Billinghurst and done correctly—can be entirely acceptable. There is no reason why this diet should not be adequate in calories, fat, and protein and, with appropriate supplements, the right balance of calcium, phosphorus, and other essential nutrients. We view the recommendation of seasonal fruits and vegetables as an especially nice touch.

But from what we observe, it takes a committed pet companion to do the BARF diet correctly. With butcher shops pretty much a thing of the past, the raw feeder has to find reliable sources of raw meaty bones. In her book for do-it-yourself raw feeders, Carina Beth MacDonald advises, "Let's hunt, gather and freeze!" She suggests that you find meat wholesalers, buy in bulk, and invest in a separate freezer. Since most bulk raw parts come frozen in large blocks, you will need a method for breaking them up (she sensibly advises against driving over them in a pickup truck). It is also a good idea to vary the sources of meat and vegetables, get the calcium and phosphorus levels right, and provide a nutrient supplement. Making sure your pet stays at an appropriate body weight can be a problem, as it is more difficult to figure out how much an animal should be eating when you don't have that information on a package label. Depending on how you view such things, doing all this could sound like a horrible burden or an exciting adventure well worth the fuss.

COMMERCIAL RAW

The time and energy needed to locate suppliers of raw ingredients and to buy, store, and prepare appropriate quantities of the foods may seem daunting to some pet owners. But any hesitation about hunting, gathering, and freezing creates a market opportunity. Suppliers and pet food companies are aware of the raw-food movement and are moving right in to create products that make life easier for raw feeders. MacDonald's book provides lists of online suppliers of frozen raw foods. One in particular caught our eye—a supplier of frozen raw mice. The company advertises its wares as the "Other White Meat," and provides order forms for "pinkies," "fuzzies," and adult mice in packages of one hundred. Another enterprising company, Hare Today, does the same for frozen rabbit meat, ground or whole. These are not specifically advertised for cats or dogs, but in 2007 we received a note from an entrepreneur in Florida asking us to consult on a new business venture: "I am shepherding some students with a new business idea: high-end cat food made from mice." We declined the offer.

Given the intense interest in raw diets for cats and dogs, we are not surprised to see companies getting into the commercial raw-food business. Dr. Billinghurst himself, for example, is one of the founders and shareholders of BARF World, a company that sells raw meat and offal patties, minces, and supplements to the BARF diet, along with his books. In June 2008, we did a casual inventory of commercial raw-food products available at our local alternative pet food stores. Table 24 gives some selected examples.

Table 24
EXAMPLES OF "RAW" COMPLETE-AND-BALANCED PET FOODS, JUNE 2008

PRODUCT	FROZEN	CLAIMS	FIRST FIVE INGREDIENTS
Nature's Variety Medallions for Dogs and Cats	Yes	USDA Organic, grain-free	Organic chicken, raw ground organic chicken bone, organic chicken liver, organic chicken heart, organic chicken eggs
Bravo! Balance Premium Turkey Formula (patties)	Yes	Grain-free, antibiotic-free	Turkey necks, turkey organs (liver, gizzards, hearts), green beans, broccoli*
Nature's Intent Beef & Veggies (patties)	Yes	Human Grade	Beef, organic beef lungs, organic beef tripe, sweet potatoes, apples
Abady Formula for Maintenance & Stress (chub)**	Yes	No vegetables	Beef lung, beef muscle meat, dressed chicken, beef tripe, white rice
Great Life Chicken (kibble)	No	Active probiotics, enzymes, vitamins and chelated minerals	*Kibble:* Whole chicken, whole barley, brown rice, oatmeal, chicken fat *Raw spray:* freeze-dried chicken, dried ground chicken necks, and chicken liver; bok choy, inulin

* The Bravo! product contains only four ingredients.

** In the context of pet foods, a chub is a roll of moist food encased in a thin plastic wrapper.

A glance at this selection makes us wonder whether "commercial raw" is an oxymoron. What, exactly, do these companies mean by "raw"? Most commercial products take raw ingredients and freeze them; these are frozen-raw. Honest Kitchen sells dehydrated raw pet food; Bil-Jac vacuum dries its foods at low temperature. These are dried-raw. Still others, Great Life kibble, for example, spray raw ingredients onto the surface of decidedly un-raw kibble (surface-raw?). The Great Life package does not explain how it does this, but Nature's Variety, which makes a similar product, does:

> Now, we've pioneered a unique and revolutionary concept called Bio-Coating™. . . . This coating greatly increases enzymes, un-altered bio-available amino acids, essential fatty acids, vitamins and minerals that may otherwise be degraded during the process-ing necessary to produce kibble diets. This cold processed, living food is made available in its natural nutritious state—ready to release its health enhancing benefits when consumed by your pet.

Nature's Variety, however, does not mention the percentage of the kibble that is raw or whether these "living food" ingredients might be subject to rapid spoilage. The package says only to store in a cool, dry place and gives a "best if used by" date.

These products also reveal considerable ideological disagreement about what raw diets ought to contain. Some are grain-free; some pro-mote grains. The Abady website says you should never feed raw vegeta-bles to pets: "raw vegetables are not digestible and may interfere with the assimilation and absorption of all other nutrients in the ration." Other companies include bok choy (Chinese cabbage) or apples (OK, a fruit) among the leading ingredients.

In mid-2008, the companies making these products were still small, and raw foods as a whole accounted for less than 1 percent of the pet food market. Nature's Variety led the field and Bravo! was number two. Although raw and frozen pet foods generated sales of just $169 million in 2007, this amount represented an increase of 38 percent over sales four years earlier. The rapidity of this growth was enough to encourage Packaged Facts, a market research company, to produce an entire study devoted to this market in 2008. Packaged Facts estimates that sales will grow to $473 million by 2012, but will still represent only about 2 percent of the expected $20 billion pet food market at that time. If these compa-nies grow the category and their own brands within it, we would not be surprised to see them bought out by Big Pet Food.

We must add one last comment about commercial raw pet foods. In June 2009, the online pet food store, PetFoodDirect.com, was selling five-pound packages of frozen raw ground vegetables—fresh green beans, romaine lettuce, and zucchini—for $37.99 plus shipping. At $7.60 a pound, we think you could manage this at home, particularly because the guaranteed analysis says the vegetables have a moisture content of 85 percent. This is expensive water, and the vegetables aren't even organic.

PET FOOD POLITICS: RAW VERSUS COOKED

We meet many proponents of raw pet diets who view themselves as part of a movement—the raw-food revolution. This movement is linked to the human raw-food movement, with raw milk as the key indicator of commitment. The FDA considers raw milk to be dangerous because it harbors disease-causing microbes, and much prefers milk to be pasteurized, a process that kills most harmful bacteria. Raw milk ("real" milk, according to proponents) is illegal to sell for human consumption in about half the states. But it can be sold for pet food. In some of those states, farmers sometimes sell raw milk to humans under the guise of marketing it to pets.

To say that the raw-food movement is not universally admired is to understate the situation. Much of the pet food industry largely considers raw-food diets to be "the domain of the hard-core holistic set." Dr. Sharon Machlik, director of technical marketing for Nutro Products (since the 2007 recalls, owned by Mars), views raw foods as "difficult and hazardous." She writes:

> As a pet nutritionist and a breeder for over 20 years, I'm concerned that in trying to do the right thing for their dogs, breeders may actually end up harming them. Those who advocate raw diets would undo much that has been done in pet nutrition over the past quarter century by the pet food industry, pet nutritionists, and veterinarians. Their combined efforts have provided new knowledge and optimal nutrition at reasonable cost while maintaining wholesomeness and quality.

We are not surprised that the pet food industry views any alternative to commercial pet foods to be a challenge to its business, but what about veterinarians? In the wake of the 2007 pet food recalls, the American Veterinary Medical Association warned owners not to feed pets raw diets as a less hazardous alternative to commercial foods. Its press release quoted Dr. Richard C. Hill, a veterinary professor at the University of Florida: "Many raw food recipes are not balanced and most owners do not allow for the risks from zoonotic enteric bacteria and parasites . . . particularly [to] the very young, very old, immunosuppressed or pregnant."

How serious are such risks? As you might expect by now, few studies have examined the benefits and risks of raw-food diets. In 2001, investigators at the Tufts School of Veterinary Medicine did one such comparison. They obtained three homemade raw-food diets donated by pet owners and two commercial raw-food diets, analyzed their nutrient composition, and compared the results to AAFCO nutrient profiles. All the raw diets had "multiple shortcomings," among them nutrient deficiencies and high bacterial counts. The authors noted that the owners feeding such diets to their dogs had "the best intentions . . . most people feeding raw-food diets are educated and research the topic before embarking on this path."

Publication of this study provoked a flurry of angry letters accusing the investigators of bias and defamation against raw-food diets, and demanding corrections to inaccuracies. The letters complained that AAFCO profiles do not apply to raw diets because such diets, like those of humans, are not meant to provide complete nutrition with each meal but instead to do so over a period of days. Of course raw pet foods will have bacteria on them; they haven't been cooked. But could those bacteria be harmful? This, alas, you have no way to know until it is too late.

SAFETY ISSUES: THE CONTAMINATION THREAT

When it comes to raw pet foods, microbial contamination is the big worry. Various kinds of *Salmonella* and other intestinal bacteria can cause disease in humans, ranging in severity from a mild annoyance to death. Dogs and cats seem much less susceptible to the ravages of *Salmonella* than people, and often shed it in their feces without showing symptoms of illness. Cooking destroys *Salmonella* and other bacteria, but uncooked foods create risks for pets and for humans. Because the extent of the risk is unknown, there is plenty of room for argument.

As one of us (Nestle) described in *Pet Food Politics,* the FDA asked Wild Kitty Cat Food early in 2007 to recall its All Natural Frozen Cat Food because of *Salmonella* contamination. The FDA does not have the authority to demand a recall, and Wild Kitty balked:

> Statistically there is zero chance your cat will get salmonellosis [*Salmonella* infection] from eating raw foods . . . The salmonella found in Wild Kitty Cat Food is not a result of poor processing, second grade product or bad sanitation . . . There is no way, short of irradiation of all food products, to excluded [*sic*] salmonella from the US food supply. . . . We question the FDA's choice of Wild Kitty Cat Food as part of the bioterrorism initiative on pet food safety.

We had no idea that the FDA had identified pet foods as priority targets of bioterrorism, but never mind. Evidence does indeed indicate that the risk of *Salmonella* illness in cats is small, although certainly greater than zero. But *Salmonella* is not an intrinsic component of the food supply. *Salmonella* means that food must have came into contact with feces at some point or with equipment or hands that were in contact with feces. *Salmonella* is a clear indication of a breach in safe food handling procedures. Even if pets do not become ill from eating contaminated foods, humans who handle these foods are at risk. Giving *Salmonella*-infested foods to dogs or cats is not a good idea for them or their humans. Eventually, Wild Kitty agreed to recall its contaminated products.

We think bacterial contamination of pet foods is worth worrying about because it is not all that rare. The FDA typically announces recalls of *Salmonella*-contaminated pet foods several times a year. A group of investigators from Colorado State University looked at 240 samples taken from twenty commercial raw meat diets for dogs and found disease-causing bacteria in 53 percent of them. Later, these investigators were asked by a Greyhound breeder to find out why puppies in his facility were getting sick with *Salmonella* and, sometimes, dying. Greyhounds bred for racing are often fed raw meat and this meat is not always of the best quality. The investigators identified *Salmonella* in 66 percent of the food samples they tested, and in 93 percent of the samples taken from dog feces. Their recommendation: "feed only a high-quality, commercial, processed dog food or ... thoroughly cook all meat prior to feeding." Cooking is a highly effective way to kill harmful bacteria.

SAFETY ISSUES: THE FDA

The FDA is no fan of raw diets for pets. In 2004, the agency stated its position on the manufacture and labeling of raw pet foods in a guidance document for the industry.

> FDA does not believe raw meat foods for animals are consistent with the goal of protecting the public from significant health risks, particularly when products are brought into the home and/or used to feed domestic pets. . . . Although there have been claims that raw meat foods are superior with respect to providing adequate nutrition than other products substantiated to be complete and balanced, FDA is not aware of scientific evidence to support such claims.

The FDA's main concern is about the microbial hazards. It notes that raw meats come from three sources: human food processing facilities, animals that have died from means other than slaughter, and animals originally intended for the human food supply but no longer fit for consumption. Of the meats that are by-products of human food processing, 10–20 percent are likely to be contaminated with infectious forms of *Campylobacter* and *Salmonella* (from poultry) and *Escherichia coli* and *Salmonella* (from meats). Meats from the other two sources are likely to carry much higher percentages.

The FDA document makes many recommendations for safety practices to avoid harm from raw pet foods. But these are just recommendations. They are nonbinding and not legally enforceable. However, as the FDA points out, manufacturers should be aware that it is against the law to "introduce into interstate commerce" any adulterated food, including food intended for pets. In this case, adulterated means contaminated with infectious microbes. So the FDA could go after raw pet foods if it decided the hazard was great enough.

The 2004 document was aimed at the makers of pet foods. In 2007, the FDA issued a safe handling guide for consumers who buy, prepare, or store pet foods. In effect, the guide recommends following the same food safety procedures for handling pet food that should be followed for human foods:

- Clean: Wash hands and surfaces often.
- Separate: Don't cross-contaminate!
- Cook: Cook to proper temperature.
- Chill: Refrigerate promptly.

For raw-food diets, the FDA once again emphasizes that it "does not advocate a raw meat, poultry or seafood diet for pets." But because the agency understands that "some people prefer to feed these types of diets to their pets," it advises special handling of raw pet foods:

- Keep raw meat and poultry products frozen until ready to use.
- Thaw in refrigerator or microwave.
- Keep raw-food diets separate from other foods. Wash working surfaces, utensils (including cutting boards, preparation and feeding bowls), hands, and any other items that touch or contact raw meat, poultry, or seafood with hot soapy water.
- Cover and refrigerate leftovers immediately or discard safely.
- For added protection, kitchen sanitizers should be used on cutting boards and countertops periodically. A sanitizing solution can be made by mixing one teaspoon of chlorine bleach to one quart of water.
- If you use plastic or other nonporous cutting boards, run them through the dishwasher after each use.

We think this is excellent advice not only for raw pet foods but for all food handling. Most raw foods will not be contaminated. Most pets will not get sick from contaminated pet foods. And most owners will not get sick from handling contaminated pet food. But some will, and especially the young, the old, and those with weak immune systems. Lots of such people exist, so why take a chance? Safe food handling procedures may take some getting used to but we think they are well worth the effort—and not only for pet food.

SAFETY ISSUES: COMMERCIAL RAW FOODS

The threat of bacterial contamination made us wonder what the makers of commercial raw products do to prevent it. We were delighted to meet Bette Loughran, the founder and director of sales for Bravo! Raw Food Diets ("join the raw diet revolution") and even more delighted when she invited us to tour the Bravo! offices and meet David Bogner, who runs the manufacturing plant that produces Bravo! products in Connecticut. Bette is an enthusiastic proponent of raw-food diets and deeply committed to growing the category. She takes great pride in the quality of the ingredients in Bravo! products. We saw enormous freezers full of frozen blocks of turkey necks, chicken racks, and beef tracheas—all unprocessed by-products of human food production. Bravo! makes treats as well as complete-and-balanced foods, and we were particularly impressed—awestruck, actually—by the company's production of yard-long "bully sticks" (penises). Such treats, made from every imaginable part of the animal, seem to be an especially efficient use of by-products that would otherwise be rendered into meat meal or fertilizer.

Our not-so-secret reason for wanting to view the manufacturing plant was to find out what commercial raw-food makers do to prevent bacterial contamination. Bravo! products are manufactured in a USDA-inspected plant that processes and packs meat for human consumption for about half the week, and pet food the rest of the time. In 2007, Bravo! recalled some frozen raw chicken chubs that the FDA had found contaminated with *Salmonella* and *Listeria*. We were relieved to hear that as a result of that experience, Bravo! now tests finished products for several kinds of bacteria, and does not release the products until the tests come back negative (the company disposes of products that test positive). We think this should be standard practice for the raw pet food industry.

Nancy Kerns, who edits the *Whole Dog Journal,* provides a lengthy list of the makers of complete-and-balanced and supplemental raw foods, and suggests that you question the companies' "level of commitment to providing clear, credible guidance for feeding your dog in an optimal way." Ask companies, she says, about their formulas, nutrient contents, and ingredient sources—and their food safety programs. Ask them what they are doing to make sure that their products are as free from harmful bacteria as possible. And, we would add, be sure to let them know that you care very much about the safety of their foods.

NUTRITION ISSUES: COOKING

Despite the testimonials of raw feeders, we are unaware of any special nutritional advantages—or disadvantages—of raw-food diets. Some foods, meats for example, are digested well whether they are cooked or raw. Yes, cooking destroys fragile nutrients like vitamin C (which dogs and cats do not need anyway), but cooking also makes other nutrients more available or digestible. Heat also destroys factors in foods that inactivate vitamins and inhibit protein digestion. A classic example is an enzyme in raw fish that destroys thiamin, a vitamin. Cats fed exclusively on raw fish have been found to develop a thiamin deficiency disorder. If the fish is cooked, the inactivating factor is destroyed. Cooking vegetables like carrots and spinach makes some of their nutrients more available to the human body, and we would expect dogs and cats to respond the same way. And studies have shown that cooking grains and potatoes makes their starches more digestible by dogs and cats. But rather than worrying about each of these nutritional problems, feeding animals a variety of raw and cooked foods (or foods made from a variety of ingredients) usually compensates for destructive factors or nutrient losses.

NUTRITION ISSUES: BONES

How safe is it to feed raw bones to cats or dogs? Raw meaty bones are at the core of raw-food diets. Dr. Billinghurst says that "whole raw bones have benefits beyond nutrition. They play a major role in maintaining the health of your pet's immune system and also its mouth, teeth, and gums.

They also provide unique psychological and physical benefits not available from any other source." Despite his claims, we find little agreement about the acceptability of feeding any bones to pets, let alone whether the bones should be raw or cooked.

Not much research has been done on the bone question, again leaving much room for opinions based on personal interpretations. Books for veterinary professionals, for example, rarely discuss the safety of feeding bones to cats or dogs. When the word "bones" appears in an index, it refers to the animals' bones, not to their food. But popular books and websites offer firm advice. The *Whole Pet Diet* is pro-bone: "raw, natural bones are often called 'nature's toothbrush' (for pets!). . . . And in case you're wondering, raw bones are good for cats, too, especially because cats have a higher incidence of tooth decay than dogs."

Other sources argue the opposite. One Internet article, illustrated with X-ray photographs of bone fragments piercing the intestinal walls of dogs, states:

> Feeding bones to dogs is not perfectly safe to do . . . For those of you who state with confidence that "wolves in the wild eat bones all the time; so it must be OK for dogs to do the same," I would ask you this . . . How many times have you ever seen a healthy wolf? How can you state with authority that wolves are not occasionally harmed by a bone splinter?

Indeed, this anonymous writer has a point. A 1997 report from the World Veterinary Dental Congress discussed the oral status of sixty-seven foxhounds that had been routinely fed whole raw carcasses—bones, muscle, and tissues. Many of the dogs exhibited signs of gum disease and tooth fractures.

Chicken bones elicit particular debate. The BARF diet recommends chicken wings, backs, and necks as sources of raw meaty bones even though some people say they should never be fed to dogs. In *The Dog Bible*, Tracy Hotchner says: "Chicken bones can splinter and pierce the dog's intestines or stomach. Cooked chicken bones are the most dangerous, but raw bones can also splinter into needle-sharp points." Still, we have no trouble finding raw chicken backs and necks offered as dried treats.

In the absence of research, making sense of all this is not easy. And do not expect research to resolve such questions. We cannot imagine that anyone could conduct a study of raw versus cooked bones if there is any chance either one might harm a cat or dog. Such a study would be unethical. But as we read the opinions, we find plenty of agreement that cooked bones splinter more easily than raw. We think if you are going to feed bones to your pet, you ought to keep an eye on how things are going. As Nancy Kerns would say, "Supervise!" If the bones start splintering, put them someplace where your pet cannot get to them. Bones are an excellent source of calcium and phosphorus but so is bone meal. Consider ground bone as an alternative. Although the risks of eating bones of any type might be small, they are finite. Why take the risk? But this too is a personal decision.

Overall, we think it is entirely possible to feed pets safely and adequately on raw-food diets, but it takes some commitment to do so without resorting to commercial products. The commitment does not necessarily need to be overwhelming. If you want to feed raw without using commercial products, you need to be careful about a few matters. You must supplement meat with other foods. You must take care of the special nutritional requirements of cats and dogs, using appropriate supplements. And you most definitely must take extra care with matters of food safety. This level of commitment is not much greater than that needed to do home-cooking for pets, as we explain next.

The Home Cooked

WE DON'T GET it. We don't understand what the big deal is about cooking for pets. Pet owners are constantly warned against cooking and preparing foods for dogs and cats: too difficult, too complicated, and too confusing. Maybe, but we assume that nearly everyone gives their pets table scraps once in a while, and we know plenty of people who cook for their pets at home. How many people do this? The American Pet Products Association reports that 23 percent of dog owners say they buy human food for their pets, but only 7 percent say they do this most of the time. The equivalent figures for cat owners are 15 percent and 3 percent, respectively. Another survey says that nearly all owners of dogs and cats, 93 percent and 98 percent, respectively, give their dog or cat some human food at least half the time. So if you do this, you are not alone.

We have good evidence that the number of home feeders increased following the 2007 recalls, when people were desperate to find safe foods for their dogs and cats. Books about home cooking for pets experienced gratifying jumps in sales. In April 2007, for example, the Associated Press observed that Moore's *Real Food for Dogs* moved into the top 200 sellers on Amazon.com and Strombeck's *Home Prepared Dog and Cat Diets: The Healthy Alternative* went from an Amazon ranking of 60,000 to a respectable 1,000 during that period, indicating a sharp increase in sales.

Yet during the height of the 2007 pet food recalls, the American Veterinary Medical Association (AVMA) warned frightened pet owners not to resort to home cooking: "pets have complex nutritional needs that are unique to their species, age and other factors, and any changes to a pet's diet could cause intestinal upset, particularly a change as significant as switching from commercial to home-cooked food." AVMA quoted Dr. Tony Buffington, a professor at the Ohio State University College of Veterinary Medicine:

> For pet owners who are having trouble finding acceptable pet food during a recall, recipes are available for home-cooked food for dogs and cats online and in many books. These recipes are all generally fine, but certainly home-cooked diets are not created with the care that these commercial pet foods are. . . . Commercial pet foods for dogs and cats are designed by Ph.D. nutritionists.

Although both of us are Ph.D.-trained nutritionists, we hardly believe you need a Ph.D. to cook for yourself or your pet. We view cooking for pets as no more complicated or difficult than cooking for yourself and your family, but we wholeheartedly agree that the advice that's out there makes cooking for pets seem like an overwhelming challenge. A review of books on feeding pets can be a bewildering experience. Many of them give thoroughly contradictory advice. To cite just a few examples:

Should pets eat grains? (For our take, review chapter 19)

> YES. "Whole grains are a very cost-effective and environmentally sensitive way to provide the mainstay of your pet's diet . . . carbohydrates may properly supply over half of the diet for dogs and cats . . . [Cooked grains] are completely utilizable by the body."
> NO. ". . . pet foods today contain many foods that dogs and cats would not normally eat. Neither dogs nor cats were designed to eat wheat, corn, rice, or other cereal grains,

yet these are the mainstay ingredients for hundreds of commercial foods."

Is it OK for pets to eat garlic? (See later in this chapter)

YES. "We all know garlic has numerous beneficial properties ... for pets, it stimulates digestion and boosts the immune system ... it's a natural antibiotic, and it's recommended by every holistic veterinarian I know. ... It helps control intestinal parasites, including tapeworms, roundworms, and hookworms, and repels the bane of some pets' existence—fleas."

NO. "... certain foods can be toxic to pets. It is very important that you follow this 'Do Not Feed' list closely: ... Garlic ... Vitamins and supplements such as garlic, brewer's yeast and vitamin B provide no protection against fleas."

Should you feed cheese to your dog? (This chapter)

YES. "Cheese is a useful source of animal protein, and most dogs like it. Serve it in chunks."

NO. "As for cheese—it's not as bad as milk, but you should avoid the processed cheeses."

Should you feed table scraps to your cat or dog? (This chapter)

YES. "When you are cleaning up after your own dinner ... Take a look at what's left over. ... Uneaten cubes of squash, a bit of the roast, a heel of the whole wheat baguette, the slab of uneaten fried egg—these things, your pet would like you to know, would look great in that very special bowl on the floor."

NO. "Just because a dog *will* eat anything does not mean that she *should* eat it—and it certainly does not mean that you should facilitate it. ... Your dog is not a living garbage can: the garbage disposal in your sink is a better place for the nasty fat you cut off a steak."

BASIC NUTRITION PRINCIPLES

What is the poor pet owner to make of all this? No wonder people are hesitant (if not terrified) to start cooking for their pets. But think about this for a minute: isn't it just amazing that most Americans—and, for that matter, most people in the world—manage to survive and do pretty well without eating AAFCO-approved, complete-and-balanced diets every day? Humans flourish whether or not we count nutrients. How do we manage this? Without having to think about it, we follow three fundamental principles of nutrition: balance, variety, and moderation. As those of us who are Ph.D. nutritionists can tell you, it is extremely difficult to induce a nutritional deficiency in animals—or people—who follow those principles. So let's take a look at how balance, variety, and moderation work for home-cooked pet foods. There is only one caveat: you must follow all three principles at the same time.

Balance

Balance means getting all needed nutrients into a diet in the right proportions. You do this automatically without thinking about it, simply by eating. Foods contain nutrients. If you eat foods, you get nutrients. Somehow you do that well enough to survive and function. Are pets any different? We don't think so, except that they are smaller and problems may show up faster.

To show how easy it is to create balance, consider the section on home cooking in the standard veterinary textbook, *Small Animal Clinical Nutrition*. You will soon see why we like this book so much, even though it is published by the Mark Morris Institute, an offshoot of Hill's Pet Nutrition. The authors, some of whom are Hill's scientists, go on for several pages about what a bad idea it is for clients to cook for their pets. Clients (and some veterinarians), they warn, may—horrors—want to use fresh, natural ingredients; avoid additives, contaminants, and by-products; or prevent disease in their pets. Or, they may simply want to cook for their pet. The authors admit that "It is possible to achieve the same nutrient balance with a homemade food as with a commercially prepared food," but doing so "largely depends on the accuracy and competence of the veterinarian or animal nutritionist formulating the food, and on the compliance and discipline of the owner. . . . [M]aking homemade foods requires knowledge, motivation, additional financial resources and careful, consistent attention to recipe detail to ensure a consistent, balanced intake of nutrients."

We cannot help but be amused by what this book does next. After all these dire warnings, the authors then provide utterly simple, generic recipes for complete-and-balanced diets for dogs and cats that meet AAFCO nutrient profiles for all life stages. Take a look at table 25 and judge for yourself how difficult it might be to manage something like this on a daily basis.

Yes, to do this right you will need a kitchen scale and measuring spoons. And yes, you will need to buy supplements at a grocery store or pet supply store. And yes, you should give the supplements to your pet every day. But beyond that, nothing is all that complicated. Cook the ingredients separately and mix them together. Mix in the bone meal and salts. Add the vitamin-mineral supplement just before serving. Your pet ought to love it, as shown in figure 10. That's all it takes, except for variety and moderation.

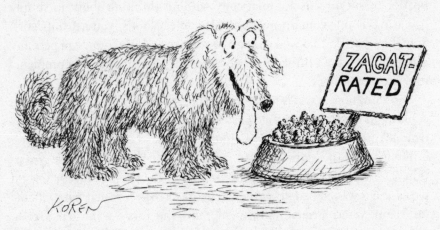

FIGURE 10
Home-cooked foods offer many pleasures to pets as well as to their owners.

Table 25

GENERIC DIETARY FORMULAS FOR HEALTHY
ADULT DOGS AND CATS, AMOUNTS PER DAY*

INGREDIENT	DOG, 40 POUNDS	CAT, 10 POUNDS
FOODS, *examples*		
Grains, cooked	8 ounces	2 ounces
Rice, cornmeal, oatmeal, potato, pasta, other grains and cereals		
Meat, cooked	4 ounces	1.5 ounces
Beef, lamb, pork, venison, chicken, turkey, fish		
Fats	2 teaspoons	2 teaspoons
Beef fat, chicken fat, vegetable oil, olive oil, fish oil		
Vegetables	1 ounce	—
Prepared high-fiber cereals (e.g., All Bran, Fiber One); raw or cooked vegetables		
SUPPLEMENTS		
Bone meal (or dicalcium phosphate supplement)	1 teaspoon	¼ teaspoon
Potassium chloride supplement (salt substitute)	¼ teaspoon	—
"Lite" salt (sodium chloride/ potassium chloride)	—	¼ teaspoon
Human adult daily multi-vitamin, multi-mineral tablet	1 tablet	½ tablet
Taurine supplement	—	⅛ teaspoon

* Adapted from *Small Animal Clinical Nutrition*, 2000:168–169. Formulas meet AAFCO nutrient profiles ("complete and balanced"). The dog and cat formulas provide about 820 and 250 calories, respectively. Food amounts must be adjusted to the size, age, and condition of the animal.

Variety

Variety may be the spice of life but it is also a basic principle of nutrition. Foods contain many essential nutrients but in different proportions. Fruits and vegetables have lots of vitamin C and folic acid, but no vitamin B_{12}. Meats don't have much vitamin C or folic acid, but do have vitamin B_{12}. And so it goes for all relatively unprocessed foods. So within the generic recipes, you should vary the sources of cereals, meat, and fiber, and do so frequently. Your pet may like some foods more than others (don't you?), so if you enjoy experimenting, here is your chance. Try different foods and ingredients. If your own diet is reasonably well balanced, your pet's diet will be too. The supplements take care of the special nutritional needs of dogs and cats. You can easily find the salt substitute, "lite" salt, and vitamin-mineral supplements at grocery stores, and get bone meal and taurine at pet supply stores. All are relatively inexpensive and last a long time as you don't need to use much of them at a time.

Note that these recipes, and most of the veterinary formulas we have seen, call for similar proportions of carbohydrate-rich foods to meat. If you want to cook a vegetarian diet, you will need to substitute tofu or beans to compensate for the protein in meat, and to increase the fat content to compensate for the reduced calories. If you are of the opinion that animals should not be fed grains or potatoes, you can use more meat. This increases the amount of fat in your pet's diet and you must compensate for the higher calories by feeding less. You should also make sure to use appropriate supplements.

Moderation

Moderation is about caloric balance. The recipes in table 25 are for a forty-pound dog and a ten-pound cat. If your pet weighs more, you will need to increase the amount you feed. If your pet is smaller, you need to feed it less. Because you will not know how many calories your pet is getting, you will have to keep a close eye on its weight.

Really, this is all there is to home cooking, except for one more concern. Is there anything your pet should not eat? Yes, indeed there is.

WHAT *NOT* TO FEED YOUR PET

When we started researching this book, we heard many warnings about long lists of foods that should never be fed to pets. Frankly, we were skeptical. Dogs in particular are omnivores. We couldn't think of any reason why they couldn't handle the same foods we do. Then we took a look at the research. We wish there were more of it, but the little there is convinces us that it really is better to avoid feeding certain foods to dogs and cats. And, since we are talking about home cooking in this chapter, we are taking the liberty of adding a few caveats of our own.

The main reason for restrictions on certain foods is that animals sometimes are more sensitive to them than we are. To cite just one example: in the 1960s, large flocks of turkeys and ducks died after eating corn contaminated with the aflatoxin-producing fungus *Aspergillus flavus*. Small amounts of aflatoxin may kill turkeys and ducks, but not chickens. Aflatoxin causes liver cancer in people, and can be lethal to dogs and cats. This is why the discovery of aflatoxin in dog foods made by Diamond Pet Foods in a factory in South Carolina triggered a recall in 2005. Several dogs died as a result of eating the contaminated food, and Diamond agreed to pay $3.1 million to settle the resulting class-action suit.

Here is another example from 2009, this one having to do with irradiation. In Australia, exceptionally high doses of irradiation were used to sterilize imported pet foods. Australian researchers linked this process to cases of severe neurological problems in more than 80 cats. Dogs were not affected by eating the irradiated food. Researchers speculate that irradiation might have caused the formation of chemicals that are especially toxic to cats or perhaps destroyed most of the vitamin A that they needed. The point here is that some animals are more sensitive to food toxins than others. Let's look at some other examples of foods that should not be fed to pets, or at least not often or in large amounts.

Chocolate

Chocolate is hardly considered a toxin by most people, but dogs react differently to it than we do. Chocolate contains two compounds that cause problems for pets: theobromine and, to a lesser extent, caffeine. Humans metabolize these chemicals—change them into something harmless or excrete them—quite rapidly. Dogs and cats do this more slowly, so the chemicals can accumulate in the body and induce vomiting, diarrhea, nervous system problems, and, if doses are high enough, death. One or two truffles is unlikely to harm a hefty dog, but a twenty-pound dog can get into trouble eating a ten-ounce bar of dark baking chocolate. While this is more than most people would eat at one time (maybe), it's best to keep chocolate in places where curious dogs can't get to it. Even sharing milk chocolate with your pet is not a good idea. Its caffeine has the same effects on dogs as it does on people, and most dogs are frisky enough without it.

Other Food No-No's

Small-animal toxicologists are uniformly negative about feeding several common foods to dogs and cats. These include:

- *Onions and garlic:* These foods may be wonders of Italian and other delicious cuisines and garlic is often used as a flavoring in premium pet foods or in recipes for home cooking. But pets seem to be sensitive to certain chemicals in garlic and onions that can damage red blood cells and cause a form of anemia. In 2008, the National Research Council (NRC) attempted to set a safe upper limit for garlic consumption in dogs and cats. The NRC committee did not say anything special about onions other than to avoid them but did say that based on the limited information available, a safe amount of garlic powder or oil should not exceed about 0.1 percent of the diet of dogs (one-tenth of a gram in 3.5 ounces of food); for cats, the percentage should be slightly less. We guess that this limit is about equivalent to one small clove of fresh garlic. Although it is difficult for us to believe that one clove of garlic could do much harm, pets don't need onions and garlic, so why take a chance?
- *Grapes and raisins:* Veterinarians have published reports of kidney toxicity and death in dogs eating large amounts (one-

half pound to two pounds) of grapes and raisins. They have no idea why these foods should cause problems, but enough such reports exist to suggest keeping more than a grape or two away from your animals.

- *Macadamia nuts:* Some research suggests that these highly expensive nuts, even in small amounts, are toxic to dogs.
- *Xylitol:* This is an indigestible form of a small sugar used to artificially sweeten "sugar-free" toothpaste, chewing gum, candy, and some baked goods. Veterinarians from the ASPCA Animal Poison Control Center have described eight cases of liver failure in dogs consuming this sweetener. We don't advise using it.

This information is based on few studies and it would be nice to have more research to know what amounts of these foods, if any, are safe to eat. An NRC committee concluded in 2008 that more research would help, but we see no signs that such research is forthcoming. In its absence, it seems best to be cautious. Eating these foods may not cause your pet to drop dead on the spot, but why do unnecessary experiments? Plenty of other foods are available for pets to eat.

Junk Food

We also think it is not a good idea to feed junk foods—sodas, salty snacks, processed hamburgers of unknown composition, hot dogs, candy, cookies, cakes, cheesy pizza, and french fries—to dogs and cats, except in very small amounts on rare occasions, if you must. These foods are high in calories for the nutrients they contain. Just as people do, your animals might love to eat them, but just as in people, high-calorie foods predispose to obesity. We don't consider cheese itself to be a junk food (quite the contrary) but it is rather high in calories. It's best to keep such foods in places where your pets can't get to them. Here's one way to think about the junk food issue: if you eat the way your dogs and cats are *supposed* to eat, you too will be eating healthfully.

THINKING ABOUT PET FOODS

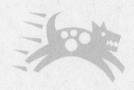

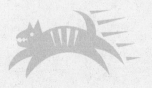

Are Commercial Pet Foods Healthy for Pets?

MOST DOGS AND cats in the United States subsist on commercial pet foods, but such foods do have their critics.
These argue that today's dry and canned foods are so full
of indigestible and toxic ingredients that they cause diseases of the skin, immune system, heart, kidney, and digestive system,
and shorten the lives of pets that eat them. Ann Martin, author of *Foods
Pets Die For,* argues this position forcefully:

> Corporations make huge profits by rendering garbage and sell-
> ing it in attractive cans and bags as food for our pets. Then they
> have the audacity to call it "balanced and nutritious." The infe-
> rior ingredients in most commercial pet foods and other legally
> acceptable—yet potentially harmful—fillers are causing untold
> health problems for pets. This translates into pain, suffering and
> sometimes death for millions of animal companions, and bil-
> lions of dollars in veterinary care.

Are pets that eat commercial foods worse off than
pets that foraged or hunted for themselves or were fed
oatmeal, sheep heads, horse entrails, or table waste? Are

they worse off than those fed raw or home-cooked diets? To our surprise, we could not find the kind of research that we hoped might help answer these questions. We wanted to see data on the average life span of cats and dogs before and after the widespread introduction of commercial pet food. We searched for studies comparing the health of pets fed commercial foods to those fed home-cooked or raw diets. We could not find them. In the absence of research, we must resort to indirect indicators, just as everyone else seems to. Based on what we have been able to discover, here is our take on the effects of commercial pet foods on pet health and longevity.

PROBLEMS WITH COMMERCIAL PET FOODS

The most obvious problems with commercial pet foods are those that result in recalls. The melamine recalls of 2007 may have affected thousands of pets (we will never know the exact number), but were not otherwise unique. *Pet Food Politics* describes multiple recalls that took place before and after that particular incident. Recalls continue to occur occasionally, most often due to bacterial contamination but sometimes to errors in manufacture. Any time an animal (or human) is dependent on just one source of food, a deficiency or excess of a nutrient or a toxin in that food can have a large effect on health.

The vulnerability of pet foods to formula errors has been known for a very long time. In 1941, veterinarians evaluated the six hundred brands of dog food (made by 250 manufacturers) then said to be on the market. Most, they said, were nutritionally adequate, but claims for nutritional adequacy were "open to doubt in a large number of cases." They pointed to frequent reports of vitamin and mineral deficiencies in dogs eating commercial pet foods. Occasional reports of such problems in dogs and cats fed commercial foods continued well into the 1970s and 1980s.

Such problems sometimes led to useful outcomes. Production failures helped scientists identify previously unknown nutrient requirements, such as that for taurine in cats. Cats fed commercial diets developed vision problems that were corrected when taurine was added to their diets. Veterinarians discovered additional needs for vitamin E in cat foods based mainly on red tuna. The cats developed "yellow fat storage" disease if not enough vitamin E had been added to protect against fat oxidation. Pet foods made with relatively unprocessed cereals and soy meals sometimes caused skin problems in dogs because the grains contained phytates and other substances that interfered with zinc absorption.

These nutrient deficiencies were corrected as soon as they were discovered. Today, foods that meet AAFCO profiles are so rarely associated with formulation problems that hardly anyone suspects them when something goes wrong. In 2009, Mars recalled Nutro cat foods that contained excessive amounts of zinc in its vitamin-mineral mix. This error occurred as a result of the loss of hands-on quality control that often accompanies our increasingly centralized and globalized food supply. But most problems with pet foods involve inadvertent contamination with *Salmonella*, aflatoxin, or other toxic substances. The melamine pet food recalls of 2007—and the subsequent introduction of melamine into Chinese food products and infant formula—were unusual examples of deliberate adulteration.

But perhaps such problems are just the tip of the iceberg. Perhaps pet foods cause "subclinical" problems in cats and dogs that are not immediately obvious but eventually lead to health conditions that shorten pets' lives. Or consider the opposite: maybe pets are healthier now that they are eating complete-and-balanced foods. We wanted to know whether the health and life span of dogs and cats was any different now than before commercial pet foods came into common use.

We discussed this question with David Fraser, a professor and former dean of veterinary medicine at the University of Sydney who has had a long and distinguished career in the field. In his view, commercial pet foods solved major nutritional problems in dogs and cats. Early in his career, Professor Fraser frequently observed signs of nutritional imbalances in dogs and cats, particularly those eating diets consisting mainly of meat. Meat is low in calcium relative to phosphorus; organ meats contain about thirty times more phosphorus than calcium and muscle meats about ten times more. The result of the imbalance was "secondary hyperparathyroidism," which caused joint pain, lameness, bone deformities, and fractures. Such problems were also seen in cats, as were signs of vitamin A toxicity in cats fed large amounts of liver. The introduction of complete-and-balanced foods largely solved these problems.

HAS PET LIFE SPAN CHANGED OVER TIME?

Perhaps the health gains from elimination of deficiencies have been offset by new kinds of problems caused by overfeeding and sedentary lifestyles. Today's pets are obese and develop degenerative diseases such as heart disease, cancers, and the like, conditions that were relatively uncommon in the old days when nutritional deficiencies and imbalances were more common. The development of diet-related chronic diseases suggests that pets must be living long enough to display signs of such conditions and, as such, must be living longer. But are they really? What were the life spans of dogs and cats before eating commercial pet food became the norm?

The Life Span of Dogs and Cats: Then

Statisticians at the U.S. Centers for Disease Control and Prevention (CDC) continuously track the dates of birth and death of human individuals, and use these data to determine trends in longevity. Their work tells us that the expected life span of Americans born today is about seventy-eight years, nine years longer than that of Americans born fifty years ago. But no agency or organization does anything like that for pets.

To estimate the length of human life in the far distant past, anthropologists can examine the fossilized, mummified, or buried remains of humans, and historians can search church records of births and deaths. No such historical sources are available for dogs and cats. The American Kennel Club, for example, records the births, but not the deaths of purebred dogs. Even today, information about pet life span depends on sporadic—not systematic—studies based on information provided by owners. Scientists consider such information to be "anecdotal"— interesting and sometimes valuable, but requiring careful interpretation to make sense of it. The lack of systematic information is so profound that we do not even know how long dogs and cats lived during the early years of the twentieth century. Newspaper accounts of dog deaths may describe accidents or problems with distemper, but these are not necessarily representative. And breeders consistently overstate how long their dogs live.

The lack of information and potential for biases explains why

Dr. Kelly Cassidy volunteers so much of her time examining dog longevity. On her website, she tracks, summarizes, and critically evaluates research studies on the longevity of dogs, by breed. She too laments the absence of scientifically valid information in a note to us:

> I only wish there were more studies of dog life span from the past. I have searched and searched and can't find any real data, not even poorly designed studies. . . . You are probably looking for studies before WW 2 [World War II], when commercial dog food became the norm. I wish. There are none that I know of and not even much anecdotal information. Even if there were, I think you would have a heck of a time separating mortality from infectious disease and parasites in that era from any influence of diet. . . . I think any good food study would need to be a long-term project with controlled diets and much larger sample sizes for the groups fed non-commercial diets.

Indeed it would. Absent science, we have speculation. Ours is that house pets undoubtedly live longer than dogs and cats running wild. They get more reliable food and are protected against predators, infectious diseases, and traffic accidents. They get better veterinary care. The CEO of Banfield pet hospitals emphasizes this point: "pets who are on wellness plans live about 25 percent longer." Perhaps they do, but Banfield does not explain how the company knows this. Banfield sells "optimal wellness plans" for pets and it is in its interest to promote the benefits of such plans.

The Life Span of Dogs and Cats: Now

Here, we are on somewhat firmer ground. Veterinarians and breeders have collected enough data on the average life span of dogs to have a pretty good idea of what to expect by breed. Information on cats is less well developed, but still suggestive. According to any number of surveys conducted by breeders, the life span of dogs varies by breed, size, how they are raised, and the country in which they are raised, and—most important for the skeptics among us—who collects the data. For any breed, the breeders say the average life span of dogs is from ten to thirteen years, but the range varies from five to seven years for short-lived dogs like bloodhounds, wolfhounds, and Great Danes, to fourteen to fifteen years for small poodles, dachshunds, and spaniels. In general, smaller dogs live longer than larger ones, and mixed-breed dogs live a year or so longer than purebred dogs. But these are just averages and generalizations, and plenty of exceptions exist in all categories.

Veterinary surveys, however, consistently report shorter life spans—by as much as 40 percent—than those reported by breeders. Why? Nobody really knows. Maybe veterinarians see sicker animals, or breeders are more optimistic. The British say their dogs live nearly a year longer than American dogs. But without systematic research designed to examine such statements, these claims are difficult to evaluate.

Most of the studies aimed at defining the dog life span have been done relatively recently—just since the 1990s. Some of them may have been designed to respond to charges that commercial foods were bad for pets. In the early 1990s, for example, Ian Billinghurst, the Australian veterinarian and enthusiastic proponent of raw-food diets, argued that commercial dog food was responsible for an extraordinary range of diseases and conditions that shortened the animals' lives. Billinghurst's book, *Give Your Dog a Bone*, elicited great public interest (see chapter 20).

Just after his book appeared in Great Britain, British investigators distributed a questionnaire to clients of a large pet insurance company asking them to report the age at which their dogs died. The investigators analyzed the results of more than three thousand responses, although they do not state the number of questionnaires distributed. From the self-reported responses, they concluded that the average dog dying of natural causes lived thirteen years, but those dying of unnatural causes (accidents, illnesses, euthanasia) lived eleven years. In this sample, only 7 percent died from natural causes. The majority—53 percent—had been euthanized, and 35 percent died from illnesses such as cancers, heart disease, kidney disease, and liver disease. The study confirmed that larger breeds died younger than smaller breeds, male dogs died earlier than female dogs, and intact females died younger than those that had been neutered.

For dogs at least one study exists but for cats, even less is known. The average life span of a neutered cat in countries with good veterinary care is generally said to be thirteen to fourteen years. But we have seen many reports of individual cats living to be much older—well into their late twenties and even early thirties. In August 2008, *Cat Fancy* reported the results of a longevity contest. Most cat contestants were in their late teens, but nineteen cats were twenty to twenty-five years old, and four were twenty-five to thirty, with the three winners aged twenty-seven, twenty-eight, and thirty-four. These ages were self-reported by owners and the article did not mention whether anyone tried to verify the reports.

Pet food companies are another source. Nestlé Purina PetCare, for example, keeps a cat colony and says that its cats live an average of twelve to fourteen years. The company considers any cat older than age twelve to be geriatric. Figure 11 presents a graphic comparison of the life span of cats and dogs, but its source provides no references. The data seem reasonable, but we cannot vouch for their accuracy.

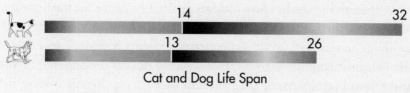

Cat and Dog Life Span

FIGURE 11
The average life span of dogs and cats. No references are given for these figures.

Source: http://catwebsite.googlepages.com/cat-lifespan.htm

Are Pets Living Longer Now?

We have been able to find only two studies attempting to answer this question, both relatively recent. In 1996, a study done in Great Britain reported that from 1960 to 1994, the average age of dogs currently alive increased from 4.8 to 6.0 years. The study also reported an increase in the proportion of older animals in the population during those years, from 24 percent to 34 percent for dogs and from 23 percent to 28 percent for cats. These increases suggest that if pets survive to be young adults, they will have many more good years left. During the period of this study, the use of commercial foods for dogs increased from 49 percent to 69 percent, and for cats from 64 percent to 90 percent, suggesting a correlation with increased longevity. But another study reported no change in longevity from 1984 to 1996.

A study in Munich also addressed this question. It found an increase in the average age of dogs and cats brought to a university pet clinic from 1983 to 1995. The average age of death was about nine years. Neutered dogs lived about one year longer and neutered cats lived four or five years longer, a benefit attributed to their more tranquil way of life and consumption of commercial pet food. But because the Munich studies were of animals brought to a veterinary clinic, these results may not be representative.

From this scanty evidence, we do not think it is possible to say much about the overall effects of commercial pet foods on pet health. Some evidence suggests that they support a longer life span. But the increase in longevity, if real, could also be due to better veterinary care, higher rates of neutering, and keeping pets indoors.

Although the studies provide only limited evidence for the benefit of commercial diets, they provide no evidence at all for harm. If pets truly are living longer, we would expect rates of heart disease, cancers, and other chronic conditions to increase with age, just as they do in humans. And just as in humans, finding out how diet affects chronic disease risk in pets requires long-term studies of large populations. Such studies have not been done or reported in cats or dogs, and we see no indication that anyone is trying to do them. Instead, researchers interested in pet longevity have focused on caloric restriction and antioxidants, the aspects of diet that we discussed in chapter 13.

And what about studies comparing the effects on pet health and longevity of commercial versus raw or home-cooked diets? If such studies exist, we have not been able to find them. They would be expensive to conduct and we cannot imagine who would fund them. The dismal lack of evidence leaves plenty of room for personal opinion and for speculation that commercial food, rather than genetics or some other environmental condition, is responsible for a pet's skin, digestive, or tooth disorders. In the absence of science, which we do not see coming soon, the best we can do is to advise dietary experimentation.

Do People Eat Pet Food?

WHEN WE TOLD people we were writing a book about pet food, we were asked two questions that at first caught us by surprise: Don't pet foods have to meet nutrient standards so poor people can eat them? And, if people eat dogs and cats, in effect aren't they eating pet foods too? Eventually, after hearing one or another version of these questions over and over again, we thought we had best see what they were about. Let's indulge in a short digression and take a look at the results of our investigation into these matters.

PEOPLE AND PET FOODS

We can't count the number of times we have been assured with great authority that poor people eat pet food because they have no other choice. When we ask for details, the answers invariably cover the same three points: "I heard this someplace. No, I have never seen anyone doing this. But I know it's true." The idea that people eat pet food to survive is an enduring story about poverty in the United States.

As far as we can tell, the modern version of this story began in the 1930s at the height of the Great Depression. In a speech, Senator Lester J. Dickinson (D-Iowa) announced that poor people consumed 20 percent of the canned dog food produced in America. He blamed this on the Agricultural Adjustment Administration, which, under the administration of President Franklin Roosevelt, was attempting to maintain farm prices by destroying millions of hogs. The government's artificial maintenance of high food prices, the senator said, caused millions of people to go hungry and resort to eating pet food. Despite the lack of evidence for this assertion, the USDA withdrew the use of its meat inspection stamp on containers of food for dogs and cats, and said that it would now only certify food intended for human consumption.

Fast-forward to 1974 when the Senate Select Committee on Nutrition and Human Needs (The "McGovern Committee") held hearings on the effects of rising food prices on consumer behavior. Among these effects, which supposedly included increases in cattle rustling, game poaching, meat smuggling, and shoplifting, was increased consumption of pet foods by the poor. The hearing record included this remarkable statement:

> Stories of human consumption of cat and dog food, while often difficult to document, appear more and more frequently in the press. Pet food sales are up 12 percent nationally, with significant increases occurring in inner city stores. Michael Jacobson, co-director of the nonprofit Center for Science in the Public Interest [CSPI] estimates that one-third of the dog food sold at inner city stores is bought for human consumption.

The statement made headline news. When questioned, Jacobson (who at the time of this writing still directs CSPI) could not remember whether he had said anything like this. Reporters tracked the statement to an interview given about his 1973 book, *Nutrition Scoreboard*, which gave Alpo dog food a high score in comparison to other meats. Jacobson had to admit that he had no real basis for the claim.

Despite the lack of evidence, Cornell Cooperative Extension felt compelled to issue a newsletter on the subject of "Pet Foods for Dinner." The Extension staff dismissed the charge as rumor but nevertheless discussed matters related to the safety of pet foods and their nutritional value.

The idea that the poor eat pet food seems so plausible that rumors quickly develop a life of their own. Louis Kohlmeier, a columnist for the *Chicago Tribune*, interviewed the manager of an inner-city Safeway about whether his customers were eating pet food. Typically, the manager said he didn't know for sure, but added "We take it for granted." Kohlmeier quotes the USDA: "There aren't enough pets to consume the amount of pet food that's going into inner-city stores."

And then there are the firsthand accounts. In 1975, the *New York Times* ran a column from Edward H. Peebles, an assistant professor of medicine at Virginia Commonwealth University, who described seeing neighbors and friends eating pet foods in his youth. He said he also ate fried dog and cat food for several weeks in the 1950s. By his estimate, up to 8 percent of men going through navy training ate pet foods, and pet foods constituted a significant part of the diet of 225,000 American households. His article cited no sources, however.

The notion persists and remains perfectly undocumented to this day. Pet food sellers tell us "yes, everyone in the business knows that people eat pet food," even though what everyone knows is second- or thirdhand. But the lack of corroborating data is easily explained away. Of course no data exist, how could they? Poor people are not going to admit they eat pet food because they can't afford anything else. We just assume they do. The collapse of the housing bubble in the United States in 2007 and the subsequent rise in food prices elicited another round of such assumptions, as shown in figure 12.

What about the price? Is pet food really that much cheaper than other kinds of canned meats? Here, we have facts: it is. We did a quick price comparison of canned tuna and beef dinners. At the time we looked, we could buy six-ounce cans of "people" tuna for about 75 cents each, but tuna cat food dinners were about half as much. We could buy a fifteen-ounce can of "people" beef stew for $1.80, but a supermarket-brand beef dinner for dogs for about 50 cents. The human tuna contained only tuna, while the pet foods contained other ingredients. Still, the difference in price was substantial. And so, we must say, was the difference in taste.

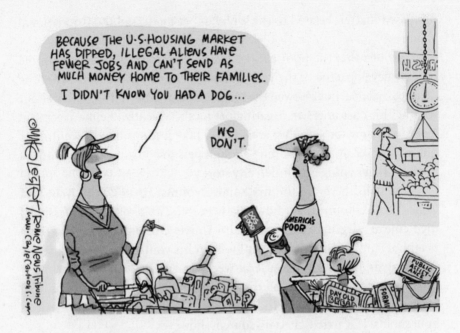

FIGURE 12
*Do America's poor eat pet food? This cartoon reflects the widespread—
but undocumented—assumption that they do.*

© *Mike Lester, 2008. Used with permission.*

We think taste is highly relevant to this discussion. Pet foods are formulated to be palatable to cats and dogs. Pets are especially fond of animal protein flavors, the ones we now call "umami." We have done occasional tastings of commercial pet foods and find them greasy, which is just what cats and dogs love about them. Pet food companies usually conduct palatability tests using cats and dogs, but some employ two-legged taste panels. Human judges generally give cat foods a score of five on a nine-point scale, meaning that they "slightly" like them. We think the judges are being kind.

People do not generally like the taste of pet food, even when they cannot tell what it is. Investigators conducted a blind taste test of Newman's Own canned Turkey & Chicken Formula for Puppies/Active Dogs (blended to a paste in a food processor) compared to four processed meat products designed for humans: duck liver mousse, pork liver paté, liverwurst, and Spam. Subjects were told in advance that one of the products was dog food. Although the eighteen tasters ranked the dog food as the least palatable of the choices, only three correctly guessed which sample was dog food.

In our view, nobody has ever described pet food better than Ray Sokolov, the restaurant critic and former food editor of the *Wall Street Journal,* who decades ago ranked the taste of several of his dogs' favorite foods on a typical restaurant scale of four stars. He gave three stars to Milk-Bone biscuits, which he liked well enough to eat two, one spread with butter. Most of the others, he said, "had a texture nigh unto that of cold cream." He particularly disliked "an inexpensive homogenized food . . . similar in effect to ipecac [an emetic]." He did not rate it, "because it was impossible to force the human subject to taste it. The dog, however, did like it." Many of today's foods with "human-grade" ingredients are made to be more appealing to human taste standards, as we discussed in chapter 12.

We are not convinced that the price difference is great enough to drive people to eat cat or dog food and we still cast our vote for urban legend. Yes, individuals do occasionally eat pet food and we are aware of many such self-reports. But as a substitute for human foods? We don't think so, but we would love to hear from readers who can provide something more convincing than anecdotes on this point.

DO PEOPLE EAT PETS?

Yes, some do. Not us, of course, but *others.* "Asians" eat dogs; "we" don't. Commenting on a directive from the Beijing Food Safety Office forbidding restaurants to serve dog meat during the 2008 Summer Olympics, Bret Thorn, the food editor of *Nation's Restaurant News,* put the "them, not us" point this way: "Sure, dogs are eaten here [in China], but not by us civilized people, but by those crazy Koreans and the yahoos from the distant southwest."

The eating of dogs and cats has a long history, and it is not difficult to find accounts of the use of such animals for food—in Asia, Africa, and the remote Pacific islands ("never us, though")—dating back to antiquity. Today, the eating of dog and cat meat is part of the culture of groups throughout Southeast Asia—Thailand, Vietnam, Indonesia, and the Philippines, as well as South Korea and China. According to reports, the dog meat industry in South Korea involves about one million dogs and six thousand restaurants, and Beijing alone is said to have 120 restaurants serving dogs as food. We have no idea if these figures are correct.

What we do know is that this practice directly confronts "Western" views of pets as beloved companions, not food. The cultural gap in views became particularly evident in 1988 during the Summer Olympics in Seoul, South Korea. Under pressure from Western visitors, the government asked restaurants not to serve dog meat. This offended South Koreans who experienced the request as the result of Western condescension and an insult to their culture. Similarly, during the 2008 Olympics in Beijing, the city government reportedly banned the serving of dog meat ("fragrant meat") in the 112 official Olympic restaurants, and asked other restaurants that specialize in cuisines of Korea and outlying provinces (*them*, again) to desist from serving dog meat. Animal welfare advocates in Great Britain perceived the Chinese government's action as cynical, because they said they had seen videos of dogs cruelly slaughtered for food.

How long the practice of eating dog meat will continue in China is uncertain. China has its own cultural clashes. The pet market in that country is booming and, like us, the Chinese do not eat pets. Instead they raise certain types of *other* dogs for this purpose. As one pet shop salesman explained, "We still eat dog but not this kind of dog . . . we eat much bigger dogs." By one estimate, China has nearly 27 million dogs and 11 million cats, but there could well be more, and the market for pet supplies is expected to approach a billion dollars in 2009, a doubling just since 2004. A reporter from *USA Today* who was covering the 2008 Olympics sent us photographs of pet foods from stores in Beijing. Whiskas and Pedigree products were well represented. The opportunities to expand sales of such products seem limitless because pet keeping is the new rage among affluent Chinese; like many Americans, the rising middle class views pets as surrogate children. Late in 2008, protesters in China's Guangdong province took to the streets to demand government intervention to stop the trading of cats for food. We predict that this trend will eventually lead to bans on the use of dogs and cats as food, or will drive the enterprise underground.

This prediction requires no crystal ball. Pressures on Asian governments to ban the practice are increasing. In South Korea, for example, concerns about conditions of slaughter and sanitation in the unregulated dog meat industry led the city of Seoul to propose that dogs be categorized as livestock "to properly regulate the trade of dog meat and strengthen sanitation inspections." In the Philippines, a law passed in 1998 banned trade in dog meat but was only selectively enforced and, by one estimate, two hundred dogs were consumed daily in the city of Baguio. In 2007, however, the Philippine Congress passed a law strengthening the earlier ban.

In the United States, the consumption of dogs and cats for human food is banned in some states, but not others. Animal welfare groups are pressing state legislatures to pass such laws, and states such as New Jersey, Georgia, and Mississippi have enacted legislation banning the sale of dog or cat meat for human consumption. In a diverse multiethnic society such as ours, the question of what is appropriate as food can lead to many different responses. Even in our pet-revering society, a Google search for dog meat recipes turns up enough examples to fill a hefty cookbook. One, for dog stew (wedding style), begins, "First, kill a medium sized dog, then burn off the fur over a hot fire." Many of us would be appalled by this thought, but we should expect to see many such cultural clashes as the conflicts among our increasingly globalized societies—both East and West—play out.

Do Pet Food Companies Influence Veterinarians?

VETERINARY PRACTICE HAS changed drastically during the last thirty years. It used to focus on large animals raised for food. Now it focuses on small animals kept as pets. We wanted to know whether nutrition instruction has kept up with this transition. One of us (Nestle) spent a decade teaching nutrition to medical students so we were well aware that most medical students get minimal nutrition instruction. Are veterinary students taught small animal nutrition? If not, where do they learn about the dietary needs of dogs and cats? We also knew that some veterinarians sell pet foods to their clients. This made us wonder whether pet food companies influence veterinarians' dietary advice in the same way that drug companies influence doctors' prescription practices. Medical schools are developing policies to limit corporate influences on medical students and faculty and we were curious to know whether veterinary schools were making similar efforts. This chapter summarizes our findings.

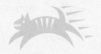

TRENDS IN VETERINARY PRACTICE

The shift from large to small animals has changed the way veterinarians are trained. Nutrition research on farm animals used to be conducted by animal scientists looking for the most efficient and profitable methods for converting feed into meat or milk. This research mostly took place in animal science departments of agricultural colleges. With the shift in focus, research on the nutrition of dogs and cats became an end in itself and animal science departments began to offer courses on dog and cat nutrition. Cornell University's animal science department, for example, continues to offer a course on the nutrition of exotic animals, a designation that includes cats and dogs. But this department is in the agriculture college, not the veterinary college.

The goals of veterinary instruction differ substantially from those of animal science. Veterinarians are interested in animal diseases and the treatment of sick animals. Even when large animal practices were common, how the animals were fed was not central to their mission. If veterinary students were taught anything about animal feeding, that instruction was likely to have come as a few lectures by animal science faculty as part of a course on animal diseases.

Perhaps more important, the shift to small animal practices occurred after the widespread introduction of complete-and-balanced pet foods. These foods take care of pets' nutritional requirements and veterinarians could recommend any complete-and-balanced product and know it would do. They could prescribe products without knowing the nutritional details. And just as is the case with human medicine, it is easier for practitioners to treat disease by prescribing drugs than by counseling pet owners about complicated dietary issues.

The American Veterinary Medical Association (AVMA) categorizes members who work with food animals at any point in the food chain as "food supply veterinarians." AVMA estimates that only 17 percent of veterinarians specialize in food animals and worries about the growing shortfall of professionals with such training. The remaining 83 percent of veterinarians are engaged in small animal practice (or are not working directly with animals). We would expect small animal veterinarians to be interested in learning about the nutritional needs of dogs and cats.

NUTRITION INSTRUCTION IN VETERINARY SCHOOLS

Nutrition is now recognized as a specialty in veterinary medicine, although one with a tiny membership. Founded in 1988, the American College of Veterinary Nutrition (ACVN) administers a nutrition certification program based on training, clinical experience, publication, and examination. By 2007, a mere 61 of 75,000 veterinarian members of AVMA had achieved this certification. Twenty years after ACVN's founding, nutrition barely registers on the veterinary radar.

Curious about what veterinary students are currently learning about nutrition, we conducted an informal telephone survey of the twenty-seven veterinary schools accredited in the United States. Administrators at twenty-two of the twenty-seven schools told us that their institution included some nutrition instruction as part of veterinary education (the other five said they taught no nutrition at all). But most of the twenty-two said their instruction was elective or minimal. About ten veterinary schools require students to take a nutrition course, usually one credit. Twelve schools said they offered elective courses, usually taught by visiting instructors. An administrator at Oregon State told us that the school used to require a nutrition course but had now made it an admission prerequisite. Only one school—Tufts—offered nutrition instruction throughout veterinary training. There, an ACVN-certified veterinary nutritionist supervises a program that includes a first-year course covering small, large, and exotic animal nutrition; third-year instruction as part of courses in small- and large-animal medicine; and clinical nutrition rounds and electives in the fourth year. A program this comprehensive is the rare exception.

We recognize that these dismal reports may exaggerate the lack of nutrition training. In our first column for *The Bark* magazine late in 2007, we asked veterinarians to write us about their experiences with nutrition education. We received several replies, one from a veterinary student who asked that we not identify her or her school. She described her nutrition training:

> As first years, we take a required 1 credit course entitled "Principles of Nutrition," which covers both small animal and large

animal nutrition. Aside from lectures, the course included a lab in which we examined pet food label claims, saw examples of the raw materials of common ingredients, and explored the differences between prescription foods for common problems. . . . Small animal people had to go through the process of calculating their pets' daily energy requirements and then comparing that to how many kilocalories they ingested each day in food and treats. . . . We had a few quizzes and also had to complete an online nutrition module from Purina (my major complaint about the course). . . . Students who track small animals will have to take a 2.5-credit nutrition course during third year and we have an option to do a clinical nutrition rotation during our fourth year. It's also easy to miss that we cover nutrition topics in classes that aren't specifically about nutrition, including in biochemistry, physiology, and pathology.

Since her school was not Tufts, there must be at least one other veterinary college that requires a significant amount of training in small animal nutrition, but most veterinary schools told us they do not offer this instruction. So where do most veterinary students and veterinarians learn about the nutritional needs of dogs and cats? Some may have studied animal science as undergraduates, but as we discovered, most get their nutrition education from pet food companies.

PET FOOD COMPANY INVOLVEMENT

Pet food companies have a vested interest in developing strong relationships with veterinarians who recommend food products as well as with veterinary students who are young, impressionable, and not taught much critical thinking about nutrition and pet feeding. These relationships raise questions of conflict of interest that do not seem to be discussed much in veterinary schools. Pet food companies are deeply entrenched in veterinary education. Consider Hill's Pet Nutrition, the maker of Science and Prescription Diets. Hill's is closely associated with the Mark Morris Institute, a separate foundation named after the company's founder. The institute offers short courses on pet nutrition to veterinary schools, free of charge. It supplies the instructors, most of whom are members of Hill's technical staff. The institute also publishes *Small Animal Clinical Nutrition,* now in its fourth edition, a weighty tome of more than 1,100 pages, which Hill's freely provides to veterinary students and practicing veterinarians.

Hill's gave us a copy of this book and we understood immediately why the company is so generous. We were impressed by the high quality of the book's review of research issues in basic and clinical nutrition, its informative case studies, and its balanced tone and opinion. We think students who take the trouble to learn the material in this book will be well grounded in the field. In saying so, we have just repaid Hill's for its gift—a good example of how the system works. You now have to judge for yourself whether our opinion of the book is truly objective or was influenced by Hill's generosity.

Hill's is by no means alone in investing resources in veterinarians and students. Many of the ways pet food companies deal with the veterinary profession are all too familiar to professionals concerned about undue corporate influence on medical practice. Attempts to influence veterinarians are not confined to the United States. In 2008, for example, Mars gave $3 million to the Ontario Veterinary College at the University of Guelph for the Royal Canin Veterinary Endowed Chair in Canine and Feline Clinical Nutrition. The university said the chair would be independent and would complement the "massive investment the company is making in the new plant in the Township of Puslinch" (which is close to Guelph). How independent? It is hard to know. With that said, let's look at some of the other ways pet food companies work with the veterinary profession.

Veterinary Students

To discover the extent of pet food company involvement with veterinary students, we examined veterinary school newsletters, websites, and bulletin boards, and sent our research assistant to collect information from current students. Pet food companies routinely give veterinary students an amazing collection of free items: textbooks, product guides, backpacks, planners, coffee mugs, pens, highlighters, scrub shirts, and lunches during orientation. They sponsor student representatives. Most impressive, they provide free or reduced price food for students' dogs and cats during the entire period of veterinary training.

We logged on to Hill's website for professionals to read about its activities for students at veterinary schools. At Cornell during the 2008–09 academic year, Hill's hosted the annual Junior Event for third-year veterinary students. This "gave students a well-deserved chance to relax and unwind after two days of exams. Over 60 students attended, plus a few faculty members came to enjoy an evening with the junior class." Hill's describes a similar event at the University of Pennsylvania: "One of the highlights of the evening took place when Dr. Schickel pitted the students against one another in a fun yet intense game of Jeopardy! Not only did students enjoy themselves, but also took home valuable information from Dr. Schickel on the nutritional benefits of Hill's Science Diet pet foods."

Hill's and Nestlé Purina are particularly generous supporters of veterinary students but all major companies participate to some extent. Canidae All Natural, for example, awards $2,500 scholarships to veterinary students who write winning essays on the theme of responsibilities of pet ownership. As far as we can determine, pet food companies sponsor such activities at *all* veterinary schools. They are not alone. Pharmaceutical companies making veterinary drugs are also actively involved in forging relationships with veterinarians-in-training.

Because we are most familiar with the situation at Cornell's veterinary college, we will use its practices as an example. Cornell permits companies to sponsor student representatives. Many do, among them Hill's, Purina, Iams, Natura, Royal Canin, and Oxbow, along with the veterinary hospital chains VCA and Banfield, and veterinary vaccine and drug companies such as Novartis, Pfizer, Bayer, Merial/Intervet, and Fort Dodge. Hill's, for example, employs two Cornell students to represent its foods; it recruits them from among first- and second-year students. Considering the cost of attending this school (tuition in 2009–10 for a New York State resident was $26,500 or $39,500 for a nonresident), the representatives are not paid much. The more senior representative received $750 a semester, while the junior student representative got $250.

In 2007, we asked our research assistant, Heather Inglis, to interview student representatives at Cornell. Her interviews made it clear why veterinary students want to represent pet food companies. The Hill's representative explained that the job entailed eight hours of work a month, mainly helping with the organization and monthly distribution of free pet foods and with events sponsored by the company. She particularly appreciated the professional contacts and training that came with the job. Hill's flies student representatives to its Kansas City headquarters for a week of lectures about nutrition in general, Hill's products in particular, and ways to communicate this information to fellow students and clients. They also get a tour of the company's factory in Topeka. This student was quite clear about the benefits: "We don't get taught much about nutrition . . . other than an optional two-credit elective so it is a huge advantage to be able to learn more about it so that I will be able to talk with my clients about nutrition in the future."

Relationships with pet food companies are attractive for other reasons. As the especially thoughtful veterinarian Patty Khuly explains on her Internet blog:

Hill's and Waltham routinely paid for our parties, our canine blood-drives, our faculty awards, our own pets' dietary needs, etc. etc . . . The list of all their contributions to US vet schools is taller than a tower of pet food cans stacked to the moon and back. I, for one, am thankful of their contributions—and not just for my reduced indebtedness. It's hard for us to imagine now . . . but pet nutrition was in the dark ages before these companies started legitimately researching pet nutrition. In fact, pets often died of nutritional diseases until Purina did its thing in the '50s and standardized pet food requirements with its Dog and Cat Chow brands.

We have no trouble understanding the attraction but one thing puzzles us. Why don't veterinary educators question these relationships? The student who responded to our query in *The Bark* was an exception. She mentioned that her school gave out copies of *Small Animal Clinical Nutrition*. These, she said, came "courtesy of Hill's (hard to complain about not having to pay for a textbook, but I didn't really feel comfortable about that either)."

Patty Khuly points out that many of her peers were skeptical of "the pet food issue." But because pet food companies seemed so supportive of what they need, students readily, if uncomfortably, accepted the assistance. But "to make matters worse, the influence of this pet food industry oligopoly on real-life veterinary practice is extreme. Not only does the modern vet practice believe in the science behind the bags of food, it has come to rely on the income these foods provide."

Practicing Veterinarians

Pet food companies like having veterinarians recommend their products to clients. At the moment, fewer than 10 percent of pet owners say they buy their food from veterinarians, so there is much room for growth in this area. Pet food companies that own veterinary practices clearly have a vested interest in selling their products through such channels. Banfield veterinary hospitals, owned in part by Mars, constitute the most obvious example. We visited the one located in the back of the PetSmart store in Ithaca, New York, where clients have to go through the store to get to and leave the clinic. We asked a technician whether the hospital did anything special to promote Mars's Royal Canin and Nutro brands. No, she said, although the clinic stocks Royal Canin, a formulary committee decides which other brands to stock. She was much more interested in other Mars products. At a Mars training facility, she had been given so many M&Ms that she thought she could never eat them again.

Hill's deliberately sells its products through veterinarians and about half the company's annual sales occur through this channel. Hill's is a subsidiary of Colgate-Palmolive, a company famous for working through professionals. As explained in a recent annual report, Colgate models its work with veterinarians on its success in selling toothbrushes and toothpaste through dentists.

> Recommendations from professionals drive product trial and long-term loyalty. Colgate's long-standing relationships with dental and veterinary professionals greatly contribute to the Company's growing market shares in oral care and pet nutrition . . . in the pet nutrition category, Hill's market shares

have risen as a result of initiatives encouraging recommendation of veterinarians. . . . Hill's sponsors numerous conferences around the world and Hill's experts make frequent presentations at veterinary colleges and gatherings. . . . As a result of initiatives like these veterinary endorsements continue to strengthen around the world.

Much of Hill's business with veterinarians is to help them use Hill's Prescription Diets. Hill's emphasizes that these products are not only useful treatment strategies but also are good for a veterinarian's business. Other companies do this too. Mars, Nestlé Purina, and Procter & Gamble (Iams) all make veterinary diets to be sold through veterinarians, but for Hill's this channel represents a much larger fraction of overall sales.

Veterinarians who sell pet foods tell us that they see nothing wrong with this practice. They consider the products they sell to be entirely suited to the needs of their dog and cat patients. They assure us that owners are going to buy food for their pets anyway. What's wrong with trying to make a little money from pet food sales? Let's let Khuly answer this question.

The problem lies in our dependence on these products for our livelihood, the same way drugs and services do. Our human tendency is to respond to manufacturer entreaties to consider their products not only for their innate benefits, but also for the income they'll drive our way . . . Pet food is so important to some practices that it's come to affect even the fundamentals of hospital design and pricing. New hospitals are physically planned for food retail and storage. It's my opinion that even the pricing of vet services is often artificially reduced so that hospitals can compete on service price while making up the difference in food and drug sales.

CONFLICTS OF INTEREST

That veterinarians who sell pet foods make money on them is a given, and this alone is sufficient to raise questions of conflict of interest. The goal of a pet food company is to sell product. The goal of a small animal veterinarian is to promote pet health. Although both goals can be achieved by recommending the most appropriate food, the profit motive muddies the waters.

The involvement of pet food, drug, and medical device companies in veterinary training and practice is strikingly similar to the involvement of drug and medical device companies in medical training and practice. The American Medical Student Association considers medical students to be so "at risk" of failing to recognize how marketing affects their practices that it started a PharmFree campaign to immunize medical students against corporate influences. In response to concerns about undue influence, at least thirty medical colleges have adopted policies governing conflicts of interest in research and some have acted to limit the ways corporate vendors interact with students and faculty. The University of Pittsburgh, for example, developed policies that address gift and consulting relationships. Its medical students and faculty are not permitted to accept personal gifts (including food) from industry representatives, no matter how small the dollar value: no pens, notepads, clocks, or office items with company logos, let alone stethoscopes or meals. The University of Massachusetts Medical Center in Worcester adopted a similar policy in 2007.

In urging such policies for physicians involved in medical education and practice, the editors of the *Journal of the American Medical Association* (*JAMA*) said:

> When integrity in medical science or practice is impugned or threatened—such as by the influence of industry—patients, clinicians, and researchers are all at risk for harm, and public trust in research is jeopardized. Ensuring, maintaining, and strengthening the integrity of medical science must be a priority for everyone.

More recently, a task force of the Association of American Medical Colleges, the trade group for academic medical centers, urged the association's members "to accelerate their adoption of policies that better manage, and when necessary, prohibit, academic-industry interactions that can inherently create conflicts of interest and undermine standards of professionalism." The task force also called on industry to "voluntarily discontinue those practices that compromise professionalism as well as public trust." Perhaps because of this last recommendation, three industry members of the task force dissented from some of the report's recommendations. In 2009, medical ethicists called for major revisions of the guidelines governing relationships between professional medical associations (PMAs) and industry: "Because PMAs receive extensive funding from pharmaceutical and device companies, it is crucial that their guidelines manage both real and perceived conflict of interests."

What most surprises us is how little discussion of such issues seems to be taking place in veterinary schools. We conducted another informal telephone poll, this time of student affairs deans, to ask them whether they had or were considering policies to restrict educational materials, sponsorships, or gifts from pet food companies. For the most part, they answered no. They said the programs were popular with students and generated support for student organizations. They argued that government support for veterinary education was so inadequate that industry funds were essential for carrying out their programs. They viewed the gifts and sponsorships as acceptable, and felt that the transparency of the corporate sponsorships was a sufficient safeguard.

If the situation in medical schools is at all relevant to veterinary training, these views are stunningly naïve. A few student affairs deans told us that their schools have made efforts to define policies for industry interactions. The Tufts veterinary school, for example, has formal policies and guidelines for student corporate representatives, but these only require disclosure; they do not call for bans on gifts or sponsorship. One dean told us that his school viewed its state's legislative efforts to address corporate conflicts in state-supported medical schools as a threat to similar practices in veterinary schools; his school opposed such legislation.

We take the liberty of quoting Patty Khuly one last time: "Much as selling drugs is unethical for a doctor, selling drugs and foods should be considered as such for vets. . . . Studies show that pet owners believe that vets and human physicians are comparable in most respects, yet our culture holds these two professions to different ethical standards. What's up with that?"

What's up with that, indeed. We think the veterinary profession needs to catch up quickly with the medical profession in addressing conflicts of interest with pet food and drug companies. Veterinary training should require open discussion of conflicts of interest in student orientation sessions and in courses on professional ethics. If such courses do not exist, the role of pet food companies is a good reason for creating them. And so are the ethical concerns about pet food research that we discuss next.

Is Pet Food Research Ethical?

THROUGHOUT THIS BOOK, we have repeatedly commented on the lack of research relevant to many key questions about pet nutrition. We have often argued for more—and better—research on those questions. Others agree. Some animal scientists view the generally inadequate funding for animal research as a crisis.

By now, the nutrient requirements of dogs and cats are so well defined that it is possible to raise these animals on highly purified mixes of nutrients (not foods) that supply everything they need to grow and reproduce. When you hear people say that more is known about the nutritional needs of pets than of people, they are referring to requirements for specific nutrients—not foods or diets. But today, much of what we want to know about dog and cat nutrition involves more subtle—and more complicated—research questions about the effects of various kinds of diets on chronic diseases, longevity, and body weight. These questions are precisely the same as those relevant to human nutrition research. In this chapter, we deal with the ethics of investigating such questions using cats and dogs as experimental animals, when they have no choice about participating and cannot give informed consent.

As with research on humans, studies of the effects of diet on the health of dogs and cats are difficult to design, conduct, and interpret. Variations in individual characteristics mean that large numbers of animals must be used in experiments in order to obtain results that are statistically meaningful. In humans, such trials are extremely expensive, costing hundreds of millions of dollars. Even so, they often produce ambiguous results that require careful interpretation. Much of the research on human diet and health is supported by government agencies such as the NIH or USDA, although some is supported by food companies with a vested interest in the outcome of such research. But unless dogs and cats can be used as models to address problems in human nutrition, government agencies do not fund pet food research.

Beyond the lack of funding, research on pet nutrition encounters one other barrier. Many Americans—some of them members of well-organized and politically effective groups—object strongly to the use of dogs and cats in experiments. One such group is People for the Ethical Treatment of Animals (PETA). Among its other activities, PETA runs a website—"Iams Tortures Animals"—devoted to pressuring that company to stop performing research on companion animals. The site advocates a boycott of Iams products and urges supporters to buy only from pet food companies that promise PETA they will not use animals in research.

In 2007, PETA owned seventy shares of common stock in Iams's parent company, Procter & Gamble (P&G), giving it the right to file shareholder petitions. One PETA petition gave the company five years in which to "conduct humane, safe, and scientifically reliable in-home testing of commercial dog and cat food . . . which has been demonstrated to work for a wide variety of test protocols, including [AAFCO] palatability, preference, and feeding trials."

The P&G board of directors recommended voting against this proposal. The board explained that P&G has "an ethical responsibility to assure the products we develop are safe and wholesome," and said that it already conducts most of its feeding studies in the homes of six hundred of its employees. The board insisted that its studies are conducted in new facilities in which "dogs and cats live in a cageless environment and have ample opportunity to interact with loving caregivers and each other . . .

All animals are eventually adopted into homes or placed into our retirement facility."

Undoubtedly, pressures from animal welfare advocates encouraged P&G to produce its state-of-the-art animal care facilities, but we worry about the chilling effect of this kind of advocacy on individual researchers. To give just one example: Professor George Fahey at the University of Illinois conducts research on the ability of dogs to digest and use pet food ingredients. When a reporter, Fredrick Kaufmann, described this work in the *New York Times Magazine* in 2007, Fahey's email in-box was overwhelmed for nearly a year by thousands of identically worded—and clearly well-organized—messages protesting his research. For busy researchers, email spam is hardly a peaceful form of protest. Fahey conducts his research in full accordance with laws governing protection of animals used in research, and he deserves protection from harassment by animal rights advocates. If they do not like the laws, they can use democratic processes to try to get them changed.

But we have some sympathy for other forms of PETA protest. For years, Iams has supported pet research at Mississippi State University. In 2006, PETA sued the university to reveal information about the number and type of animals used in Iams's experiments, the conditions under which the animals were housed, and whether they had been subjected to surgical procedures. Two years later, the Mississippi Supreme Court ruled that PETA had no right to this information—not because the organization's requests were unreasonable, but because these details were Iams's trade secrets protected under state laws.

What? Since when is research carried out at state-supported universities not public information? The idea that proprietary research could be carried out in a public university without publishing the research protocols and results is inconsistent with the ethics of scientific inquiry. This incident constitutes one more example of the lack of transparency in corporate-sponsored research.

Between funding problems and animal welfare advocacy, few universities are willing to house research programs on small animals. Those that do run such programs can be counted on the fingers of one hand. In addition to the University of Illinois, the Universities of Kentucky, Texas, and Florida house active programs on small animal nutrition, as does the

University of California at Davis. Investigators at some other universities also publish research on small animal nutrition but few maintain dog or cat colonies.

This means that the most extensive research facilities are run by major pet food companies or private animal testing facilities. Nestlé-Purina, Iams, Hill's, and Mars all support animal research facilities. One of us (Nesheim) toured the Hill's animal research facilities in Kansas, and both of us visited Mars's Waltham Centre in England. These are handsome new facilities with clean and well-managed housing for dogs and cats, run by a large staff of people who care for and routinely play with the animals. The dogs and cats seemed relaxed, cheerful, and interested in strangers.

But in our experience, Hill's and Mars were exceptional in allowing us access to their facilities. These companies take pride in how well they treat the animals and are not afraid to show outsiders what they are doing. In contrast, as noted earlier, we were denied access to the Nestlé-Purina facilities in Missouri (even with "pull") and to the private testing facility, Summit Ridge Farms, in Pennsylvania. Our attempts to tour facilities run by Procter & Gamble also failed (also despite "pull"). We understand why these places would be concerned about animal welfare advocacy or client protection, but cannot help wondering what it is they want to hide from people like us with no particular axe to grind.

One result of the lack of funding, the limited number of research sites, the vested interest of pet food companies, and the atmosphere of secrecy is that the research that does get published—and we wish we knew a more diplomatic way of saying this—is not always of the highest quality. Some studies from company-owned facilities do appear in peer-reviewed journals, but more often appear in sponsored journal supplements paid for by the companies themselves. Mars Pet Foods, for example, describes its studies in its in-house publication, *Veterinary Nutrition* (formerly *Waltham Nutrition*) and pays for publication of the proceedings of symposia run by its Waltham Center for Pet Nutrition in supplements to the *Journal of Nutrition*.

Because much of the research conducted by pet food companies is designed to produce evidence for the benefits of ingredients that can be promoted for marketing purposes, the studies can be difficult to interpret. In standard scientific practice, high-quality reports of research studies must provide sufficient detail for other investigators to repeat them. If companies consider their diet formulas to be proprietary and do not disclose their nutritional composition, independent investigators cannot confirm the results. A study designed to compare the effects of adding or not adding an antioxidant supplement to a commercial formula cannot be reproduced without knowing what else was in the diet.

To find out whether nondisclosure of dietary composition is typical of pet food research, we did a quick online search for "diets" in recent studies published in the *Journal of the American Veterinary Medical Association* and the *Journal of Veterinary Research*. Among the first one hundred papers retrieved by this search, we found thirty-five that compared the effects of one kind of diet to another. Of these, about half (seventeen) provided enough details to reproduce the diets. The other half used commercial diets and reported the guaranteed analysis but not much else. Pet food companies sponsored twenty-four of the thirty-five studies, and these included nearly all of the papers that lacked dietary details. In contrast, the papers disclosing dietary composition mostly came from university investigators in the United States or Japan.

But undefined diets are just one of the problems we encountered as we delved into pet food research. Many studies use too few animals to get statistically significant results. Many have not been repeated or confirmed by other investigators. We worried about the quality of studies in which the control and experimental animals were not well matched. In one weight-loss trial involving carnitine supplementation of obese cats, for example, the control group weighed 6.5 kilograms at the start of the study, whereas the carnitine-supplemented group weighed 7.3 kilograms. The already lighter control group could well have been expected to lose weight less rapidly during the course of the trial.

Another example: in a study of the effects of a dietary supplement on the learning ability of aging dogs, the control group was seven months older than the treatment group. Did the control group learn less well because it lacked the supplement or because of its more advanced age? We can't tell. Studies like these need to be repeated, often with larger numbers of animals, for us and for pet owners to have any confidence in their conclusions. If the effects of diets on dogs and cats are going to be studied at all, the standards of pet food research and publication should be much higher than much of what we have observed. Research quality is as much of an ethical issue as is the nondisclosure of proprietary results.

PET FOOD RESEARCH: ETHICAL CONCERNS

As a result of pressures by animal welfare advocates, all of the major pet food companies have developed—and prominently display—their policies on animal research. Hill's, for example, says, "We do not participate in studies that jeopardize the health of dogs and cats. All Hill's-supported studies are designed to maintain and improve the animals' health. No study will be performed on dogs or cats which requires euthanasia."

Researchers are extraordinarily sensitive to questions about the welfare of animals participating in their experiments. They have to be. Universities require researchers to obtain advance approval from animal care committees and to conduct their studies in strict compliance with federal legislation on animal welfare, policies of the Public Health Service, and guidelines for use of animals in research and teaching. Most professional journals require disclosure of animal welfare committee approvals as well as funding sources.

Researchers must think twice before they undertake experiments on dogs and cats, no matter how urgent the need for the study. During the melamine recalls of 2007, for example, a team of researchers at the University of California, Davis, designed an elaborate, three-part, dose-response experiment to demonstrate that only a few milligrams of melamine and its by-product, cyanuric acid, were enough to damage the kidneys of cats. The study used a total of just four cats, all euthanized at the end of the trial. The lead author explained: "We had to make some sacrifices but I hope a large population of pets will benefit from it."

As we keep saying, we think high-quality feeding studies are needed to sort out the benefits and risks of various kinds of diets and to settle questions about whether dogs and cats fare better with or without supplements or particular diet ingredients. For reasons of ethics, many types of human nutrition research cannot be done on children. Do feeding studies on dogs and cats raise the same kinds of ethical concerns? As it happens, one of us (Nestle) knows four animal ethicists who have devoted careers to dealing with such questions. We asked them to help us think through whether there could be circumstances under which feeding studies on dogs and cats might be appropriate, and what those circumstances might be. All responded and gave permission to quote their opinions.

We began with Peter Singer, the Ira W. DeCamp Professor of Bioethics at Princeton University, whose book *Animal Liberation* provides a theoretical basis for the animal welfare movement. He said:

> If it is possible to do this research in a way that inflicts no serious distress on the dogs or cats, then yes, it would be OK. If, for example, you could have well-cared-for animals (perhaps actual pets?) randomized to receive the commercial food to be tested, or an improved one, and the health of the animals was closely monitored (by vets blind to what the animal is receiving), I see no problem with that, especially since some pets would be getting the commercial food anyway.

Next, we asked Bernard Rollin, University Distinguished Professor (of Philosophy, Animal Science, and Biomedical Sciences) and University Bioethicist at Colorado State University. He began with some comments on the "checkered history" of pet feeding studies. These, he says, were sometimes done with no regard for the animals, which typically ended up euthanized or used in toxicology studies.

> Some of the big dog food companies got into serious trouble when such studies were exposed. . . . The dog food companies are currently paranoid about being identified with invasive studies. . . . As far as I am personally concerned, a well-run, noninvasive nutrition study that culminates in the animals' being adopted could be exemplary animal research, as no suffering nor death is involved and the animals find homes. Minor procedures such as blood draws can be viewed as a small cost to the animal for being placed in a good home.

Alan Goldberg is Professor of Toxicology and Director of the Center for Alternatives to Animal Testing at the Bloomberg School of Public Health, Johns Hopkins University. His view (slightly edited):

I have no difficulty using dog and cats in feeding studies to improve animal health. The conditions that I would require are that the control group is fed the current optimal diet, all test ingredients are added in anticipation of an improved diet, and the anticipated outcome is improved health or quality of life. The measures should include non-invasive approaches and observations. Additionally, [the studies] should be done with the animal in its home environment . . . informed consent provided by the pet's owner (oops . . . human companion) and the experimental design overseen by an NIH-approved Animal Care and Use Committee.

Finally, we queried Neal Barnard, who is president of the Physicians Committee for Responsible Medicine, a Washington, DC–based group that advocates vegetarian and vegan diets and alternatives to animal experimentation:

Some companies . . . use animals in tests of animal food products. It is disturbing to see animals confined, experimented on in various ways, and ultimately killed for such purposes. . . . Nutritional research can be ethically done in animals in much the same way it is done in humans—by maintaining records on diets while the animals remain in their home environments. The same applies when animals' diets are altered for health reasons: It is possible to alter their diets and track the benefits that result. Regarding more invasive experiments, a case can be made for such experiments when the intended result is a benefit for the individual animal involved—as in the case of an experimental cancer therapy given to an animal who has no other treatment option.

We are reassured by the consistency of the views of people who have thought long and hard about such issues. They view feeding studies as appropriate when the animals are well treated and cared for (preferably in their home environments), the studies do no harm, the procedures are largely noninvasive, the animals are eventually adopted into good homes, and the experiments are well designed and monitored.

We agree. We believe that it is more ethical to test pet foods to make sure they really are complete and balanced than to put a "complete" food on the market that no cat or dog has ever eaten. We think AAFCO feeding trials could be conducted in homes although we worry a bit about how well the diets can be controlled in such situations. Cats and dogs are clever at finding food wherever it is hidden and treats are always a temptation. This kind of cheating, however, may be a small risk worth taking for the greater good of the animals. We think that AAFCO should examine this possibility and develop protocols for in-home testing.

Nevertheless, we still believe that some research needs to be carried out in controlled environments. At the Hill's and Mars facilities we visited, we saw cats and dogs housed in groups, cared for and played with by employees who look after the health and well-being of relatively small numbers of animals. The devices for collecting data were precise and the animals trained and rewarded for participating. We think these animals are no worse off than pets left alone and confined indoors all day while owners are at work.

Early in our scientific careers, both of us were involved in studies on animals; some of these studies were invasive or resulted in the death of the animals. These animals were not dogs or cats, although that no longer matters. Today, the rules for studying animals have changed. The changes represent a major shift in how society views animal research and are a tribute to the successful efforts of animal welfare advocates.

We especially agree with Professors Singer and Goldberg that pet feeding trials should be conducted under the highest possible standards of study design, monitoring, and publication. We are not suggesting that pet food research should be viewed as a national priority, but we do believe that if the research is going to be done at all, it should be done well. If companies are conducting research to establish a basis for marketing, they must make the details of the research available to the greater scientific community for independent evaluation. Anything less is disrespectful of the animals and, in our view, unethical.

Concluding Thoughts

WE BEGAN TO write this book without knowing much about where it would lead us. Pet food was close to our fields of expertise but enough out of our usual paths of reading and researching to present challenges. We took on this project as we would any other academic pursuit and entered into our research with open minds and much curiosity. We already were familiar with the depth of affection people have for their pets, and that bond was one of the reasons we were so interested in this topic. Nevertheless, much of what we discovered surprised us. We had not known that pets formed the core of an industry that generated more than $40 billion a year in U.S. sales of products and services, with pet foods accounting for nearly half that amount. Until the 2007 melamine recalls, we had not realized how tightly the system for producing pet foods is linked to the food systems for farm animals and for people. For these reasons alone, but also because people so deeply treasure their dogs and cats, we believe the pet food industry merits the serious examination we have given it here.

In researching this book, we dealt with a wide range of topics related to foods for dogs and cats. Our investigations led us to several conclusions, some of them expected, some not. These, in turn, led us to some obvious and not-so-obvious recommendations that we think might be helpful to the pet food industry and its government regulators, as well as to pet owners. We begin this final chapter with the findings that we found most surprising, and end it with some recommendations for future action.

OUR CONCLUSIONS

No One Method Is Best for Feeding Dogs or Cats

Pets can flourish eating just about any foods (with a few caveats). In mulling over this conclusion, we realize that we should not have been surprised to make this discovery. After all, we know perfectly well that humans grow, reproduce, and live to ripe old age on diets that differ enormously in what is considered normal and acceptable to eat. As long as the diet includes sufficient amounts of a variety of minimally processed foods—meat, dairy, fruit, vegetables, grains (or their substitutes)—the needs for essential nutrients and energy will be met. The same goes for dogs and cats.

As we have said, it is extremely difficult to induce a nutrient deficiency in a person or animal eating enough of a variety of foods. This means that you have lots of options for feeding pets healthfully. You can choose a feeding method that not only meets the nutritional needs and preferences of your particular animal, but also—and we think this is an important consideration—one that fits comfortably with the way you live and with your personal dietary beliefs and preferences.

If this concept seems as surprising to you as it did to us, it is because nobody would ever know this from surveying current books on how to care for pets. The books that are out there tend to cite every bit of research or experience they can muster to argue that you must feed your pet only one kind of diet—only commercial pet food, only one or another alternative pet food, only meat, only grains and vegetables, only raw foods, or only home-cooked foods. Humans don't eat only one way. Pets don't need to either. Any or all of those methods, singly or together, can promote excellent health in a dog or cat.

Commercial Pet Foods Are Adequate and Appropriate for Many Pets

We suspect that many readers will consider this statement to be either blatant heresy or evidence that we drank the Kool-Aid. If you are one such reader, we understand your skepticism. We expected to be appalled by the contents of commercial foods. But by the end of our explorations, we didn't think they were all that bad. We appreciated their convenience, their low cost, and the public service they perform.

Commercial pet foods are the ultimate convenience food. If by opening a can or a bag of dry food you can provide a diet that meets your pet's nutrient requirements, you have solved a major problem in pet care. Dogs and cats must be fed. The pet food industry provides an easy and inexpensive way to do that. A high proportion of dogs and cats in America are fed commercial pet foods, either exclusively or for a good part of their diet. We found no evidence that these foods routinely cause nutrient deficiencies or other health problems or shorten pets' lives (except for the accidental contaminations or errors that we wish occurred less frequently). In the absence of real research, our version of personal observation suggests that plenty of cats and dogs appear to be living long and healthy lives eating commercial pet foods.

Commercial Pet Foods Are Pretty Much Alike, Nutritionally Speaking

Pet food regulations, no matter how confusing or weak, require all foods labeled as complete and balanced to meet nutrient profiles that are generous for the requirements of most pets. In this sense, pet foods are like infant formulas; they provide complete nutrition in one food product and are nutritionally indistinguishable. Like infant formulas, the nutritional content of pet foods is governed by regulations.

For human infants, formula is a substitute for breast milk. But for pets, complete-and-balanced foods are about convenience. There are other ways to feed pets that meet nutritional requirements, although these methods may be less convenient. If pet food companies claim that their products do more for owners than other methods, we think they need to prove it. If they claim they are providing one-stop nutrition, they need to prove that too. That is why we prefer nutritional adequacy to be confirmed by feeding trials rather than by nutrient profiles.

By-Products Are By-Products, and Not Necessarily Bad

If you buy any commercial pet foods at all, you are buying ingredients that humans do not want to eat. The by-products of meat, poultry, and fish processing—rendered or not—represent a major portion of the protein and fat in most pet foods. These ingredients may be disgusting for us to think about—that's why we don't eat them—but they do not disgust dogs and cats and they have plenty of nutritional value. Even nonrendered, "human-grade" ingredients are still by-products of human food production; they are the backs, necks, wings, "racks," kidneys, spleens, lungs, and other organs and parts that humans do not usually eat.

By the time we finished this book, we had come to believe that the pet food industry performs an essential public service by providing an outlet for by-products, one far more nutritionally and environmentally friendly than any of the alternatives: burial, incineration, composting, or biofuels. As we mentioned earlier, from the standpoint of calories the 172 million dogs and cats in the United States are equivalent to 42 million people. If we fed them the same foods we ate, we would be competing fiercely with pets for the same food sources and wasting those valuable by-products.

Dogs and Cats Can Eat Grains

Ancestral dogs and cats may not have eaten grains, but after thousands of years, their progency can do so quite efficiently. Pets can use and thrive on a wide variety of plant foods, including grains that have been properly cooked. We do not expect humans to eat the way our hunter-gatherer forebears did, and we do not think pets need to be fed their primordial diet. One reason why dogs and cats have survived their long associations with humans is their adaptability. Grains and other starchy foods have their place in pet food. They supply calories and fiber along with nutrients. But if you don't want to feed grains to your pet, you don't have to. Plenty of other ingredients are available.

The Most Important Guideline for Feeding Pets Is Not to Feed Them Too Much

As it is with humans these days, obesity is the most important public health nutrition problem in pets. And just as with humans, obesity is the result of too much food and too little physical activity. Moderation applies. Foods and treats both count as sources of calories. Whenever you are tempted to give extra food or treats to your dog or cat, remember: thinner pets live longer.

Balance, Variety, and Moderation Work for Pet Food as Well as for Human Food

Whatever feeding method you choose should include ingredients that provide all necessary nutrients (balance), and a variety of different kinds of foods or ingredients in appropriate amounts. Commercial foods do this for you, but you can do this yourself at home too, as we explained in chapter 21. If you don't want to use commercial complete-and-balanced products, be sure to vary the foods you use and add the supplements that take care of the special nutritional needs of your cat and dog. Like humans, dogs and cats respond in different ways to different foods, and you can try different methods until you find one that works as well for you as it does for your pet.

Alternative Feeding Methods Are about Values, Not Nutrients

Do not misunderstand us; we value values. We prefer our own foods to be natural and organic; free of pesticides, antibiotics, and hormones; and fairly, humanely, sustainably, and locally grown and raised. And we are willing to pay more for our food to support those values. You too may be willing to pay more for pet food to accommodate your own value system, personal dietary preferences, or lifestyle. The pet food industry is more than willing to accommodate your personal choices. If you want all meat, vegetarian, kosher, or raw pet foods, the industry has a product just for you. If you live in an urban apartment, the industry makes premium products to make your life easier. Any of these alternatives can work for a pet as long as its nutritional needs are being met. So can raw and home-cooked diets. But pets, like people, are individuals. Some will respond better to some diets than others. We favor experimentation, especially because it can be quite gratifying to discover what a dog or cat likes to eat and the diet on which it best thrives.

Really, It's OK to Cook for Your Pet

Despite warnings about the dangers of do-it-yourself pet feeding, cooking for your pet doesn't have to be a big deal. If you cook for your family and enjoy preparing food, cooking for pets should pose no additional problems. Just follow the principles of balance, variety, and moderation, use recipes, and measure out the supplements to provide some nutritional insurance. Don't be afraid to add some kibble now and then, but watch the amount of food you are giving, and monitor your animal's weight. Go easy on the treats and be sure to count them in. See what your pet likes and thrives on, and do be careful to follow safe food handling procedures just as you would for any human you cook for.

Really, It's OK to Do What Works Best for You

Pets don't live long and we assume that you want to keep them as healthy as possible for as long as possible. This means doing four things: you must make sure their nutritional needs are met, they are not under- or overfed, they are willing to eat what you feed them, and you are comfortable with what they are eating. We think all four of these requirements matter. As long as whatever you do takes good care of the first three, the fourth is up to you. If by-products horrify you, you don't have to use them. If you want to feed your pet a raw diet, go ahead. If you want to mix and match different methods, that's fine too. Varying ingredients and foods is always a good idea. Just as food forms a central part of family life, feeding pets should strengthen the bonds of affection and companionship that come with living with a cat or dog.

SOME RECOMMENDATIONS

We did not intend this book to be one of those ghastly government reports with long lists of recommendations that nobody ever reads. But we are academics. We can't resist making a few final suggestions for improving pet food production, marketing, regulation, and use. We have commented on these issues throughout the book, but thought it would be useful to summarize our recommendations in a more organized way at this point.

For the Pet Food Industry

We are well aware that the pet food industry does not exist solely as a public service but must sell products and generate profits to exist. But pet foods can no longer be considered an insignificant but profitable sideline to much greater enterprises; pet foods now generate loads of money on their own. As industries mature, they must behave differently, and this industry is maturing quickly. Today's pet food industry is dominated by large, thoroughly mature consumer product companies and it is time that this segment of the industry behaved the way mature companies are expected to. The pet food industry should:

- *Adhere to AAFCO and FDA guidelines in spirit as well as letter.* High standards promote consumer confidence. In the absence of federal legislation, pet food companies have a great deal of leeway in their interpretation of guidelines for product labeling, health claims, and marketing. We have seen all too many violations of AAFCO labeling regulations on pet food packages. These confuse customers and elicit skepticism about the quality of the products. While waiting for federal legislation, the industry as a whole would be well served by a higher level of voluntary compliance with existing guidelines.
- *Make transparency the norm.* The industry seems unnecessarily secretive about its ingredient sourcing, quality controls, testing methods, and research results. We understand

that some of this secrecy may stem from perceived competitive pressures or threats from animal rights advocates, but if companies are doing what they are supposed to, greater transparency can only instill greater confidence. Animal ethicists tell us that research on pet feeding is acceptable if done appropriately, and we think more openness might help resolve the concerns of responsible groups that care about animal welfare. We are particularly concerned about secrecy in research. With human studies, investigators put research subjects at risk for the benefit of the larger human community. We think the same ethic can apply to research using dogs and cats. If research methods and results are not made available for the benefit of all pets, we view it as unethical to use that research as the basis of marketing campaigns. High-quality research, published in high-quality journals, should be standard practice for the industry and should be good for business.

- *Establish standard food safety systems—with testing for pathogens and toxins—as the industry norm.* The frequent recalls of pet foods contaminated with *Salmonella,* the 2007 recalls of those deliberately adulterated with melamine, and the mistake in manufacturing a vitamin mix in 2009 are clear indications of the inadequacy of current systems for producing safe pet food. Although no system can guarantee 100 percent safety, implementation of well-designed and faithfully followed HACCP (hazard analysis and critical control point) systems with pathogen reduction demonstrably reduces risks. HACCP systems simply require companies to identify places where contamination can occur (hazard analysis), take steps to prevent hazards at those places (critical control points), and monitor and test to make sure the procedures were followed and are effective (pathogen and hazard reduction). We think *all* pet foods should be produced according to HACCP plans and that doing so would provide a firm basis for consumer confidence in this industry.

- *Establish an industry-wide funding source for independent research.* Many important questions about the effects of diets on the health of pets remain unanswered and in need of further investigation. Without an independent source of funding, those questions are unlikely to be addressed satisfactorily. High-quality research is necessarily independent of the commercial interests of any one company. Sponsored research, especially research that is impossible to evaluate or to repeat independently, raises conflicts of interest and issues of scientific ethics. This is a problem for all pet food companies, which is why development of a common research fund, to which independent researchers can apply, might be worth serious consideration. If researchers were given absolute independence from corporate influence and complete freedom to publish, they might be able to design more objective experiments and their results might be more useful to veterinarians, owners, and the animals themselves. In the long run, independent research should benefit pet food companies, as well.

For the Rendering Industry

Whether cats and dogs, diseased animals, and other unsavory meat sources end up in pet food continues to be a source of concern to pet owners. We think this concern should be taken seriously and addressed directly by the rendering industry and by pet food companies. As we have stated throughout this book, we think the rendering industry serves society by providing a use for nutritious by-products that would otherwise be wasted. The rendering industry should:

- *Separate animal by-products of human food production from the carcasses of dogs, cats, diseased animals, and roadkill.* It makes sense to us to separate and label the rendered animal by-products of human food production (to which nobody objects) from the rendered carcasses of dogs, cats, diseased and euthanized animals, and roadkill (to which there is substantial distaste and objection).

- *Develop an independent certification program for rendered ingredients in pet foods.* Our understanding is that renderers are already separating the by-products of human food production from other such sources of rendered material. In that case, the rendering industry might benefit from creating a third-party certification program to establish standards for the composition of rendered products destined for pet foods.

For AAFCO

The role of AAFCO is a complicated one, as it mediates between state and federal regulators and the pet food industry. Even so, we think AAFCO model regulations could be strengthened in several areas. As we have stated repeatedly, we think AAFCO model regulations should:

- *Require calorie labels on pet food packages.*
- *Require sell-by dates on package labels.*
- *Provide more complete guidelines and models for the use of health claims on pet food labels.*
- *Provide more complete guidelines for the content and labeling of dietary supplements for pets.*
- *Require animal testing as the basis for determination of nutritional adequacy.*
- *Develop protocols for in-home testing as a means to establish nutritional adequacy.*

For the FDA

The FDA deals with foods intended for people, farm animals, and pets. It currently regulates pet foods as feed for farm animals. We think it is time to reconsider this approach, especially with respect to food labels. People do not generally eat pet foods, but they do buy foods for their pets. The public views pet foods as distinct from foods intended for farm animals. Congress also recognized this distinction when it instructed the FDA to work with the industry to establish federal standards for pet food contents and to develop a surveillance system for pet illnesses. Because of inconsistencies in state feed control regulations and the ambiguous role of AAFCO, we think distinct federal standards are needed for pet foods, and the sooner the better. The FDA should:

- *Establish, monitor, and enforce federal standards for ingredient definitions, contents, labeling, and the safety of pet foods.*
- *Consider developing a pet food facts label for pet foods, similar to the nutrition facts panel on human foods or the supplement facts panel on dietary supplements.*
- *Until that label is implemented, require calorie labels on pet foods.*
- *Develop standards for "truthful and not misleading" health claims on pet foods.*
- *Develop standards for the contents, labeling, and marketing of pet supplements, and require appropriate disclaimers of federal approval.*
- *Work with the pet food industry and veterinary community to establish an early warning and surveillance system for identifying episodes of adulteration and outbreaks of illness associated with pet food.*

For the USDA

The National Organic Program resides in the USDA, so that agency also is involved in pet food regulation. To resolve the lingering ambiguities in the organic status of pet foods, the USDA should move quickly to:

- *Implement, monitor, and enforce organic standards for pet foods similar to those for human foods.*

For Veterinary Schools

We are dismayed by the cozy relationship of pet food companies to veterinary schools and think some serious self-examination of conflicts of interest is much in order. To meet the needs of practicing veterinarians, the owners of dogs and cats, and pets themselves, veterinary schools should:

- *Require small animal nutrition instruction in the veterinary curriculum, with courses taught by veterinary school faculty.*
- *Promote independent small animal nutrition instruction in continuing education courses for veterinarians.*
- *Include discussions of the relationship of pet food (and other) companies to veterinary education and practice in courses in nutrition and in professional ethics.*
- *Develop, publicize, and enforce school policies regarding conflicts of interest of students and faculty with pet food (and other) companies.*
- *Insist that research sponsored by pet food companies be published and the methods and results of such research be made fully available to the veterinary science community.*

For Pet Owners

A democratic society depends on an informed citizenry willing to take responsibility for its opinions and actions. The melamine recalls of 2007 were a wake-up call to an industry that had managed to stay below the public radar for nearly a century. They also were a wake-up call to pet owners who had not given much thought to what was in the cans and bags of food they routinely fed to their dogs and cats.

Just as you have the right to know what is in your own food, where it comes from, and how it is produced—and to make food choices based on that information—your pets deserve no less. As an informed citizen in a democratic society, exercise your rights! Take responsibility, and tell the makers and sellers of the foods you buy for your pets that you care about what you are feeding them and want to know:

- *What is in pet food.*
- *Where the ingredients come from.*
- *How they were produced or made.*
- *The science behind the health claims.*
- *The truth behind marketing claims.*
- *Any conflicts of interest that might exist.*
- *How well product contents adhere to personal values.*

We think these questions matter, not only to the health and welfare of dogs and cats, but to the functioning of our democratic society. An active, informed community of pet owners can only strengthen the pet food industry and lead to better lives for all concerned, human as well as animal.

Acknowledgments

As with any research project of this scope, we received valuable and much appreciated help from colleagues, friends, and experts. For their generous sharing of information, research materials, anecdotes, or advice, we especially want to thank Elinor Blake, Mike Blanchard, Bill Bookout, Wendel Brunner, Dave Carter, Liz Clancy, Rebecca Davies, Kelly Donohue, George Fahey, Emily Fishwick, Laura Gargano, Elizabeth Hodgkins, J. Paul Jennette, Amy Johnson, Fred Kaufman, Dorothy Laflamme, Alexandra Lewin, David Lummis, Anna McCarthy, Janet McDonald, Deb McGregor, Anne Mendelson, Morten Strunge Meyer, Linda Meyers, Marie Moody, Eliza Moore, Quinton Rogers, Eva Saks, John Sauer, Michael Schaffer, Aria Sloss, Abigail Smith, Alan Stewart, Sue Tasa, Jon Tienstra, Bret Thorn, Megan Watland, Bob Weaver, Kurt Weingand, Elizabeth Weise, Jim Wirth, Frank Wu, Shiguang Yu, and Ted Zittell.

We were assisted at various times by summer interns Barbara Linhardt and Juliana Weinstein, NYU students Lauren Ercole, Maggie Lynch, Brelyn Johnson, and Lauren Roth, and most of all by Heather Catherine Inglis, then at Cornell.

We freely drew on the work of Patricia Khuly, Kelly Cassidy, and Tim Phillips and Debbie Phillips-Donaldson. For special help with library research, we thank Barbara Kolk of the American Kennel Club, Roger Gambrel of the Joliet Public Library, and the staff of the Flower Veterinary Library at Cornell and the Bobst Library at New York University.

Our deepest thanks and admiration go to the members of the pet community who welcomed us into their midst: Claudia Kawczynka of *The Bark*, Nancy Kern of *Whole Dog Journal*, Heidi Hill of Holistic Hound in Berkeley, Michael Levy and Terry Lim of Pet Food Express in the Bay Area, Tracie Hotchner of *The Dog Bible* and Dog Talk radio, Celia Sack and Paula Harris of Noe Valley Pet Co. and Omnivore Books in San Francisco, and Gina Spadafori and Christie Keith of Pet Connection.

We owe much to the pet food companies that permitted us access to their manufacturing or research facilities, and we particularly thank Bette Loughran of Bravo!, Catherine Woteki and John Rowlings of Mars, and the staffs of Hill's and of Chenango Valley for their hospitality and candor.

We also acknowledge the tolerance of the staff of other stores in which we did our research, principally Whiskers Holistic Pet Care in Manhattan; the Agway, Wegmans, and PetSmart stores in Ithaca; and Ithaca Grain & Pet Supply. Our conversations with Mary Ellen Burris and Dwight Battles about Wegmans private label pet foods were particularly enlightening.

For an education in animal welfare and the ethics of pet food research, we thank Neal Barnard and Peter Singer, as well as Alan Goldberg, Bernard Rollin, and other members and staff of the Pew Commission on Industrial Farm Animal Production.

We are grateful for the contributions of our NYU colleagues Steve Burden, Ellen Fried, Ruth Lehmann, Domingo Piñero, Lisa Sasson, Marcia Thomas, Fred Tripp, and Lisa Young. Special thanks to Sheldon Watts for computer life support and to Dean Mary Brabeck of NYU's Steinhardt School for her unfailing support of our work.

We greatly appreciate the help of Cornell colleagues Fran Kallfelz, Don Smith, Christina Stark, Sue Travis and Walter Lynn. We especially valued our many conversations with David Fraser of the University of Sydney during his annual summer visits to Cornell, and his thoughtful comments on a draft of our manuscript.

We owe much to Rebecca Saletan for her detailed comments on early versions of the book, and even more to our agent, Lydia Wills of Paradigm. Much appreciation to Maya Joseph and Rebecca Nestle for sharp-eyed proofreading. And last but not least, we thank our editor, Leslie Meredith, Donna Loffredo, and everyone else at Free Press and Simon & Schuster who made the production of this book such an extraordinarily seamless and pleasant experience.

Appendix 1

The U.S. Pet Food Industry: Facts and Figures

CATEGORIES AND SALES OF PET FOODS, U.S., 2007

PET FOOD CATEGORY	SALES, $ MILLIONS	PERCENT
Dry	8,100	48
Wet (cans and pouches)	4,700	27
Snacks and treats	2,400	14
Nonedible treats (rawhide chews)	980	6
Other pet foods	720	4
Semi-moist (patties)	130	<1
Frozen	70	<0.5
Total	17,100	100

Source: Mintel Reports, *Pet Food and Supplies—US*, August 2007.

AMOUNTS ($) AMERICANS SAY THEY SPENT
FOR THE CARE OF DOGS AND CATS, 2008

CATEGORY	DOGS	CATS
Surgical veterinary visits	532	278
Kennel boarding	273	255
Routine veterinary care	225	203
Food	229	203
Grooming, grooming aids	65	22
Vitamin supplements	61	28
Treats	64	37
Flea/tick products	76	57
Toys	40	19
Chews	32	—
Shampoo/conditioner	21	16

Source: American Pet Products Association, 2009–10 APPA *National Pet Owners Survey*.

Appendix 2

Recent History of the Pet Food Industry

SELECTED EVENTS IN THE MODERN HISTORY OF
THE U.S. PET FOOD INDUSTRY, 1953 TO 2009

YEAR	EVENT
1953	National Research Council (NRC) recommends nutrient standards for dogs.
1954	Ralston Purina develops extruded X-24 product (renamed Dog Chow in 1957). Puss 'n Boots adds thiamin (vitamin B₁) to canned fish formula.
1955	Pet food members of American Feed Manufacturers Association (AFMA) hold first convention.
1956	AFMA forms American Pet Food Manufacturers.
1957	Ralston Purina introduces Dog Chow extruded dry food. AAFCO establishes Pet Food Committee.
1958	Carnation introduces Friskies dry cat food. General Mills acquires Spratt's Patent (American). American Pet Products Manufacturers Association formed.
1959	Pet Food Institute formed.
1960	Spillers acquires Spratt's U.K., ending that company after nearly a century in business.

(continued)

YEAR	EVENT
1962	Quaker Oats establishes research facilities in Barrington, Illinois. AAFCO Pet Food Committee issues first report.
1963	H.J. Heinz acquires StarKist Foods (9Lives).
1965	PETCO opens first store.
1967	Royal Canin established.
1968	Mark Morris creates Science Diet. AAFCO Pet Food Committee issues model pet food label standards.
1969	StarKist Tuna (9Lives) introduces marketing campaign involving the tomcat Morris.
1972	Iams introduces Eukanuba line.
1973	Atlantic and Pacific Tea Co (A&P) introduces private-label pet foods.
1976	Colgate-Palmolive acquires Hill's Pet Nutrition.
1978	NRC recommends nutrient standards for cats.
1982	Clayton Mathile acquires Iams. Nestlé introduces Fancy Feast in 3-ounce cans.
1984	Anderson acquires Gaines from General Foods.
1985	Nestlé acquires Carnation (Friskies). NRC issues recommended allowances for dogs.
1986	PetSmart founded. Quaker (Ken-L-Ration, Kibbles 'n Bits) acquires Anderson-Clayton (Gaines), thereby acquiring Gainesburgers, Cycle, and Gravy Train. NRC issues recommended allowances for cats.
1987	Quaker sells Anderson-Clayton (Gaines) to Kraft.
1989	Dick Van Patten founds Natural Balance Pet Foods.
1992	AAFCO establishes dog food nutrient profiles.
1993	AAFCO establishes cat food nutrient profiles.
1994	Nestlé acquires Alpo.
1995	H.J. Heinz acquires the North American pet food businesses of Quaker Oats (Kibbles 'n Bits, Cycle, Gravy Train, Ken-L Ration).
1998	Nestlé acquires Spillers.
1999	Procter & Gamble acquires Iams.
2000	Nestlé acquires Cargill Argentina.
2001	Ralston Purina merges with Nestlé's Friskies business to create Nestlé Purina Pet Care.

(continued)

YEAR	EVENT
2002	Mars/Masterfood acquires Royal Canin. Del Monte Foods acquires pet foods of H.J. Heinz.
2006	Del Monte Foods acquires Meow Mix from Cypress Group and Milk-Bone from Kraft. Mars acquires S&M Nu Tech, maker of Greenies dog snacks; also acquires U.S. operations of Doane Pet Care. NCR issues recommended allowances for dogs and cats.
2007	Mars acquires Nutro Products, Inc. Menu Foods recalls 60 millions units of nearly 100 brands of pet foods potentially contaminated with melamine. FDA issues Food Protection Plan to ensure the safety of imported foods. Congress says AAFCO, the FDA, and pet food manufacturers must establish processing and labeling standards and an early warning and surveillance system for pet food adulteration and pet illnesses.
2008	Melamine found in human and pet food products throughout Asia and the Pacific; nearly 300,000 Chinese infants become ill from consuming melamine-tainted infant formula.
2009	*Salmonella* in products made with peanut butter sicken more than 700 people and cause at least nine deaths; Peanut Corporation of America recalls pet foods and treats made with its peanut butter. Mars recalls Nutro cat foods containing high levels of zinc.

Principal sources: 100 years of the petfood industry, *Petfood Industry*, October 2007:6–58; K. C. Grier, *Pets in America* (Chapel Hill: University of North Carolina Press, 2006), 281–291. Other sources are contemporary newspaper accounts, as well as G. Gruber, The exciting history of the pet food industry, *Petfood Industry*, September/October 1982:43–49; V. Lazar, Dog food history, *Petfood Industry*, September/October 1989:40–43; K. C. Grier, Provisioning "man's best friend": the hidden early years of the American pet food industry, in: R. Horowitz and W. Belasco, *Food Chains* (Philadelphia: University of Pennsylvania Press, 2009), 126–141.

Appendix 3

The History of Pet Food Regulation

Although you might not think so from looking at packages of pet foods in supermarkets, what goes into those packages—and what their labels say—is thoroughly determined by rules and regulations. These rules date back to the early years of the twentieth century when federal and state officials responsible for the safety and accurate labeling of feed for farm animals decided to lump rules for pet foods together with those for animal feed in efforts to prevent fraud in the feed industry. In a way, this made sense; pet foods and animal feed both serve as a means for disposing of the by-products of human food production, and some of the original pet food makers were feed manufacturers for whom the business was a profitable sideline. Both pet foods and animal feed were—and are—subject to the same kinds of fraud. For these reasons, we provide some history to describe how the present ingredients and labels on pet foods got that way.

In the United States, the need to oversee feed for farm animals became all too evident in the late 1800s. Before then, farmers fed their animals whatever foods they could grow or obtain cheaply. Commercial feeds existed but were mainly peddled to city dwellers who kept horses. Beginning in the 1870s, researchers at the USDA and universities began to study the effects of different kinds of feeds on the growth and development of farm animals. These studies demonstrated that by-products of the production of human food were rich in nutrients and had great value as feed for animals.

Wheat bran, for example, contains most of the vitamins, minerals, and fiber in wheat grains (white flour provides calories and protein but is so nutritionally depleted that it must be enriched with vitamins and iron). But because they had no use for the bran, Minneapolis flour millers routinely dumped it into the Mississippi river. Some enterprising millers figured out that it would be profitable to rescue the bran and mix it with grains to form "concentrated feeding stuff" rich in energy, protein, and other nutrients. This was soon shown to improve the production of milk by dairy cattle and of meat by cattle, pigs, and poultry. Concentrates could also be made from cottonseed meal (a by-product of cottonseed oil production), linseed meal (from linseed oil, used in paints), middlings and shorts (fine particles produced by flour milling), hominy and corn germ (from corn milling), and tankage (the residues from meat slaughter).

A commercial feed industry soon developed to sell these by-product mixtures to farmers. But the possibility that unscrupulous feed sellers could put nonnutritious materials—sawdust, for example—into these mixtures was of great concern, and for good reason. This happened so often that states soon enacted feed laws to prevent such adulteration. Connecticut passed the first state law regulating the sale of commercial feeds in 1895, and other states quickly enacted similar laws. In 1906, in the wake of Upton Sinclair's revelations of unsafe and unsanitary conditions in the meatpacking industry, Congress passed the Pure Food and Drug Act. The act was designed to prevent "the manufacture, sale, or transportation of adulterated or misbranded or poisonous or deleterious foods, drugs, medicines, and liquors, and for regulating traffic therein, and for other purposes." Although the law itself said nothing special about food for animals, let alone pets, it was widely interpreted as applying to animal feed. In effect, the 1906 Act made it illegal to produce, transport, mislabel, or sell adulterated animal feed and, by implication, pet food.

By this time, many states had passed laws governing the content and labeling of feedstuffs. Although some of these laws had similar provisions, others differed substantially. As noted earlier, AAFCO formed in 1909 to attempt to reconcile the inconsistencies. In 1913, AAFCO joined with feed manufacturing groups to propose a uniform federal feed law. This did not pass. Despite many subsequent attempts, it still has not passed.

In the early years of the twentieth century, the feed industry grew rapidly. In 1914, American farmers bought slightly less than 70,000 tons of manufactured feed; five years later, they bought more than 200,000 tons. This rapid increase made fraud a particularly acute problem. By 1918, Congress was so concerned about the widespread adulteration of animal feed that it proposed (but did not pass) federal laws to control the practice. At congressional hearings, one witness after another testified that animal feeds were commonly mixed with useless materials—sawdust and water were particular favorites—and that their animals suffered as a result. Then, as now, congressional committees were tough on federal officials. Committee members pressed Dr. John Haywood, chief of the USDA's oddly named Miscellaneous Division, Bureau of Chemistry (the forerunner of the FDA), to reveal his opinion of the nutritional value of common feed adulterants:

The Chairman: In that you would not include sawdust, would you, doctor?
Dr. Haywood: No, sir; that has no feeding value.
The Chairman: What are ivory-nut turnings?
Dr. Haywood: I believe they make buttons from ivory nuts, and they get turnings from these, which are very hard and woody and very low in protein and fat, but they have carbohydrates in them. There is considerable value in ivory-nut turnings.
The Chairman: Then would you regard it as concentrated feed?
Dr. Haywood: I would not call it concentrated feed by itself, no sir.
Representative Haugen: How about cottonseed hulls?
Dr. Haywood: They have some feeding value.

The director of New York's agricultural experiment station told the committee that 41 percent of feed samples tested in 1912 "contained what we would class as inferior ingredients; I would not use the term 'worthless,' but 'inferior.' " Since then, he said, the situation had only gotten worse; nearly 60 percent of feed samples tested poorly. But the American Feed Manufacturing Association (AFMA) sent telegrams to its members, urging them to oppose the proposed antiadulteration laws:

> [The] amendment to House bill 11949 makes it unlawful to ship or transport . . . feeding stuffs containing mill, elevator, or other sweepings or dust, buckwheat, cottonseed, oats, or other hulls, clippings, screenings, chaff, or offal from any seed or grain when separated from standard product or from cleaning or milling, peat, flax, straw, hay, etc. . . . This infamous measure will practically prohibit the shipment of every commercial mixed feed. Wire your Senators and Congressmen immediately to stop this bill.

In effect, AFMA argued that since *all* feed was adulterated with such materials, the bill was unenforceable. The hearing record makes instructive reading. It has much to say about early agricultural politics—in a classic example of the "revolving door" between government and industry, a former state official in charge of food regulation resigned to become the executive secretary of AFMA. It also reveals much about the rural nature of the United States at that time. The members of this congressional committee were extraordinarily well versed in the day-to-day details of producing and feeding farm animals. Most of them had grown up on farms and owned farms or feed businesses.

By 1918, forty-two states had passed laws to protect farmers against inferior feedstuffs and to require the contents of feeds to be listed on labels. Most states with such laws required feeds to be registered by name and brand; to provide a guaranteed analysis giving the minimum percentages of protein and fat and the maximum percentage of fiber (measures to protect against fraud); and to list the common names of the ingredients in the feed, although not necessarily in order by weight. The state feed laws also applied to pet foods, and the labels of early-twentieth-century pet foods looked much like those on feed sacks. But because the laws varied, manufacturers had to prepare different labels if they wanted to sell their products in different states.

In 1938, Congress passed the Food, Drug, and Cosmetic Act, which amended the 1906 law but retained its provisions dealing with adulteration and misbranding of foods and drugs for people and animals. The new law again said nothing specific about pet foods. Pet foods were assumed to be covered by the same statutes that applied to farm animals. The 1938 act also established the basis for forming a section on veterinary medicine within the FDA, although this did not happen until 1953. That year, 1953, marked the publication of the first recommendations of the National Research Council (NRC) for the nutrient content of dog foods—the beginning of the scientific era of pet foods.

Driving the development of these standards was widespread recognition that fraud was as much of a problem for the pet food industry as it was for the animal feed industry. Many small manufacturers were unaware of regulatory requirements (which, in any case, varied by state or were voluntary), and feed control officials often noted that pet foods in their states did not meet label guarantees.

In 1958, an industry leader, Gilbert Gruber, discussed tensions between manufacturers and regulators in an address to an AAFCO annual meeting. Gruber had founded the first commercial pet food association in 1935. At the time of his speech, he was president of the Eastern Pet Food Canners Association and editor of the trade magazine *Petfood Industry*. His message: the industry needed to do something about its public image as "dog food manipulators in a racket." Gruber, who apparently liked using capital letters for emphasis, told his audience that they must explain that "we ARE legitimate people in business and must so convince the public AND ALL CONTROL OFFICIALS." How? By making sure that pet food manufacturers were familiar with AAFCO and state standards. Yes, state regulations varied but the appropriate way to deal with this problem was quite simple: aim for the highest possible standards:

> It is generally recognized that the "most stringent" state regulation is the BELLWETHER—the rest don't count—To be safe, a manufacturer must take the lowest common denominator country-wide—and these "most stringent" regulations FROM SEVERAL STATES, gives you the UNIFORM PETFOOD LAW IN EXISTENCE RIGHT NOW.

Gruber urged pet food manufacturers to find the laws of the states that most firmly enforced rigorous standards of nutrient content and labeling and to follow those rules in both letter and spirit. By following this advice, he suggested, manufacturers would encounter no problems with state regulators. He did not mention—perhaps it was obvious—that high standards are also essential for inducing public trust in the integrity of pet food products.

In 1966, Congress passed the Fair Packaging and Labeling Act, which required the labels on all consumer products to be honest and informative. State laws continued to address labeling issues, each in its own fashion. California, for example, passed a Pure Pet Food Act in 1969; this mandated product registration, prohibited adulteration and false advertising, and required labels to provide information about the manufacturer and to list ingredients in descending order of prominence. The federal government, however, did not address the labeling of animal feed until 1976, and the first national rules for Animal Food Labeling appeared in the Code of Federal Regulations only in 1977. The 1977 Code remains in force today with only minimal changes, and continues to govern the FDA's rules for regulation of animal feed and pet food. We think this situation requires an update.

Appendix 4

Estimating Pet Food Calories

Even though most pet foods do not disclose calories, you can guess what they are from the guaranteed analysis. The guaranteed analysis lists only two components—fat and protein—that are sources of calories. It does not list carbohydrates ("nitrogen-free extract") because carbohydrates are not required in the diet of pets. Dogs and cats are perfectly able to digest, absorb, and use carbohydrates, but they also can make the sugars they need in their blood from the metabolism of amino acids and fatty acids.

The guaranteed analysis of the Whiskas dry cat food discussed in chapters 7 and 10 lists minimums of 13 percent fat and 31 percent protein, which translate into 13 grams of fat and 31 grams of protein in 100 grams of food (3.5 ounces). The guarantees also list moisture (12 percent), fiber (4.5 percent), and calcium and phosphorus (1.8 percent), none of which provides calories. The product may also contain another percent or two of unstated ash residue, but this won't make much difference and can be ignored. The only other component listed is taurine; this can be a source of calories but is present in such a small amount (0.1 percent) that it also can be ignored. The noncalorie guarantees add up to about 18 percent. We can then assume that everything other than the 13 percent fat, 31 percent protein, and 18 percent noncalorie matter is carbohydrate—38 percent or 38 grams. Now let's do the calories using the standard values for metabolizable energy for animal feed:

Fat: 13 grams × 8.5 calories per gram = 111 calories
Protein: 31 grams × 3.5 calories per gram = 109 calories
Carbohydrate: 38 grams × 3.5 calories per gram = 133 calories

This adds up to 353 calories per 100 grams of food. For this particular product, we can check our rough guess because the Whiskas website provides calorie information for this product—367. Our estimate is not bad, but a bit low, perhaps because the fat content of the food is higher than the minimum guarantee, or the fiber content is lower than its maximum.

Appendix 5

Food Needs of Alaskan Sled Racing Dogs

POUNDS OF VARIOUS KINDS OF FOOD NEEDED TO
MEET THE CALORIC REQUIREMENTS OF SIXTEEN
ALASKAN SLED DOGS RUNNING A 1,000-MILE RACE.

POUNDS	TYPE OF FOOD
FOR ALL 16 DOGS	
700	High-quality (high-fat, high-protein) dog kibble
200	Lamb, high-fat
200	Beef, medium-fat
200	Fish
100	Meat or tripe, freeze-dried
50	Beaver
50	Beef by-products
FOR THE PICKY EATERS	
30	Chicken
30	Horse
30	Turkey
30	Eggs
FOR TREATS	
120	Fats: lard, fish oil
50	Chicken or turkey skins
50	Liver

This diet is also supplemented with vitamins, minerals, bone meal, and psyllium and other sources of fiber.

Adapted from M. Collins and J. Collins, *Dog Driver: A Guide for the Serious Musher*, 2nd ed. (Crawford, CO: Alpine, 2009), 309.

Appendix 6

Resources

In researching this book, we relied upon a wide range of government, professional, and popular sources cited in the notes about the nutrition and health of cats and dogs, the ingredients in pet foods, the development of the pet food industry and its regulation, and advice to owners about what to feed their animals. On this last point, we were surprised to find that books aimed at complete pet care had so little to say about feeding issues. We attribute this omission to the existence of complete-and-balanced pet foods that take care of the vast majority of feeding issues. Even the most comprehensive books provide just a few pages on feeding dogs or cats, and these mostly tell readers to stick with dog food brands manufactured by major pet food companies. With few exceptions, we found few discussions of nutrition principles or analysis that might help owners navigate through supermarket aisles filled with competing brands and marketing claims. In contrast, other books, articles, and magazines proved to be invaluable resources. Here, we provide a short list of our personal favorites among the many resources we consulted.

Grier, K. C. *Pets in America: A History.* Chapel Hill, NC: University of North Carolina Press, 2006. Only one chapter is devoted to pet foods in this excellent history of the experience of American pet owners from colonial times to the present, but it is well worth reading. Professor Grier was the curator of a museum exhibition based on this book and provides materials from it, including a superb collection of pet food labels (alas, undated) at www.petsinamerica.org.

American Association of Feed Control Officials. *AAFCO Official Publication.* Oxford, IN: AAFCO, 2009. This publication, updated every year, is *the* resource for finding out about ingredient definitions, labeling requirements, nutrient profiles, and testing protocols; identifying the nutrient content of pet food ingredients; and learning who's who on AAFCO committees.

National Research Council. *Nutrient Requirements of Dogs and Cats.* **Washington, DC: National Academies Press, 2006.** The pet equivalent of the human *Dietary Reference Intakes* (formerly *Recommended Dietary Allowances*), this 398-page summary of research on the nutrient needs of cats and dogs is well referenced and authoritative. Readers may disagree with some of the conclusions—this is, after all, a committee report—but it is the starting place for anyone interested in the research basis of AAFCO model regulations.

Even better, the committees that prepared this report took the trouble to summarize its most important take-home messages in pamphlets for dog and cat owners and to make them available online at no cost. See: *Your Dog's Nutritional Needs: A Science-Based Guide for Pet Owners,* at http://dels.nas.edu/dels/rpt_briefs/dog_nutrition_final.pdf, and *Your Cat's Nutritional Needs: A Science-Based Guide for Pet Owners,* at http://dels.nas.edu/dels/rpt_briefs/cat_nutrition_final.pdf.

Hand MK, Thatcher CD, Remillard RL, Roudebush P. eds. *Small Animal Clinical Nutrition,* **4th ed. Topeka, KS: Mark Morris Institute, 2000.** This tome includes nearly 1,200 pages devoted to the principles of nutrition for cats and dogs as well as clinical applications. The Mark Morris Institute is an offshoot of Hill's Pet Nutrition (Colgate-Palmolive) and some of its editors work for Hill's, but the book gets the facts right and the opinions seem fair and well balanced. We adapted the basic recipes for home-cooked meals for cats and dogs in chapter 21 from this book.

MacDonald ML, Rogers QR, and Morris, JG. Nutrition of the domestic cat, a mammalian carnivore. *Annual Review of Nutrition* **1984;4:521–62.** Although getting on in years, this review of basic cat nutrition remains a standard reference in the field.

Kvamme JL, Phillips TD, eds. *Petfood Technology.* **Mt. Morris, IL: Watt Publishing, 2003.** This is the basic reference—an encyclopedia, really—on how to make pet food: wet, semi-moist, or dry.

Meeker DL, ed. *Essential Rendering—All about the Animal By-Products Industry.* **Alexandria, VA: National Renderers Association, 2006,** available online at http://national renderers.org/assets/essential_rendering_book.pdf. Questions about rendering and byproducts are so controversial that it is refreshing to find the National Renderers Association taking them on in such a candid and enlightened way. The book is written from the perspective of the industry but the information is fascinating and difficult to obtain anywhere else.

Petfood Industry. **Watt Publishing, Rockford, IL,** at www.petfoodindustry.com. This is *the* trade publication for this industry. Appearing monthly, the magazine works hard to keep the industry informed about current events likely to affect competition and sales. The articles are interesting and well edited, and pitched at a thoughtful readership.

Whole Dog Journal. **Belvoir Media Group, Norwalk, CT,** at www.whole-dog-journal .com. Described as a "monthly guide to natural dog care and training," this publication focuses occasionally on feeding issues, and when it does it becomes the *Consumer Reports* of alternative and unconventional dog foods and feeding practices.

Bark: *The Modern Dog Culture Magazine.* **Berkeley, CA:** The Bark, at www.thebark .com. We love its slogan, "Dog is my co-pilot," and think this bi-monthly magazine deserves its reputation as *The New Yorker* of dog publications. We are not exactly objective about this; we occasionally contribute to it.

List of Tables and Figures

FIGURES   PAGE

Notes

Abbreviations

Am	*American*
AAFCO	Association of American Feed Control Officials
APPA	American Pet Products Association (until 2009, APPMA)
APPMA	American Pet Products Manufacturers Association (now APPA)
AVMA	American Veterinary Medical Association
FDA	Food and Drug Administration
J	*Journal, Journal of*
JAMA	*Journal of the American Medical Association*
JAMVA	*Journal of the American Veterinary Medical Association*
NRC	National Research Council
NYT	*New York Times*
U	University
USDA	U.S. Department of Agriculture
WSJ	*Wall Street Journal*

Note: all Internet links were accessible in September 2009.

Chapter 1. Introduction

8 *Let's begin by:* The store has 7.5 center aisles, each 120 feet long, devoted to packaged foods. The 13 percent overestimates the proportion of pet foods as some of its shelves are devoted to foods for birds, fish, and small reptiles, and the store also has peripheral sections for produce, meat, dairy, frozen foods, bakery goods, prepared foods, candy, supplements, consumer products, and a restaurant.

Chapter 2. What Pets Ate

14 *It makes no:* Wang X, Tedford RH. Evolutionary history of canids, and Savolainen P. Domestication of dogs. In: Jenson P, ed. *The Behavioural Biology of Dogs.* Wallingford, UK: CABI International, 2007:3–37.

14 *The fossil history:* Breeds have to do with appearances ("stereotypes") as well as behavioral characteristics. Some aspects of the genetic basis of size, shape, and breed have been defined. See Sutter NB, et al. A single IGF1 allele is a major determinant of small size in dogs. *Science* 2007;316:112–15, and Jones P, et al. Single-nucleotide-polymorphism-based association of dog stereotypes. *Genetics* 2008;179:1033–44. Coppinger R, Coppinger L. *Dogs: A Startling New Understanding of Canine Origin, Behavior & Evolution.* New York, Scribner, 2001.

15 *During the 7,000:* Petrie WMF. *Social Life in Ancient Egypt.* New York: Houghton Mifflin, 1923:42,139–40. James TGH. *An Introduction to Ancient Egypt.* New York: Farrar, Straus & Giroux, 1979:31,112.

16 *The best guess:* Driscoll CA, et al. The Near Eastern origin of cat domestication. *Science* 2007;317 (July 27):519–23. Vigne J-D et al. Early taming of the cat in Cyprus. *Science* 2004;304:259.

16 *As is the:* Langton N, Langton B. *The Cat in Ancient Egypt.* London: Kegan Paul, 2002. Montet P. *Everyday Life in Ancient Egypt.* New York: St. Martin's Press, 1958:64–68.

16 *The precise role:* Morrison-Scott TCS. The mummified cats of ancient Egypt. *Proceedings of the Zoological Society London* 1952;121:861–67.

17 *Following the:* Donalson MD. *The Domestic Cat in Roman Civilization.* Lewiston, NY: Edwin Mellen Press, 1999:1–19.

18 *Let's start with:* Jesse E. *Anecdotes of Dogs.* London: H.G. Bohn, 1858:483–84. See Anderson J. *Recreations in Agriculture, Natural-History, Arts, and Miscellaneous Literature,* Vol. III. London: John Cumming, 1800:90. Comstock AB. *The Pet Book,* 2nd ed. Ithaca, NY: Comstock Publishing, 1915:11–13.

18 *The natural food:* Jesse E. *Anecdotes of Dogs.* London: H.G. Bohn:1858:483–84.

18 *Besides meat:* Herbert HW. *Frank Forester's Field Sports of the United States and British Provinces of North America,* Vol. 1. New York: W.A. Townsend & Co., 1860: 346–347. Fernandez A. Dinner is served: a history of dog food. *Dogs in Review,* December 2004:8–12.

19 *Sheep-heads:* Hill JW. *The Management and Diseases of the Dog,* 5th ed. London: Swan Sonnenschein & Co, 1900:1–8.

19 *In the fourth:* Stonehenge. *The Dog in Health and Disease.* London: Longman, Green, Longman, and Roberts, 1859:204–5.

19 *And what about:* James RK, ed. *The Angora Cat: How to Breed, Train, and Keep It.* Boston: James Bros, 1898:16–18. Buckworth-Herne-Soame E. *Cats: Long-Haired and Short: Their Breeding, Rearing & Showing.* London: Methuen, 1933:8–11.

Chapter 3. What Pets Need

23 *We mentioned:* Carpenter KJ. A short history of nutritional science: parts 2 (1885–1912) and 3 (1912–1944). *J Nutrition* 2003;133:975–84 and 3023–32. MacDonald ML, Rogers QE, Morris JG. Nutrition of the domestic cat, a mammalian carnivore. *Annual Review of Nutrition* 1984;4:521–62.

24 *Humans and dogs:* Meat is a good source of vitamin A. Liver is a better source but vitamin A is toxic at high doses. Only small amounts should be fed to cats and kittens. See
Seawright AA, English PB. Hypervitaminosis A and deforming cervical spondylosis
of the cat 1967. *J Comparative Pathology* 77:29–39.

24 *Human skin:* Unless dogs and cats are outdoors for many hours a day, they will not
make enough vitamin D. How KL, Hazewinkel HAW, Mol JA. Dietary vitamin D de-
pendance of cat and dog due to inadequate cutaneous synthesis of vitamin D. *General
and Comparative Endocrinology* 1994;96:12–18.

25 *By the early:* Earle IP. Nutritional Requirements of Dogs. In: *USDA Yearbook of Agriculture*, 1939:844–55. Speelman SR. Feeding Dogs. In: *USDA Yearbook of Agriculture*,
1939:856–70. Baird J. *The Standard Book of Household Pets*. Garden City, NJ: Halcyon
House, 1948:114–202.

26 *Many cat owners:* Advertisement *NYT*, November 5, 1953.

26 *Since 1953:* The other organizations are the National Academy of Sciences, the Institute of Medicine, and the National Academy of Engineering. The National Academies are at www.nationalacademies.org/about.

27 *The NRC established:* Ullrey D. Landmark and historic contributions of NRC's Committee on Animal Nutrition. In: Committee on Animal Nutrition, National Research Council. *Scientific Advances in Animal Nutrition: Promise for the New Century*.
Washington, DC: National Academy Press, 2002:7.

27 *The NRC's first:* The committee chair, H. E. Robinson, worked at Swift and Co. Other
members were G. R. Cowgill, a physiologist from Yale; P. H. Phillips, a biochemist
from U Wisconsin; R. H. Udall from Cornell; and Agnes Fay Morgan.

28 *Difficulties associated:* Committee on Animal Nutrition, National Research Council.
Nutrient Requirements of Dogs, rev. 1972.

28 *In this revision:* Letter from Tony J. Cunha, chair, Committee on Animal Nutrition,
National Research Council. In: *Nutrient Requirements of Dogs*, rev. 1974. Washington, DC: National Academy of Sciences, 1974. The report suggested amounts of protein ranging from 1.6 (adult maintenance) to 13 (lactation) g/kg body weight$^{0.73}$ per
day. For adult dogs, this worked out to 4.8 g protein per kg body weight.

29 *As for cats:* The 1986 cat subcommittee was chaired by Quinton Rogers, UC Davis.
Other members were David Baker, U Illinois; K. C. Hayes, Brandeis U (who discov-
ered the requirement for taurine in cats); Peter Kendall, Pedigree Foods, and James
Morris, UC Davis.

29 *In 2006:* National Research Council. *Nutrient Requirements of Dogs and Cats*. Washington, DC: National Academies Press, 2006. Institute of Medicine. Dietary Reference Intake Research Synthesis, at www.iom.edu.

30 *The European:* FEDIAF. *Nutritional Guidelines for Complete and Complementary Pet
Food for Cats and Dogs*. Brussels: European Pet Food Industry Federation, February 2008. National Research Council. *Your Dog's Nutritional Needs: A Science-Based
Guide for Pet Owners*. Washington, DC: National Academies, 2006. It and the parallel
report for cats are at http://dels.nas.edu.

30 *AAFCO did not:* AAFCO. *Official Publications*, 1957, 1962, 1968, and Report of the
Pet Food Labeling Committee, October 1961, AAFCO, 1962.

Chapter 4. Inventing Commercial Pet Foods

33 *Everyone who writes:* The history of kibble. Online, unreferenced and unexplained at http://jenniferlennon.com/home.html. Gruber G. The exciting history of the pet food industry. *Petfood Industry,* September/October 1982:45–49. Also see *Petfood Industry,* January/February 1975. The date for Spratt's patent is usually cited as 1860 but the application is dated November 15, 1861; he obtained provisional protection on November 29. See Agricultural Patents for the year 1861, in: *J Royal Agricultural Society of England,* Vol. 23. London: John Murray, 1862:495. For information about Spratt's pet food company, see Myers WS, ed. *The Story of New Jersey,* Vol. 5. New York: Lewis Historical Publications, 1945:667–68 (reprinted as *Prominent Families of New Jersey,* Vol. 1. Baltimore: Clearfield, 2000); the entry is unreferenced.

34 *Decades before: Sporting Magazine.* London: Rogerson and Tuxford, 1792:250, and 1826:163.

34 *By the 1850s:* Simmonds PL *Dictionary of Trade Products: Commercial, Manufacturing and Technical Terms.* London: G. Routledge & Co., 1858: 129. Timbs J. *Curiosities of London.* London: David Bogue: 1855:741. Hassall AH. *Food Adulterations; Comprising the Reports of the Analytical Sanitary Commission of "The Lancet," for the Years 1851 to 1854 Inclusive.* London: Longman, Brown, Green & Longmans: 177.

34 *Spratt took full:* Woodcroft B. *Chronological Index of Patentees and Applicants for Patents of Invention.* London, Office of the Commissioners of Patents for Inventions, 1868. Cobbold TS. *The Internal Parasites of Our Domesticated Animals.* London: The Field Office, 1873:145. The testimonial is dated 15 May 1873. *Baily's Magazine: Sports and Pastimes,* Vol. 32. London: A.H. Baily & Co, 1878:246–47.

35 *Spratt also made:* Stables WG. *The Domestic Cat.* Gordon Stables, 1876:61. Jennings J. *Domestic or Fancy Cats.* London: L. Upcott Gill, 1893:52–57.

35 *In the 1870s:* Grier KC. Provisioning "Man's best friend": the hidden early years of the American pet food industry. In: Horowitz R, Belasco W. *Food Chains.* Philadelphia: U Pennsylvania Press, 2009:126–41. Advertisement. Westminster Kennel Club. Catalogue: Sixth Annual New York Bench Show, April 18, 19, 20, 21, 1882.

36 *Spratt's soon:* What to feed your dog. In: *The St. Louis Exposition: World's Work.* New York: Doubleday, August 1904.

36 *But by the:* Some examples: "I consider professor Woodroffe Hill's Biscuits are model ones, and fully deserve the title 'perfect' " (advertisement in *Western Field,* February 1907:26). "Dear Sirs, I have used your [*Champion*] Dog Biscuit in my kennels for several years and find my dogs relish it, and thrive on it better than any food I have ever used." Champion Dog Biscuits were advertised in dog, sports, and literary magazines at least as late as 1938 (*The Literary Digest,* 1938:902). Comstock AB. *The Pet Book,* 2nd ed. Ithaca, NY: Comstock Publishing, 1915:12. Speelman SR. Feeding Dogs. In: *USDA Yearbook of Agriculture,* 1939:860.

36 *Today, vitamin:* Advertisement in the *NYT,* October 13, 1930.

36 *If your dog:* Advertisement in the *NYT,* April 14, 1940. Vitamin G referred to riboflavin, later understood to be a B-vitamin.

37 *Until the early:* Grier KC, *Pets in America: A History.* Chapel Hill: University of North Carolina Press, 2006. Grier K. Provisioning "man's best friend": the hidden early years of the American pet food industry. In: Horowitz R, Belasco W. *Food Chains.* Philadelphia: U Pennsylvania Press, 2009:126–41.

37 *From the beginning:* Ralston Purina originated in 1894 with William H. Danforth's Purina Mills farm feed. In 1898, his Robinson-Danforth Commission Company added Ralston cereal. The company name changed to Ralston Purina in 1902. Ralston cereal, the invention of health guru Webster Edgerly, was an acronym of Regime. Activity, Light, Strength, Temptation, Oxygen, and Nature. The origins of Chappel Bros. are discussed in Marquette AF. *Brands, Trademarks and Good Will: The Story of the Quaker Oats Company.* New York: McGraw-Hill, 1967:174–91.

38 *The history of:* The A&P advertisement on June 16, 1932, listed other prices: bananas 5¢/lb, oranges 15 for 25¢.

38 *A 1935 advertisement:* A dog's life to be pretty nice with food guarded by code. *Washington Post,* April 9, 1934. Sails to kill sea lions; Pacific skipper expects to get 1,200 for dog and cat food. *NYT,* February 13, 1938.

38 *In 1939, the:* Speelman SR. Feeding Dogs. In: *USDA Yearbook of Agriculture,* 1939: 856–70.

39 *During the 1940s:* Grier KC. Pets in America (Museum Exhibit), 2005–2008. Her label collection is at www.petsinamerica.org/petfoodlabels.htm.

39 *Horse meat continued:* New curb on horse meat. *NYT,* August 11, 1943. Horne LS. Horse meat fraud found widespread. *NYT,* January 28, 1952.

40 *But some American:* Goodman M. Those "pets" sure eat an awful lot of horsemeat. *Los Angeles Times,* August 3, 1973.

40 *Indeed, "this mental:* In 1980, 270,000 horses were slaughtered in the United States, largely for food for export. The numbers dropped to 92,000 in 2005. In 2006, the courts required the USDA to stop inspecting horse slaughterhouses, which effectively shut them down. Some, however, reopened under private inspection, and horses continue to be shipped to Mexico for slaughter. In the face of proposed legislation to abolish horse slaughter entirely, the numbers dropped to about 1,500 a month in 2007. See USDA. National Agricultural Statistics Service. Equine slaughter at www.nass.usda .gov. For information about the current state of legislation, see "End horse slaughter permanently," Humane Society of the United States at www.hsus.org.

Chapter 5. Pet Foods as an Industry

41 *Since the days:* APPA. *2009–2010 APPA National Pet Owners Survey.* Greenwich, CT: APPA, 2009.

41 *The industry that:* APPA. Pet pampering and pet health insurance drive pet industry sales to another all time high (press release), February 15, 2008, at www.appa.org.

42 *Pet foods account:* Countries of the world. *Gross National Product distribution—2005.* at www.studentsoftheworld.info/infopays/rank/PNB2.html. U.S. Census Bureau. Annual Survey of Manufacturers, Sector 31, 2006, at http://factfinder.census.gov.

43 *The growth of:* Nelson T. The billion dollar pet food market. *Feedstuffs,* July 19, 1969:38. The quotation is from "Irrationality in the pet food business." *Fortune,* October 8, 1990, at http://money.cnn.com/magazines/fortune/fortune_archive.

44 *Indeed, pet food:* It is not easy to identify products owned by a specific company. Del Monte, for example, lists most—but not all—of its foods and treats on its website, www.delmonte.com. The site does not include Skippy or Cycle foods although the websites of these products (www.skippydog.com, www.cyclenatural.com) clearly identify Del Monte as their parent company.

46 *Milk-Bone played:* Authors were investigative reporters Bryan Burrough and John Helyar. Nestle M. *Food Politics* (U. California Press, rev. ed., 2007) provides a chronology of the events leading up to Philip Morris's purchase of Nabisco Holdings in 2000. The company subsequently changed its name to Altria, and divested Kraft in 2007.

46 *One final point: Colgate-Palmolive Company 2008 Annual Report,* at www.colgate .com. Also see Funding Universe: Colgate-Palmolive at www.fundinguniverse.com.

47 *If you want:* Global Market Information Database. *Global Market for Pet Food and Pet Care Products.* Chicago: Euromonitor International, 2007.

47 *Virtually all:* Pet Food Institute. What is PFI?, 2006, at www.petfoodinstitute.org. What foods are imported from China? Cattle Network, July 8, 2009, at www.cattle network.com.

48 *As we discussed:* Packaged Facts. *Pet Food in the U.S.* MarketResearch.com, September 2006.

50 *Nestlé Purina PetCare:* PetfoodIndustry.com e-newsletter, June 17, 2008.

Chapter 6. Pet Foods: Wet and Dry

57 *Because the processes:* Nestle M. *Pet Food Politics: The Chihuahua in the Coal Mine.* Berkeley, U California Press, 2008.

59 *Preconditioning and extrusion:* Kvamme JL, Phillips TD. *Petfood Technology.* Mt. Morris, IL: Watt Publishing, 2003.

60 *Semi-moist foods:* Christopher MM, Perlman V, Eaton JW. Contribution of propylene glycol–induced Heinz body formation to anemia in cats. *JAVMA* 1989;194:1045–56. Mintel Reports. *Pet Food and Supplies.* Chicago: Mintel International Group, August 2007.

60 *Wet foods are sold:* Edley D, Moss J, Plant T. Wet petfood manufacture. In: Kvamme JL, and Phillips TD, eds., *Pet Food Technology.* Mt. Morris, IL: Watt Publishing, 2003:382–88.

Chapter 7. The Ingredients

66 *The amount of salt:* Hand MS, et al., eds. *Small Animal Clinical Nutrition.* Topeka, KS: Mark Morris Institute, 2000:1081–82.

68 *CBC: Old boots:* Canadian Broadcasting Corporation. A Dog's Breakfast (video-script), December 12, 2007.

70 *If the meat:* Aldrich G. Chicken first: marketing ploy or quality enhancement? *Petfood Industry,* May 2007, at www.petfoodindustry.com.

72 *How nutritious:* Murray SM, et al. Raw and rendered animal by-products as ingredients in dog diets. *J Animal Science* 1997;75:2497–505. Zuo Y, et al. Digestion responses to low oligosaccharide soybean meal by ileally-cannulated dogs. *J Animal Science* 1996;74:2441–49. Yamka U, et al. Evaluation of low-ash poultry meal as a protein source in canine foods—1. *J Animal Science* 2003;81:2279–84.

73 *If the notion:* Greenberg P. Cat got your fish? *NYT,* March 22, 2009:WK10. Food and Agriculture Organization of the United Nations. *Fishmeal Market Report,* May 2007, at www.globefish.org/index.php?id=4098.

75 *As mentioned:* McDonald ML, Rogers QR, Morris JG. In: Nutrition of the domestic cat, a mammalian carnivore. *Annual Review of Nutrition* 1984;4:521–62. Kvamme JL, Phillips TD, eds. *Pet Food Technology.* Mt. Morris, IL: Watt Publishing, 2003.

77 *The Whiskas label:* Coelho M. Vitamins and carotenoids in pet care. In: Kvamme JL, Phillips TD, eds. *Pet Food Technology,* Mt. Morris, IL: Watt Publishing, 2003:101–20.

77 *AAFCO model:* Required minerals are calcium, phosphorus, sodium, chlorine, iodine, potassium, magnesium, iron, copper, selenium, zinc, and manganese. Evidence suggests that some animals also require molybdenum, chromium, arsenic, boron, silicon, arsenic, vanadium, and nickel.

78 *The fats sprayed:* Phillips T. Antioxidant options. *Petfood Industry,* October 2008: 32–33.

78 *The FDA considers:* Coast Guard, Department of Homeland Security. Carriage of solid hazardous materials in bulk, fishmeal or scrap, ground or pelletized. *Code of Federal Regulations,* 46CFR148.04–9, October 1, 2008.

78 *In the 1980s:* Dzanis DA. Safety of ethoxyquin in dog foods. *J Nutrition* 1991;121:163s–64s. Ethoxyquin is approved for use in human food for preserving spices, such as cayenne and chili powder, at a level of 100 ppm, but humans do not eat much chili powder. FDA finds no adverse health effects from ethoxyquin, November 2, 1989, at www.fda.gov.

79 *In 1997, even:* FDA requests that ethoxyquin levels be reduced in dog foods, August 14, 1997, at www.fda.gov.

79 *Potentially cancer-causing:* Get the facts: What's really in pet food, at www.api4 animals.org.

79 *Some authors of:* Weiskopf J. *Pet Food Nation.* New York: Collins, 2007:68. Strombeck DR. *Home-Prepared Dog & Cat Diets.* Ames, IA: Blackwell Publishing, 1999:55.

80 *No doubt as:* The Whiskas website is at www.whiskas.com.

Chapter 8. The Rendered Ingredients

81 *Much concern about:* See Frederick LD, Robinson HE. Canine nutritional deficiency diseases. *JAVMA* 1941;98:288–94.

81 *Consider the numbers:* USDA. Livestock slaughter, 2007 annual summary, March 2008, and USDA. Poultry slaughter, 2007 annual summary, February 2008, at http:// usda.mannlib.cornell.edu/usda. Breitmeyer RE, Hamilton CR, and Kirstein D. The rendering industry's contribution to public and animal health. In: Meeker DL, ed. *Essential Rendering: All About the Animal By-Products Industry.* Alexandria, VA: National Renderers Association, 2006:82.

82 *Instead, practically:* Meeker DL, Hamilton CR. An overview of the rendering industry 2006. In: Meeker DL, ed. *Essential Rendering: All About the Animal By-Products Industry.* Alexandria, VA: National Renderers Association, 2006:1–17. In this same book, also see Aldrich G. Rendered products in pet food, 159–77.

82 *In researching:* Thixton S. Could risky meat by-products be turned into energy? AmericanChronicle.com, August 4, 2008. The Cornell Veterinary College is building just such a facility and expects it to go into operation in 2009.

84 *Cows are ruminants:* See Nestle M. *Safe Food: The Politics of Food Safety,* rev. ed. Berkeley: U California Press, 2010 (last chapter), and *What to Eat.* New York: North

Point Press, 2006 (chapter on meat safety). Also see Rampton S, Stauber J. *Mad Cow U.S.A.* Monroe, ME: Common Courage Press, 2004; and Schwartz M. *How the Cows Turned Mad.* Berkeley: U California Press, 2004. For BSE in cats, see Cornell U College of Veterinary Medicine. Veterinary information brief: mad cow disease and cats, November 15, 2006, at www.vet.cornell.edu. U.K. statistics on cat prion disease are from the British Department for Environment, Food and Rural Affairs, March 3, 2008, at www.defra.gov.uk.

84 *BSE is an unusual:* Department for Environment, Food and Rural Affairs. Review of the origin of BSE, July 5, 2001, at www.defra.gov.uk.

84 *In the United:* FDA. Substances prohibited in animal food or feed: proposed rule. *Federal Register,* October 6, 2005:58569–58601. USDA. Agriculture secretary Ed Schafer announces plan to end exceptions to animal handling rule (news release), May 20, 2008, at www.usda.gov.

85 *Federal agencies cite:* Stecklow S. Porous borders: despite assurances, U.S. could be at risk for mad cow disease. *WSJ,* November 28, 2001.

85 *That was in 2001:* General Accounting Office. Mad cow disease: improvements in the animal feed ban and other regulatory areas would strengthen U.S. prevention efforts (GAO-02–183), January 2002:3. FDA Science Board. Science and Mission at Risk: Report of the Subcommittee on Science and Technology, November 2007, at www .fda.gov.

85 *So where does:* Lysek DA, et al. Prion structures of cats, dog, pigs, and sheep. *Proceedings of the National Academy of Sciences* 2005;102:640–45.

86 *As this third:* Martin AN. *Foods Pets Diet For: Shocking Facts about Pet Food*, 3rd ed. Troutdale, OR: NewSage Press, 2008:25.

86 *Yes this is:* Franko DA. Animal disposal. The environmental, animal disease, and public health related implications: an assessment of options, April 8, 2002, at www .rendermagazine.com. Ockerman HW, Hansen CL. *Animal By-Product Processing.* Chichester UK: Ellis Horwood, 1988.

87 *Considerable evidence:* Simon S. Outcry over pets in pet food. *Los Angeles Times,* January 6, 2002. Parish, N. County facility begins cremating animals; facility is for dogs and cats, usually strays, that are euthanized. *St. Louis Post Dispatch,* October 2, 2003. Berry K. Export ban leads to pileup of dead beasts at rendering facility. *Los Angeles Business J,* March 22, 2004.

87 *Gruesome, definitely:* Kibbles and bits. *St. Louis Post Dispatch,* December 26, 2001.

87 *At about that time:* FDA/CVM. Report on the risk from pentobarbital in dog food, February 28, 2002, at www.fda.gov.

88 *The FDA concluded:* Myers MJ, et al. Development of a polymerase chain reaction–based method to identify species-specific components in dog food. *Am J Veterinary Research* 2004;65:99–103.

89 *As for the alternatives:* Lazaroff C. Euthanized animals can kill wildlife. *Environment News Service,* October 10, 2002, at www.ens-newswire.com. Rourke K. Euthanized animals can poison wildlife. *JAMVA* 2002;220:146–47.

Chapter 9. Who Sets Pet Food Rules?

 90 *The pet food industry:* Pet Food Institute. Pet food report: regulation and safety test-ing (undated), at www.petfoodreport.com.
 91 *Individual states:* AAFCO. Syverson D. Questions and answers concerning pet food regulations (undated, but probably 2007) at www.aafco.org.
 92 *As we mentioned:* AAFCO. *Official Publication* 2009.
 93 *AAFCO also works:* The group advocates for improved pet food regulations, labeling, and inspection at www.defendourpets.org.
 94 *In 2008 alone:* FDA. Pet food, at www.fda.gov.
 95 *ConsumerAffairs.com filed:* Nutro Products. Nutro products announces voluntary recall of limited range of dry cat food products, May 21, 2009 at www.nutproducts .com. McCormick LW. Tests find "ski high" zinc levels in Nutro cat food, June 18, 2009 at www.consumeraffairs.com. Keith C. Lax oversight of pet food safety hurts us all, May 14, 2009 at www.sfgate.com. Pet Food Products Safety Alliance. News updates, June 14, 2009 at www.pfpsa.org/news.html.

Chapter 10. What's on Those Labels?

 99 *Reading a pet food:* AAFCO. *AAFCO Pet Food and Specialty Pet Food Labeling Guide.* Oxford, IN, 2008. Dzanis DA. Interpreting pet food labels. FDA, at www.fda.gov.
 99 *Even so, hardly:* Haberl A, Kilgos K, Buffington T. Comparison of owners' and vet-erinarians' perceptions, knowledge, and use of nutritional information on pet food labels [research abstract]. *Proceedings, 2001 Purina Nutrition Forum,* 2002;24(9a):84.
103 *The AAFCO label:* Federal Trade Commission. *Report of the Federal Trade Commis-sion on Commercial Feeds.* Washington, DC, March 29, 1921.
103 *The guaranteed analysis:* Hill RC, et al. Comparison of the guaranteed analysis with the measured nutrient composition of commercial pet foods. *JAMVA* 2009;234: 347–51.
105 *The amount of:* The essential amino acids for dogs and cats are arginine, histidine, isoleucine, leucine, lysine, methionine, phenylalanine, threonine, tryptophan, and valine.
106 *Dogs and cats can:* Fat chemistry: Fats are triglycerides made up of three long-chain fatty acids bound to a small sugar (glycerol). Fatty acids that are fully hydrogenated are saturated; those with one unsaturated double bond are called unsaturated; and those with more than one unsaturated double bond are polyunsaturated. Two unsat-urated fatty acids, linoleic acid (omega-6) and alpha-linolenic acid (omega-3) cannot be made in the body and must be consumed from food. The term "fat" usually refers to more highly saturated food fats; these tend to be solid at room temperature. Oils have a higher proportion of unsaturated and polyunsaturated fatty acids and tend to be liquid at room temperature. Solid fats usually come from animals (beef tallow, lard) although tropical oils are exceptions. Oils generally come from seeds (corn, soybean, rapeseed, nuts) or, sometimes, fruits (olives, avocados).
106 *All food fats:* McAlister KG, et al. Canine lipoproteins and lecithin: acyl transferase activities in dietary oil supplemented dogs. *Veterinary Clinical Nutrition* 1996;3:50–56. NRC. *Nutrient Requirements of Cats and Dogs.* Washington, DC: National Acad-emies Press, 2006.

111 *All of this:* Morris JG, Rogers QR. Assessment of the nutritional adequacy of pet foods through the life cycle. *J Nutrition* 1994;124:2520s–34s.

Chapter 11. The Pet Food Marketplace: Segments

116 *Much has been:* See special issue of *J Business Research*, Vol. 61, 2008. Lancendorfer KM, Atkin JL, Reece BB. Animals in advertising: love dogs? Love the ad! (pp. 384–91). Kennedy PF, McGarvey MG. Animal-companion depictions in women's magazine advertising (pp. 424–30). Dotson MJ, Hyatt EM. Understanding dog-human companionship (pp. 457–66). Jones D. You're not sick, you're just in love. *NYT*, February 12, 2006. Mostly, see Schaffer M. *One Nation Under Dog.* New York: Henry Holt, 2009.

116 *Pet humanization:* Dale S. Hugs and a little help from our four-legged friends (undated), at www.goodnewsforpets.com.

116 *As a vastly:* Holbrook MB, Woodside AG. Animal companions, consumption experiences, and the marketing of pets—transcending boundaries in the animal-human distinction. *J Business Research* 2008;61:377–81.

116 *Pets, according to:* Ehart T. "Humanization" top trend fueling growth in $43 billion global pet food market, June 4, 2007 at www.sys-con.com.

117 *Companies state:* Fass A. Marketing animal house. Forbes.com, February 12, 2007, at www.forbes.com. 100 leading national advertisers. *Advertising Age*, June 22, 2009.

117 *One strategy for:* Packaged Facts. *Pet Food in the U.S.: Cat Food*; and *Pet Food in the U.S.: Dog Food*, January 2009.

119 *These figures do not:* Letter from Melissa Hillyer, Media Coordinator, Starcom, November 13, 2007. The recipient requested anonymity.

119 *Whatever sums:* Colgate-Palmolive Annual Report, 2007. 100 leading national advertisers. *Advertising Age*, June 22, 2009.

119 *We must now:* Trade commission cases: orders issued on ads for dog food and tooth powder. *NYT*, January 3, 1940.

120 *In 1969, the:* Federal Trade Commission. Request for comment concerning guides for the dog and cat food industry. *Federal Register*, 64 FR 13368, March 18, 1999. The guides were originally published at 34 FR 3619, February 28, 1969. FTC issued the rescission in 1999.

120 *Today, problems:* Neff J. NAD rejects P&G pet-food claim. *Advertising Age*, August 28, 2007.

121 *Trying to feed:* Email from Anne Mendelson to M. Nestle, February 2, 2008. Used with permission.

124 *In judging prices:* Woon E. Is petfood recession-proof? *Petfood Industry*, September 2008:28–33.

128 *This is brilliant:* Royal Canin. The Poodle, at www.royalcanin.us.

Chapter 12. Products at a Premium

129 *Pet product trade:* Banasiak K. Pampering your pet. *Food Technology*, November 2006:34–42.

129 *In turn, the:* APPMA. *2007–2008 APPMA National Pet Owners Survey.* Greenwich, CT: APPMA, 2008.

130 *Among the alternatives:* Organic Trade Association. *2006 Manufacturer Survey*, at www.ota.com. Sales of organic, natural pet food skyrocket after 2007 recall. *Nutrition Business J*, March/April 2008:34–35.

131 *AAFCO is able:* Crowley L. HFCS is natural, says FDA in a letter, July 8, 2008, at www.foodnavigator-usa.com. USDA. FSIS issues advance notice of proposed rulemaking on use of the voluntary claim "Natural," September 11, 2009, at www.fsis .usda.gov.

132 *In part to fill:* Natural Pet Nutrition. *Quality Systems Manual for Natural Pet Nutrition*. Quality Assured Verification Program, Nestlé Purina PetCare, June 2007.

133 *In the odd:* USDA National Organic Program. NOP Guidance Statement, April 13, 2004.

133 *In 2005, the NOSB: Interim Report of the National Organic Program*, Organic Pet Food Task Force, April 7, 2006, at www.ams.usda.gov.

133 *As the NOSB:* USDA. Adoption of genetically engineered crops in the U.S., July 1, 2009, at www.ers.usda.gov/Data/BiotechCrops. The figure on cattle hormones is from ML Thonney, Cornell U, personal communication, May 13, 2008.

134 *Developing new organic:* National Organic Standards Board (NOSB). Formal recommendation to the National Organic Program (NOP) on organic pet food standards, November 19, 2008, at www.ams.usda.gov.

134 [1] *The NOP:* AAFCO. *Pet Food and Specialty Pet Food Labeling Guide*, February 2008:68–69.

135 *For an explanation:* California Department of Public Health. Organic Processed Product Registration Requirements (undated) at www.dhs.ca.gov.

137 *Another certifying:* Quality Assurance International. QAI Organic Pet Food Addendum, at www.qai-inc.com. Oklahoma Department of Agriculture, Food, and Forestry. Certified Organic Food (brochure) at www.oda.state.ok.us.

138 *Hormones, antibiotics:* Pew Commission on Industrial Farm Animal Production. *Putting Meat on the Table: Industrial Farm Animal Production in America*. Baltimore, MD: The Pew Charitable Trusts and Johns Hopkins Bloomberg School of Public Health, 2008.

138 *In 2004, they:* Pet Promise is (or was) at www.petpromiseinc.com. Nestle's sustainable agriculture initiatives are at www.nestle.com.

139 *Others prefer:* NAD [National Advertising Division of the Better Business Bureau] refers Blue Buffalo's advertising to Federal Trade Commission, May 11, 2009, at www.petproductnews.com.

139 *Whether you consider:* Dogs (78 million) require about 1,000 calories a day, and cats (94 million) about 300. If we assume that the average human requires 2,500 calories a day (probably an overestimate), the needs of dogs are at least equivalent to those of 31 million humans, and of cats to about 11 million, or 42 million people in total.

140 *AAFCO's unease:* The Honest Kitchen. The Honest Kitchen wins its battle for commercial free speech (news release), November 8, 2007, at www.thehonestkitchen .com. The Back to Basics quotation at is at http://beowulfs.com/dog_food.html.

141 *Although only:* Eagle Pack is at www.eaglepack.com.

141 *Q: Does Newman's:* Newman's Own Organics is at www.newmansownorganics.com/ pet/faqs.

142 *In 1985, we:* Harrington-McGill S. Proof that Solid Gold continues to produce the best and safest dog food in the world (advertisement). *The Bark*, January/February, 2008:95.

142 *The meaning of:* Dzanis DA. Superpremium: What does it mean? Should AAFCO establish an official definition? *Petfood Industry*, May/June 1999, at www.vibclub.com/articles/index.tpl.

143 *We are not alone:* Sanderson SL, et al. Owner impressions of three premium diets fed to healthy adult dogs. *JAVMA* 2005;227:1931–36. APPMA. *2007–2008 APPMA National Pet Owners Survey.* Greenwich, CT: APPMA, 2008.

145 *Meat produces less:* Corbin J. A decade of dog food developments. *Dogs, USA Annual*, 1995:91–94.

148 *Nancy Kerns, who:* Kerns N. Top dog foods for total wellness [pamphlet]. *Whole Dog J*, 2007. Also: Choosing good foods. *Whole Dog J*, February 2009:3–9.

Chapter 13. For Young and Old

151 *Pet food companies:* APPA. *2009–2010 APPA National Pet Owners Survey.* Greenwich, CT: APPA, 2009.

151 *Puppies and kittens:* NRC. *Nutrient Requirements of Dogs and Cats.* Washington, DC: National Academies Press, 2006.

152 *The feeding guidelines:* Demko J, McLaughlin R. Developmental orthopedic disease. *Veterinary Clinics of North America Small Animal Practice* 2005;35(5):1111–35.

152 *Let's hear applause:* Omega-3 refers to the position of the first double bond from the methyl end of the fatty acid carbon chain; this double bond links the #3 and #4 carbons in all fatty acids in the omega-3 series. EPA (eicosapentaenoic acid) and DHA (docosahexaenoic acid) are long and highly polyunsaturated: EPA has twenty carbons (eicosa) and five (penta) double bonds (enoic), and DHA has 22 carbons (docosa) and six (hexa) double bonds (enoic). Alpha-linolenic acid is shorter and somewhat less polyunsaturated; it has eighteen carbons and three double bonds.

153 *How much is optimal* Uauy R, Dangour AD. Nutrition in brain development and aging: role of essential fatty acids. *Nutrition Reviews* 2006;64(5):24s–33s.

153 *In one typical:* Starling S. DHA boosts children's brain power, says Martek. Nutra Ingredients.com, Europe, June 30, 2008, at www.nutraingredients.com. Ryan AS, Nelson EB. Assessing the effect of docosahexaenoic acid on cognitive functions in healthy, preschool children: a randomized, placebo-controlled, double-blind study. *Clinical Pediatrics* 2008;47:355–62.

153 *Pet food companies:* Bauer JE. Responses of dogs to dietary omega 3 fatty acids. *JAVMA* 2007;231:1657–1661. Heineman K., et al. Long-chain (n-3) polyunsaturated fatty acids are more efficient than α-linolenic acid in improving electroretinogram responses of puppies exposed during gestation, lactation, and weaning. *J Nutrition* 2005;135:1960–66.

154 *At this point:* Iams. DHA (Docohexaenoic acid), at http://us.iams.com.

155 *Others would like:* FDA. Agency response letter to Martek Biosciences, May 17, 2001, at www.cfsan.fda.gov.

155 *The scientific evidence:* FDA. Q and A about DHA in infant formula, at www.cfsan.fda.gov.

156 *Caloric restriction as:* Heilbronn LK, Ravussin E. Calorie restriction and aging: review of the literature and implications for studies in humans. *Am J Clinical Nutrition* 2003;78:361–69.

156 *Studies like these:* Mattison JA, et al. Dietary restriction in aging nonhuman primates. *Interdisciplinary Topics in Gerontology* 2005;35:137–58. Ancel Keys and his colleagues at the U of Minnesota studied the effects of voluntary starvation on conscientious objectors in World War II. See Keys A, et al. *The Biology of Human Starvation* (2 volumes). Minneapolis: U of Minnesota Press, 1950. Also see Tucker T. *The Great Starvation Experiment. Minneapolis:* U of Minnesota Press, 2008. The Calorie Restriction Society is at www.calorierestriction.org.

157 *What about cats:* Kealy, RD, et al. Effects of age restriction on life span and age related changes in dogs. *JAVMA* 2002;220:1315–20. Lawler DF, et al. Influence of lifetime food restriction on causes, time, and predictors of death in dogs. *JAVMA* 2005;226:225–31. *The Purina Pet Institute Symposium: Advancing Life Through Dietary Restriction*, September 20–21, 2002, St. Louis, MO. Wilmington, DE: The Gloyd Group, 2002.

157 *One theory of:* Muller FL, et al. Trends in oxidative aging theories. *Free Radical Biology and Medicine* 2007;43:477–503.

158 *Epidemiology provides:* Bjelakovic G, Gluud C. Surviving antioxidant supplements. *J National Cancer Institute* 2007;99:742–43. Luchsinger JA, Noble J, Scarmeas N. Diet and Alzheimer's disease. *Current Neurology and Neuroscience* 2007;7:366–72. Chong EW-T, et al. Dietary antioxidants and primary prevention of age related macular degeneration: systematic review and meta analysis. *British Medical J* 2007;335:755. Kamel NS, et al. Antioxidants and hormones as antiaging therapies: high hopes, disappointing results. *Cleveland Clinic J Medicine* 2006;73:1049–56.

158 *As in people:* Dimakopoulos A, Mayer RJ. Aspects of neurodegeneration in the canine brain. *J Nutrition* 2002;132:1579–82. Milgram NW, et al. Learning ability in dogs is preserved by behavioral enrichment and dietary fortification: a two-year longitudinal study. *Neurobiology of Aging* 2005;26:77–90.

159 *Nestlé Purina:* Cupp CJ, et al. Effect of nutritional interventions on longevity of senior cats. *International J Applied Research in Veterinary Medicine* 2006;4:34–50.

159 *All the major:* Devlin PS, et al. Effect of antioxidant supplementation on the immune response in weaned puppies [abstract]. *Veterinary Internal Medicine* 2000;14(3):361. Koelsch S, Smith B. Strengthening barriers against feline infectious diseases: the benefits of antioxidant rich diets. *Waltham Focus* 2001;11(2):32–33.

160 *Given the limited:* Marshall RJ, et al. Supplemental vitamin C appears to slow racing greyhounds. *J Nutrition* 2002;132:1616s–1621s. Teare JA, et al. Ascorbic acid deficiency and hypertrophic osteodystrophy in the dog: a rebuttal. *Cornell Veterinarian* 1979;69(4):384–401.

Chapter 14. For Special Health Problems

162 *The NLEA put:* See Nestle M. *Food Politics: How the Food Industry Influences Nutrition and Health.* Berkeley: U California Press, rev. ed., 2007.

162 *Even with a disclaimer:* FDA rules about label claims are at www.cfsan.fda.gov.

162 *The NLEA and:* FDA. Animal food (feed) product regulation, October 25, 2005, at www.fda.gov.

163 *You might think:* FDA. Dietary Supplement Health and Education Act of 1994, Public Law 103–417, Approved October 24, 1994, at www.fda.gov.

164 *How this murky:* Pszczola DE. Polly wants a . . . neutraceutical? *Food Technology* 1998;52(10):66–72.

164 *The FDA particularly:* Hill's Prescription Diet is at www.hillspet.com.

166 *In all fairness:* Hill's describes the company's history at www.hillspet.com. Medline Plus. Diet-chronic kidney disease, at www.nlm.nih.gov. Jacob F, et al. Clinical evaluation of dietary modification for treatment of spontaneous chronic renal failure in dogs. *JAMVA* 2002;220:1163–70.

167 *Veterinarians, of course:* Therapeutic pet food requires no veterinarian prescription, pharmacy board rules. *DVM Newsmagazine*, May 20, 2008, at www.dvmnews.com.

167 *Most pet owners:* Naidenko O, Sutton, R, Houlihan J. Polluted pets: high levels of toxic industrial chemicals contaminate cats and dogs. Environmental Working Group, April 2008, at www.ewg.org/reports/pets.

168 *Food allergies are:* Kennis RA. Food allergies: update of pathogenesis, diagnoses, and management. *Veterinary Clinics Small Animal Practice* 2006;36:175–84.

169 *Once the source:* California Natural (Natura Pet Products), at www.california naturalpet.com. McNeill L, et al. Hydrolyzed proteins—hypoallergenic or hype? *Waltham Focus* 2001;11(1):32–33.

170 *An independent:* What's Greenies, at www.greenies.com.

170 *The Greenies site:* Roudebush P, Logan E, Hale FA. Evidence-based veterinary dentistry: a systematic review of homecare for prevention of periodontal disease in dogs. *J Veterinary Dentistry* 2005;22(1):6–15. The authors work for Hill's. Greenies dog food treats and dog deaths, February 24, 2006, at www.lawyersandsettlements.com/case/greenies_dog_treats.html.

170 *To deal with:* Veterinary Oral Health Council is at www.vohc.org.

171 *We would expect:* The Glycemic Index and GI Database, at www.glycemicindex.com, lets you look up the index of specific foods. Coca-Cola has a GI of 63; ice cream is 36. The Glycemic Research Institute, which runs the certification program, is at www.glycemic.com. De-Oliveira LD, et al. Effects of six carbohydrate sources on cat diet digestibility and postprandial glucose and insulin response. *J Animal Science*, May 9, 2008, online at doi:10.2527/jas.2007–0354.

171 *Cats do lick:* APPA. *2009–2010 APPA National Pet Owners Survey.* Greenwich, CT: APPA, 2009.

172 *Purina ONE Advanced:* Purina ONE Advanced Nutrition Hairball Formula, at www.purinaone.com.

172 *Hip problems and:* Beale BS. Use of nutraceuticals and chondroprotectants in osteoarthritic dogs and cats. *Veterinary Clinics Small Animal Practice* 2004;34:271–89.

172 *Cats evolved from:* Dzanis, DA. Interpreting pet food labels—special use foods, updated, at www.fda.gov.

173 *The acidity of:* Funaba M, et al. Evaluation of effects of dietary carbohydrate on formation of struvite crystals in urine and macromineral balance in clinically normal cats. *Am J Veterinary Research* 2004;65(2):138–42. Biourge V. Urine dilution: a key factor in the prevention of struvite and calcium oxalate uroliths. *Veterinary Focus* 2007;17:41–44. Houston DM. Epidemiology of feline urolithiasis. *Veterinary Focus* 2007;17:4–9.

173 *But getting pets:* Markwell PJ, Buffington CT, Smith BH. The effect of diet on lower urinary tract diseases in cats. *J Nutrition* 1998;128:2753s–57s.

Chapter 15. For Weight Loss

175 *The label of:* The BMI for adults is defined as weight in kilograms divided by height in meters squared. One kilogram is 2.2 pounds. A BMI of 25 is considered overweight; 30 is considered obese. German AJ. The growing problem of obesity in dogs and cats. *J Nutrition* 2006;136:1940s–46s. Purina provides articles on the topic at www.purina.com.

175 *Veterinarians do not:* Butterwick RF, et al. A study of obese cats on a calorie controlled weight reduction programme. *Veterinary Record* 1994;134:372–77. Purina. Understanding your cat's body condition, and Understanding your dog's body condition, are at www.purina.com. Royal Canin. S.H.A.P.E. body condition guides, at www.pet-slimmers.com/shapedog.htm.

176 *Several studies have:* Kienzle E, Bergler R, Mandernach A. Comparison of the feeding behavior of the man-animal relationship in owners of normal and obese dogs. *J Nutrition* 1998;128:2779s–82s.

176 *Studies of cat:* Kienzle E, Bergler R. Human-animal relationship of owners of normal and overweight cats. *J Nutrition* 2006;136:1947s–50s. Donoghue S, Scarlett J. Diet and feline obesity. *J Nutrition* 1998;128:2776–78.

176 *These studies form:* German AJ. The growing problem of obesity in dogs and cats. *J Nutrition* 2006;136:1940s–46s.

177 *When you see:* Scientists measure food energy in kilocalories (kcal), sometimes called Calories with a capital C (as on food labels). One food-label Calorie (kcal) is the amount of energy required to heat one liter of water 1°C under defined conditions of ambient temperature and pressure; it is 1,000 times larger than a calorie spelled with a small c. Everyone uses calories with a small c even though they mean kilocalories or Calories; we do too.

179 *Capitalize on:* Hill's Science Diet Brand. Start the year strong with one amazing promotion and two great foods [advertising flyer]. Hill's Pet Nutrition, 2008.

182 *We began by:* The Iams website for this diet product in August 2008 was at http://us.iams.com.

182 *Something did not:* Dick Van Patten's Natural Balance Pet Foods is at www.naturalbalanceinc.com.

182 *We like to think:* Mugford RA. External influences on the feeding of carnivores. In: Kare MR, Maller O, eds. *The Chemical Senses and Nutrition.* New York: Academic Press, 1977:32. Spadofori G, Pion P. *Cats for Dummies.* Foster City, CA: IDG Books Worldwide, 1997.

183 *The National Research:* NRC. *Nutrient Requirements of Dogs and Cats.* Washington, DC: National Academies Press, 2006. Metabolizable Energy (ME) in kcal needed for daily maintenance can be estimated using a calculator that does exponents. For active dogs, the formula is 130 x body weight in $kg^{0.75}$; for inactive dogs, 95 x body weight in $kg^{0.75}$; for lean domestic cats, 100 x body weight in $kg^{0.67}$.

183 *Activity levels make:* Sled dogs in the Iditarod race are said to require 10,000 to 14,000 calories per day, depending on weight. See Iditarod preparation—food drops, at www.ultimateiditarod.com. and Collins M, Collins J. *Dog Driver: A Guide for the Serious Musher,* rev. ed. Crawford, CO: Alpine, 2009.

185 *It makes no sense:* Wong, Q. Vets have advice for Congress about fat cats (dogs too), 2008, at www.mcclatchydc.com/homepage/story/36931.html.

Chapter 16. Snacks, Treats, Chews, and Bottled Waters

190 *The reason exhibitors:* Mintel Reports. *Pet Food and Supplies.* Chicago, IL: Mintel International Group, August 2007.

191 *Many small companies:* APPA. *2009–10 APPA National Pet Owners Survey.* Greenwich, CT: APPA, 2009. Sundale Research. *State of the Dog Food Industry,* April 2007, at www.sundaleresearch.com.

194 *So do the calories:* Barking Dog Pet Bakery is at www.barkingdogbakeryokc.com.

194 *In advertising the:* Phillips T. Functional treats take off. *Pet Food Industry,* June 2008:20–23. Dogswell is at www.dogswell.com.

195 *We found an Authority:* Dobernecker B, Beetz Y, Kienzle E. A placebo controlled double blind study on the effect of nutraceuticals (chondroitin sulfate and mussel extract) in dogs with joint diseases as perceived by their owners. *J Nutrition* 2002;132: 1690s–91s.

195 *We cannot resist:* Funaba M, Yamate T, Narukawa Y, et al. Effect of supplementation of dry cat food with D, L-methionine and ammonium chloride on struvite activity product and sediment in urine. *J Veterinary Medical Science* 2001;63: 337–39.

196 *On its website:* The company's website is at www.himalayandogchew.com.

197 *Natural chews:* Barber T. Manufacturing rawhides and animal part treats. In: Kvamme, JL, Phillips TD, eds. *Pet Food Technology.* Mt. Morris IL: Watt Publishing, 2003:400–402.

197 Whole Dog Journal's: Kerns N. Finding the right rawhide. *Whole Dog J,* May 2009: 8–11.

198 *At a time when:* See discussions of these issues in Nestle M. *What to Eat.* New York: North Point Press, 2006:401–15, and Royte E. *Bottlemania: How Water Went on Sale and How We Bought It.* New York: Bloomsbury, 2008. APPA. *2009–10 APPA National Pet Owners Survey.* Greenwich, CT: APPA, 2008.

199 *Yes, bottled water:* Hiltzik M. Hoping canines will lap it up. *Los Angeles Times,* June 2, 2005. Toulemonde A. Bottled water in meaty flavors? Dogs lap it up. Sawf News, July 13, 2006 at http://news.sawf.org. Zmuda N. Fortified water has gone to the dogs. *Advertising Age,* February 25, 2008:4, 30. Also see: Cordeiro A. Health food is going to the dogs—literally. *WSJ,* April 9, 2008.

199 *If you like:* Weiskopf J. *Pet Food Nation.* New York: HarperCollins, 2007:40.

Chapter 17. Dietary Supplements

200 *Dietary supplements are:* Kurtzweil P. An FDA guide to dietary supplements. *FDA Consumer Magazine,* September–October 1998, at www.fda.gov. Centers for Disease

Control and Prevention. National Health and Nutrition Examination Survey 1988–1994, at www.cdc.gov.

201 *Category growth:* Pet Naturals. Advertisement. *Whole Health,* Winter 2006:31.

201 *As we noted:* FDA. Overview of dietary supplements, January 3, 2001, at www.cfsan.fda.gov.

202 *For anyone other:* Radimer KL, Subar AF, Thompson FE. Nonvitamin, nonmineral dietary supplements: issues and findings from NHANES III. *J Am Dietetic Association* 2000;100:447–54.

202 *One additional:* Commission on Dietary Supplement Labels. *Final Report,* November 24, 1997, at http://web.health.gov/dietsupp.

202 *Finally, DSHEA:* Office of Dietary Supplements. Dietary supplement fact sheets, at http://ods.od.nih.gov. American Botanical Council. Herbal supplement sales in the United States show growth in all channels. *HerbalGram* 2008:78:60–63.

203 *The AAFCO models:* AAFCO. *AAFCO Pet Food and Specialty Pet Food Labeling Guide.* Oxford, IN, 2008.

203 *Here comes the:* Dzanis DA. Interpreting pet food labels—special use foods, at www.fda.gov.

203 *We have reason:* Howie M. AAFCO outlines strategy for unapproved feed ingredients. *Feedstuffs* 2002;74 (February 11):19.

204 *It is time:* Wynn SG. FDA/AAFCO set to remove animal supplements from sale, at www.geocities.com.

204 *The NASC, which:* National Animal Supplement Council. Regulation of animal health supplements—a historical summary, at http://nasc.cc.

204 *These pressures:* Nolen RS. Facing crackdown, dietary supplement companies promise changes. *JAMVA* online, August 15, 2002, at www.avma.org.

205 *The "threat" of:* JAVMA News. Board approves policy changes on pet food, dog shows, June 11, 2008, at www.avma.org.

205 *Without national:* National Animal Supplement Council. Regulating supplements for non-human chain animals, at http://nasc.cc.

205 *One question worth:* Marchione M. Tests reveal some pet supplements skimp on meds, July 9, 2009, at www.google.com/hostednews/ap/article. Consumer Lab is at www.consumerlab.com. Bragg RR, et al. Composition, disintegrative properties, and labeling compliance of commercially available taurine and carnitine dietary products. *JAMVA* 2009;234:209–13.

206 *Reliable data on:* APPA. *2009–2010 APPA National Pet Owners Survey.* Greenwich, CT: APPA, 2009. Supplements still top dog in U.S. pet nutrition sales. *Nutrition Business J,* August 2009.

Chapter 18. Do Supplements Work?

210 *We doubt that:* NRC. *Safety of Dietary Supplements for Horses, Dogs, and Cats.* Washington, DC: National Academies Press, 2008.

211 *Carnitine is a:* NIH, Office of Dietary Supplements. Fact sheet: Carnitine, at http://ods.od.nih.gov.

211 *Do carnitine supplements:* NRC. *Nutrient Requirements of Dogs and Cats.* Washington, DC: National Academies Press, 2006. Milgram NW, et al. Acetyl-L-carnitine

and α-lipoic acid supplementation of aged beagle dogs improves learning in two landmark discrimination tests. *FASEB J* 2007:21:3756–62.

211 *On the basis:* Center SA, et al. *J Veterinary Internal Medicine* 2000;14:598–608. Ibraham WH, et al. Effects of carnitine and taurine on fatty acid metabolism and lipid accumulation in the livers of cats during weight gain and weight loss. *Am J Veterinary Research* 2003:64:1265–77. Roudebush P, Schoenherr W, Delaney S. An evidence based review of the use of nutraceuticals and dietary supplementation for the management of obese and overweight pets. *JAMVA* 2008;232:1646–55. Phillips T. Functional fixes. *Petfood Industry,* August 2008:24.

212 *Because these:* Roush JK, McLaughlin RM, Radlinsky MG. Understanding the pathophysiology of osteoarthritis. *Veterinary Medicine* 2002;97:108–117. Clarke SP, et al. Prevalence of radiographic signs of degenerative joint disease in a hospital population of cats. *Veterinary Record* 2005: 157,793–99. Mlacnik EB, et al. Effects of calorie restriction and a moderate or intense physiotherapy program for treatment of overweight dogs with osteoarthritis. *JAMVA* 2006;229:1756–60.

212 *Everyone agrees:* Samson DJ, et al. *Treatment of Primary and Secondary Osteoarthritis of the Knee. Evidence Report/Technology Assessment No. 157* (AHRQ Publication No. 07-E012). Rockville, MD: Agency for Healthcare Research and Quality, September 2007. Beale BS. Use of nutraceuticals and chondroprotectants in osteoarthritic dogs and cats. *Veterinary Clinics Small Animal Practice* 2004;34:271–89. Clegg DO, Reda DJ, Harris CL, et al. Glucosamine, chondroitin sulfate, and the two in combination for painful knee arthritis. *New England J Medicine* 2006;354:795–808.

213 *Pets do not:* Dobenecker B, Beetz Y, Kienzle E. A placebo controlled double blind study on the effect of nutraceuticals (chondroitin sulfate and mussel extract) in dogs with joint diseases as perceived by their owners. *J Nutrition* 2002;132:1690s–91s.

213 *Investigators conducted:* Aragon CL, Hofmeister EH, Budsberg SC. Systematic review of treatments for osteoarthritis in dogs. *JAMVA* 2007;230:514–21.

214 *Do natural meals:* Purina ONE Lamb and Rice Formula is at www.purinaone.com.

214 *Neither humans nor:* See Start AH, Crawford MA, Reifen R. Update on alphalinolenic acid. *Nutrition Reviews* 2008;66:326–32. NIH, Office of Dietary Supplements. Health Information: Omega-3 fats, at http://ods.od.nih.gov.

215 *Much of the evidence:* American Heart Association. Our 2006 diet and lifestyle recommendations, at http://americanheart.org. Nesheim MC, Yaktine A, eds. *Seafood Choices, Balancing Benefits and Risks.* Washington, D.C.: National Academies Press, 2007.

216 *The research in dogs:* Brown SA, et al. Beneficial effects of chronic administration of dietary ω-3 polyunsaturated fatty acids in dogs with renal insufficiency. *J Laboratory and Clinical Medicine* 1998;131:447–55. Bauer JE. Responses of dogs to dietary omega 3 fatty acids. *JAVMA* 2007;231:1657–61.

216 *As for arthritis:* Cross AR, et al. Effects of feeding omega-3 fatty acids on force plate gait analysis in dogs with osteoarthritis—a three-month feeding study. *Hill's Nutritional Research Review* 2005;4(1):3–4.

216 *Veterinarians sometimes:* Watson TDG. Diet and skin disease in dogs and cats. *J Nutrition* 1998;128:2783s–89s. Kirby NA, Hester SL, Bauer JE. Dietary Fats and the skin and coat of dogs. *JAVMA* 2007;230:1641–44.

216 *One other complicating:* FDA and EPA. What you need to know about mercury in fish and shellfish, March 2004, at www.cfsan.fda.gov.

217 *In 2008, the:* Naidenko O, Sutton R, Houlihan J. Polluted pets: high levels of toxic industrial chemicals contaminate cats and dogs, April 2008, at www.ewg.org/reports/pets.

218 *Probiotic bacteria:* Van Neil CW, et al. *Lactobacillus* therapy for acute infectious diarrhea in children: a meta-analysis. *Pediatrics*, 2002;109:678–84. Adolfsson O, Meydani SN, Russell RM. Yogurt and gut function. *Am J Clinical Nutrition* 2004;80:245–56. The authors say that the National Yogurt Association requested this "critical and objective review" for which they were paid an unspecified honorarium. Schrezenmeir J, de Vrese M, Heller K, eds. International symposium on probiotics and prebiotics. *Am J Clinical Nutrition* 2001;73 (suppl 2):361s–498s. Sponsors included the International Dairy Federation, Danone, Nestlé, Nordmilch, Yakult, and several other international companies selling dairy foods.

218 *As for prebiotics:* Willard M, et al. Effects of dietary fructooligosaccharide on selected bacterial populations in feces of dogs. *Am J Veterinary Research* 2000;61: 820–25.

218 *Because the physiology:* Benyacoub J, et al. Probiotics as tools to improve health: perspectives for pets. *Proceedings, 2006 Nestlé Purina Nutrition Forum* 2007;29 (2A): 11–24. Baillon M-L, Marshall-Jones Z, Butterwick R. The benefits of probiotics for dogs and cats, in health and disease. *Waltham Focus* 2004;14:35–39. Baillon M-L, Marshall-Jones ZV, Butterwick R. Effects of probiotic *Lactobacillus acidophilus* strain DSM13241 in healthy adult dogs. *Am J Veterinary Research* 2004;65:338–43. Marshall-Jones ZV, et al. Effects of *Lactobacillus acidophilus* DSM 13241 as a probiotic in healthy adult cats. *Am J Veterinary Research* 2006;67:1005–12.

219 *One study sponsored:* Sauter SN, et al. Effects of probiotic bacteria in dogs with food responsive diarrhea treated with an elimination diet. *J Animal Physiology and Animal Nutrition* 2006;90(7–8):269–77. Wynn SG. Probiotics in veterinary practice. *JAMVA* 2009;234:606–13.

219 *We suspect that:* The Yogurt Association criteria are at www.aboutyogurt.com.

220 *Although the Yogurt:* Probiotics: are enough in your diet? *Consumer Reports,* 2005;7:34–35.

220 *It is unfortunate:* Weese JS. Microbiologic evaluation of commercial probiotics. *JAVMA* 2002;220:794–97.

220 *High and low:* The lactic acid-forming bacteria included in the count are *Lactobacillus acidophilus, Lactobacillus casei, and Enterococcus faecium.* Eagle Pack Hairball Formula is described at www.holisticselect.com.

Chapter 19. Unconventional Diets

225 *At this point:* Michel KE, et al. Attitudes of pet owners toward pet foods and feeding management of cats and dogs. *JAMVA* 2008;233:1699–703.

225 *Ask clients about:* Michel KE. Unconventional diets for dogs and cats. *Veterinary Clinics Small Animal Practice* 2006;36:1269–81.

226 *The label on:* Chicago Rabbinical Council. CRC passover foods for your pets, 2008, at www.crcweb.org.

227 *Given the multiple:* Newman AA. Seder fare for pets that keep kosher. *NYT,* April 9, 2009:B9.

227 *According to Rabbi:* Weinbach M. Kosher keeping pets. Ohr Somayach International, June 25, 2005, at http://ohr.edu. Silberberg N. Can I feed my pet non-kosher food? Ask Moses, at www.askmoses.com.

227 *in general, the laws:* Danziger E. Do I need to feed my pet kosher pet food? Chabad .com, at www.chabad.org.

228 *Because application* Kosher Pets is at http://kosherpets.com. Knudson WA. The pet food market. Strategic Marketing Institute working paper, December 2003, at www .aec.msu.edu. Top (kosher) dog. Ohr Somayach International, at http://ohr.edu.

228 *This means, as:* Regenstein JM, Chaudry MM, Regenstein CE. The kosher and halal food laws. *Comprehensive Reviews in Food Science and Food Safety* 2003;2: 111–27.

230 *Even with government:* Veterinarian Society UK. Dogs—a vegetarian diet? at www.vegsoc.org/info/dogfood1.html.

230 *Animal rights groups:* People for the Ethical Treatment of Animals (PETA). Meatless meals for dogs and cats: factsheet, at www.peta.org. Vegan Cats Cruelty-Free Alternatives. Online shopping, at www.vegancats.com.

230 *If the animal-rights:* Knight A. The author responds [letter]: *JAVMA* 2005;226:1047.

231 *Evolution Diet has:* Weisman E. Why use Evolution Diet pet food? at www.petfood shop.com.

231 *Testimonials like:* Christiansen W. *The Humane Society of the United States Complete Guide to Cat Care.* New York: St. Martin's Press, 2002:198.

232 *But are they?:* Gray CM, Sellon RK, Freeman LM. Nutritional adequacy of two vegan diets for cats. *JAVMA* 2004;225:1670–75. Kienzle E, Engelhard R. A field study on the nutrition of vegetarian dogs and cats in Europe [abstract]. *Supplement to Compendium on Continuing Education for the Practicing Veterinarian* 2001;23(9):81. Leon A, Bain SAF, Levick WR. Hypokalemic episodic polymyopathy in cats fed a vegetarian diet. *Australian Veterinary J* 1992;69:249–54.

233 *The answer to:* Mowll W. Feeding for proper canine nutrition. *Popular Dog,* January 1945:11. Murray SM, et al. Evaluation of selected high-starch flours as ingredients in canine diets. *J Animal Science* 1999;77:2180–86. Clapper GM, et al. Ileal and total tract nutrient digestibilities and fecal characteristics of dogs as affected by soybean protein inclusion in dry, extruded diets. *J Animal Science* 2001;79:1523–32.

233 *What about cats?:* De-Oliveira LD, et al. Effects of six carbohydrate sources on cat diet digestibility and postprandial glucose and insulin response. *J Animal Science,* May 9, 2008 (online at doi:10.2527/jas.2007–0354). Wakefield LA, Shofer FS, Michel KE. Evaluation of cats fed vegetarian diets and attitudes of their caregivers. *JAVMA* 2006;229:70–73.

233 *From this limited:* Rosenthal C. A matter of meat: why cats can't be vegetarians. *Cat Fancy,* May 2008:40–41. Wakefield LA. The authors respond [letter]. *JAVMA* 2006;229; 498.

235 *Today's companion:* Innova Evo: Brochure. The ancestral diet meets modern nutrition. Natura Pet Products, 2007, at www.evopet.com.

Chapter 20. The Raw

237 *The fiercest arguments:* Levi-Strauss C. *The Raw and the Cooked.* Chicago: U of Chicago Press, 1983. And see Keith C. Picking the bones of the raw diet debate. *The Bark,* Jan/Feb 2006:41–43. PRO: Billinghurst I. *The BARF Diet: Raw Feeding for Dogs and Cats Using Evolutionary Principles.* Bathurst, Australia: Warrigal Publishing, 2001:3. CON: Martin AN. *Foods Pets Diet For: Shocking Facts about Pet Food.* Troutdale, OR: NewSage Press, 2008:137.

238 *Given the sharp:* Billinghurst I. *Give Your Dog a Bone.* Ian Billinghurst, Australia, 1993. Milner C, Knowslety J. Dogs on pet food "risk early death." *Sunday Telegraph* (London), October 1, 1995.

239 *But from what:* MacDonald CB. *Raw Dog Food.* Wenachee, WA: Dogwise Publishing, 2004.

240 *The time and energy:* Zoological Pet Food, at www.miceonice.com. In mid-2008, 100 mice fuzzies cost $34.00; pinkies were $32.50. Hare Today is at www.hare-today .com. See Forelle C. How do cats like rabbits? Very much, and preferably raw. *WSJ,* July 30, 2007.

240 *Given the intense:* BARF World, at www.barfworld.com.

241 *A glance at:* Bil-Jac is at www.bil-jac.com. Honest Kitchen is at www.thehonest kitchen.com.

242 *Now, we've pioneered:* Nature's Variety explains the coating at www.naturesvariety .com. Great Life is at www.1doctorschoice.com/GreatLifeDogFood.html.

242 *These products also:* The Robert Abady Dog Food Co. is at http://therobertabady dogfoodcoltd.com.

242 *In mid-2008:* Packaged Facts. *Fresh Pet Food in North America: The Raw/Frozen, Refrigerated and Homemade Wave,* January 2008. This company charges $2,500 for this report.

243 *We must add:* PetFoodDirect.com is at www.petfooddirect.com.

243 *We meet many:* FDA. The dangers of raw milk, October 2006, and On the safety of raw milk, May 12, 2005, at www.cfsan.fda.gov. Kessler J. Got (raw) milk? Consumers go to great lengths for unpasteurized milk. *Atlanta Journal-Constitution,* September 7, 2007. What's happening with real milk, at www.realmilk.com.

243 *To say that:* Packaged Facts. *Pet food in the U.S.,* September 2006:198.

243 *As a pet nutritionist:* Machlik S. Raw risks, 2008, at www.vibclub.com.

244 *We are not surprised:* AVMA. Homemade and raw diets are trendy, but are they hurting pets? (press release), July 17, 2007, at www.avma.org.

244 *How serious are:* Freeman LM, Michel KE. Evaluation of raw food diets for dogs. *JAVMA* 2001;218:705–9. The authors wrote a popular account of this study for the *AKC Gazette,* April 2001:39–41. Letters are in *JAVMA* 2001;218:1553–54, and corrections are at pages 1582 and 1716. An additional letter is at 219:173.

244 *When it comes:* Finley R, Reid-Smith R, Weese JS. Human health implications of *Salmonella*-contaminated natural pet treats and raw pet food. *Clinical Infectious Diseases* 2006;42:686–91.

245 *statistically there is:* FDA. Wild Kitty Cat Food issues nationwide recall of cat food due to *Salmonella* contamination, February 16, 2007, at www.fda.gov. Wild Kitty Cat Food responds to FDA recall, February 21, 2007, at www.syscon.com.

245 *We think bacterial:* The FDA recall information is at www.fda.gov. Strohmeyer RA, et al. Evaluation of bacterial and protozoal contamination of commercially available raw meat diets for dogs. *JAMVA* 2006;226:537–42. Morley PS, et al. Evaluation of the association between feeding raw meat and *Salmonella enterica* infections at a Greyhound breeding facility. *JAVMA* 2006;228:1524–32.

246 *FDA does not:* FDA. Guidance for industry: manufacture and labeling of raw meat foods for companion and captive noncompanion carnivores and omnivores, May 18, 2004 (revised November 9, 2004), at www.fda.gov.

247 *The 2004 document:* FDA. Safe handling tips for pet foods and treats, August 6, 2007, at www.fda.gov. Partnership for food safety education. Safe food handling, at www.fightbac.org.

248 *The threat of:* Bravo! is at www.bravorawdiet.com.

248 *Our not-so-secret:* FDA. Bravo! issues nationwide recall of select poultry products for dogs and cats. September 18, 2007, at www.fda.gov.

249 *Nancy Kerns:* Kerns N. Cold standard: commercial frozen diets have proliferated but range in quality. *Whole Dog J,* June 2008:3–8.

249 *Despite the testimonials:* Gershoff SN. Nutritional problems of household cats. *JAVMA* 1975;166:455–58. Rock S, et al. Bioavailability of β-Carotene is lower in raw than in processed carrots and spinach in women. *J Nutrition* 1998;128:913–16. NRC, *Nutrient Requirements of Dogs and Cats.* Washington, DC: National Academies Press, 2006:56.

249 *How safe is it:* Billinghurst I. *The BARF Diet: Raw Feeding for Dogs and Cats Using Evolutionary Principles.* Bathurst, Australia: Warrigal Publishing, 2001:3.

250 *Not much research:* Brown A. *The Whole Pet Diet.* Berkeley: Celestial Arts, 2006:186.

250 *feeding bones to:* Anonymous. Raw or cooked bones. . . . Are either safe? July 31, 2008, at www.thepetcenter.com.

250 *Indeed, this anonymous:* Robinson JGA, Gorrel C. The oral status of a pack of foxhounds fed a "natural" diet. In: *Proceedings World Veterinary Dental Congress.* Birmingham, England, 1997:35–37.

250 *Chicken bones:* Hotchner T. *The Dog Bible.* New York: Gotham, 2005:462.

Chapter 21. The Home Cooked

252 *We don't get it:* APPA. *2009/2010 APPA National Pet Owners Survey.* Greenwich, CT: APPA, 2009. Laflamme DP, et al. Pet feeding practices of dog and cat owners in the United States and Australia. *JAMVA* 2008;232:687–94.

252 *We have good:* Associated Press. Pet owners making own dog and cat food, April 4, 2007, at http://wjz.com. Moore, A. *Real Food for Dogs.* North Adams, MA: Story Publishing, 2001. Strombeck DR. *Home Prepared Dog and Cat Diets The Healthy Alternative* 1999. Ames, IA: Iowa State U Press, 1999. An Amazon ranking of 60,000 means that 59,999 books are selling better on that site at that particular moment.

253 *Yet during the:* AVMA. Home madefood requires study of nutrition, AVMA warns, March 20, 2007, at www.avma.org.

253 *Should pets eat grains* YES: Pitcairn RH. *Dr. Pitcairn's Complete Guide to Natural Health for Dogs & Cats.* Rodale, 2005:39. NO: Palika L. *The Ultimate Pet Food*

Guide: Everything You Need to Know about Feeding Your Dog or Cat. Philadelphia, PA: Da Capo Press, 2008:46.

254 *Is it OK:* YES: Brown A. *The Whole Pet Diet: Eight Weeks to Great Health for Dogs and Cats.* Berkeley, CA: Celestial Arts, 2006:80. NO: Rees WN, Schlanger K. *Natural Pet Food Cookbook.* New York: Wiley, 2008:xvi, and Hotchner T. *The Dog Bible: Everything Your Dog Wants You to Know.* New York: Gotham Books, 2005:382.

254 *Should you feed cheese:* YES: Meadows G, Flint E. *The Complete Guide to Caring for Your Dog.* London: New Holland, 2005:56. NO: Weiskopf J. *Pet Food Nation.* New York: Collins, 2007:75.

254 *Should you feed table:* YES: Weiskopf J. *Pet Food Nation.* New York: Collins, 2007:93. NO: Hotchner T. *The Dog Bible: Everything Your Dog Wants You to Know.* New York: Gotham Books, 2005:443.

255 *To show how:* Hand MK, et al. *Small Animal Nutrition,* 4th ed. Topeka, KS: Mark Morris Institute, 2000:169.

259 *The main reason:* FDA. Diamond pet food recalled due to aflatoxin, December 20, 2005, at www.fda.gov. Welcome to the Diamond Pet Food settlement website, at www.recalledpetfoodsettlement.com.

259 *Here is another:* Child G, et al. Ataxia and paralysis in cats in Australia associated with exposure to an imported gamma-irradiated commercial dry pet food. *Australian Veterinary J* 2009;87:349–51.

259 *Chocolate is:* Hornfeldt CS. Chocolate toxicity in dogs. *Modern Veterinary Practice* 1987;68:552–54.

260 *Onions and garlic:* Lee KW, et al. Hematologic changes associated with the appearance of eccentrocytes after intragastric administration of garlic extract to dogs. *Am J Veterinary Research* 2000;61:1446–50. NRC. *Safety of Dietary Supplements for Horses, Dogs, and Cats.* Washington, DC: National Academies Press. 2008.

260 *Grapes and raisins:* Gwaltney-Brant S, et al. Renal failure associated with ingestion of grapes and raisins in dogs. *JAVMA* 2001;218:1555–56.

261 *Macadamia nuts:* Hansen SR. Macadamia nut toxicosis in dogs. *Veterinary Medicine* 2002;97:274–75.

261 *Xylitol:* Dunayer EK, Gwaltney-Brant SM. Acute hepatic failure and coagulopathy associated with xylitol ingestion in eight dogs. *JAVMA* 2006;229:113–17. Food toxins are summarized by the ASPCA, at www.aspca.org.

261 *We also think:* Jowit J. Junk food diet fuels epidemic of pet obesity. *The Observer* (London), July 20, 2008, at www.guardian.co.uk.

Chapter 22. Are Commercial Pet Foods Healthy for Pets?

265 *Corporations make:* Martin A. *Food Pets Die For: Shocking Facts about Pet Food,* 3rd ed. Troutdale, OR: New Sage Press, 2008. The quotation is from Martin A. Recalling commercial pet food, *The Bark, Unleashed,* April 9, 2007, at www.thebark.com.

266 *The most obvious:* Nestle M. *Pet Food Politics: The Chihuahua in the Coal Mine.* Berkeley: U California Press, 2008.

266 *The vulnerability:* Frederick LD, Robinson HE. Canine nutritional deficiency diseases *JAVMA* 1941;98:288–94.

266 *Such problems:* Fascetti AJ, et al. Taurine deficiency in dogs with dilated cardiomy-
     opathy: 12 cases (1997–2001). *JAVMA* 2003;223:1137–41. Gershoff SN, Norkin SA.
     Vitamin E deficiency in cats. *J Nutrition* 1962;77:303–8. Ohlen B, Scott DW. Zinc
     responsive dermatitis in puppies. *Canine Practice* 1986;13:6–10. Sousa CA, et al.
     Dermatosis associated with feeding generic dog food: 13 cases (1981–1982). *JAVMA*
     1988;192:676–80.

267 *We discussed this:* Bennett, D. Nutrition and Bone disease in the dog and cat. *Veteri-
     nary Record* 1976;98:313–20. Secondary hyperparathyroidism occurs when deficient
     calcium leads to release of parathyroid hormone, which causes bones to release cal-
     cium to maintain normal blood levels. Gershoff SN. Nutritional problems of house-
     hold cats. *JAVMA*;166:455–58. Scott PP, Greaves JP, Scott MG. Nutrition of the cat:
     4. Calcium and iodine deficiency on a meat diet. *British J Nutrition* 1961;15:35–51.
     Seawrite AA, English PB. Hypervitaminosis A and hyperostosis of the cat. *Nature*
     1965;206:1171–72.

268 *Statisticians at:* Americans living longer than ever, September 12, 2007, at www
     .cbsnews.com.

269 *I only wish:* Email message to M. Nestle, June 5, 2008. Quoted with permission.

269 *Indeed it would:* Lofflin J. Dr. Scott Campbell: how the CEO of Banfield has rewritten
     the rules of veterinary practice. *Veterinary Economics*, April 2007:36. Banfield is at
     www.banfield.net.

269 *Here, we are:* See Wikipedia entries on *Dogs* and *Aging in Dogs* at http://en.wiki
     pedia.org.

270 *Veterinary surveys:* For well-referenced comparative life span tables and analysis,
     see Cassidy KM. Dog longevity, 2007, at http://users.pullman.com/lostriver/long
     home.htm.

270 *Most of the:* Billinghurst I. *Give Your Dog a Bone.* Ian Billinghurst, Australia, 1993.

270 *Just after his:* Michell AR. Longevity of British breeds of dog and its relationships
     with sex, size, cardiovascular variables and disease. *Veterinary Record* 1999;145:
     625–29.

270 *For dogs at:* See *oldest cats* at www.messybeast.com/longevity.htm, and Cat's maxi-
     mum lifespan, How long is a cat's lifespan, at http://catwebsite.googlepages.com. The
     oldest living cat. *Cat Fancy*, August 2008:8–9.

271 *Pet food companies:* Perez-Camargo G. Cat nutrition: What is new in the old? Sup-
     plement to *Compendium on Continuing Education for the Practicing Veterinarian*
     2004;26(2A):February 2004 (*Nestle-Purina Nutrition Forum Proceedings* 2003:5–10).

271 *We have been able:* Watson D. Longevity and diet (letter). *Veterinary Record* 1996;
     138:71.

272 *A study in Munich:* Kraft W. Geriatrics in canine and feline internal medicine. *Euro-
     pean J Medical Research* 1998;3:31–41.

Chapter 23. Do People Eat Pet Food?

273 *As far as we:* Holds AAA drove poor to dog food. *NYT*, April 28, 1936. Human pure
     food label is barred from dog food. *NYT*, November 17, 1936.

274 *Stories of human:* Select Committee on Nutrition and Human Needs, U.S. Senate.
     Reference material to Part I. Food price changes, 1973–1974. Washington, DC: U.S.

Government Printing Office, 1974:197–99. This incident is discussed in: The media misled. *The Public Interest* 1975;38:129–32; and Johnston L. Are humans eating canned pet food: the growth of a rumor. *NYT*, November 26, 1974. Michael Jacobson still directed CSPI in 2009 (see www.cspinet.org).

274 *The statement made:* According to Frost & Sullivan (*U.S. Pet Products and Service Market*, January 1976), the interview appeared in the *Washington Star-News*, July 25, 1973. Jacobson's book was published by CSPI in 1973. A second edition gives Alpo dog food (fortified) a score of 30 on a protein scale ranging from 172 (beef liver) to 2 (bologna). See Jacobson MJ. *Nutrition Scoreboard: Your Guide to Better Eating.* New York: Avon, 1975:159.

274 *Despite the lack:* Travis S. Pet foods for dinner. *News and Views.* Cornell Cooperative Extension, Cornell U, 1974. Kohlmeier L. The awful truth about dog food. *Chicago Tribune*, November 18, 1974.

275 *And then there:* Peeples EH. . . . Meanwhile, humans eat pet food. *NYT*, December 16, 1975.

275 *The notion persists:* Barbaro M, Dash E. Recession just one way to tighten belt. *NYT*, April 27, 2008.

276 *People do not:* Bohannon J, Goldstein R, Herschkowitsch A. Can people distinguish pâté from dog food? AAWE Working Paper No. 36. American Association of Wine Economists, April 2009, at www.wine-economics.org.

277 *In our view:* Royal Canin. Dietary preferences of dogs and cats. *Watham Focus Special Edition*, 2005. Boatman K. Human panel judges cat food. News Channel 5 online, 2008, at www.newschannel5.com. Sokolov RA. Taste of dog foods appraised by a dog and his best friend. *NYT*, November 9, 1972. For Ipecac, see Wikipedia at http://en.wikipedia.org.

277 *The eating of:* Olsen SJ. Dogs. In: Kiple KF, Ornelas KC, eds. *The Cambridge World History of Food.* Vol. 1. Cambridge: Cambridge U Press, 2000:508–16. Food writer Andrew Coe is dubious about some of these accounts. See his *Chop Suey: A Cultural History of Chinese Food in the United States*, Oxford U. Press, 2009. Saletan W. Wok the dog. *Slate*, January 16, 2002, at www.slate.com.

278 *What we do know:* Wu FH. The best "chink" food: Dog eating and the dilemma of diversity. *Gastronomica* 2001;2:38–45. Goldkorn J. Dog meat ban for Olympics. Danwei, July 10, 2008, at www.danwei.org. Sky News Undercover Reporter. Restaurants serving dog meat in Beijing have been ordered to close for fear of upsetting thousands of western tourists arriving for this year's Olympic games, March 11, 2008, at http://news.sky.com. Dunlop F. It's too hot for dog on the menu. *NYT*, August 4, 2008.

278 *How long the:* Chaney J. As China rises, pets take a higher place. *International Herald Tribune*, March 17, 2008. Foreman W. Protests in China over cats on the menu. L.A. Unleashed, December 22, 2008, at http://latimesblogs.latimes.com.

279 *This prediction:* Kim Tae-jong. Seoul categorizing dogs as livestock. *The Korea Times*, March 24, 2008, at www.koreatimes.co.kr. Panares JP. Ban on sale of dog meat now a law. *Manila Standard Today*, June 1, 2007, at www.manilastandardtoday.com.

279 *In the United:* Feeney, J. Stewed dog. Recipe Source, at www.recipesource.com. The recipe, in the category of "ethnic Philippine," is said to require three hours preparation time and to serve thirty.

Chapter 24. Do Pet Food Companies Influence Veterinarians?

281 *The American Veterinary:* AVMA. Solving a critical shortage in food supply veteri-
      nary medicine, at www.avma.org.

282 *Nutrition is now:* The American College of Veterinary Nutrition is at www.acvn.org.

284 *Hill's is by:* O'Flanagan R. Pet-food maker steps up quality control. GuelphMercury
      .com, May 24, 2008, at http://news.guelphmercury.com.

285 *We logged on:* Hill's website for professionals can be accessed with registration. The
      Cornell information is at www.hillsvet.com/hillsvet/students.

286 *Hill's and Waltham:* Khuly P. How do vets recommend pet foods? (Part 2: education)
      Vet P.O.V., June 14, 2007. It and the first part of this series (Part 1: industry), June 11,
      2007, are at www.dolittler.com.

287 *Pet food companies:* APPMA. *2007–2008 APPMA National Pet Owners Survey.* Green-
      wich, CT: APPMA, 2008.

287 *Recommendations from:* Colgate-Palmolive Company. Creating smiles for 200 years:
      2006 annual report, 2007:8–9.

289 *The involvement of:* Research summaries and recommendations of drug company–
      free medical schools and practitioners are at No Free Lunch, at www.nofreelunch
      .org. See Sierles, FS, et al. Medical students' exposure to and attitudes about drug
      company interactions. *JAMA* 2005; 294:1034–42. The American Medical Student As-
      sociation PharmFree campaign is at www.amsa.org. Ehringhaus SH, et al. Responses
      of medical schools to institutional conflicts of interest. *JAMA* 2008;299:665–71.
      U Pittsburgh Medical Center. Policy on conflicts of interest and interactions between
      representatives of certain industries and faculty, staff, and students of the Schools of
      the Health Sciences and personnel employed by UPMC at all domestic locations, is-
      sued November 12, 2007, effective February 15, 2008, at www.coi.pitt.edu/Industry
      Relationships. U Massachusetts. Memorial Medical Center Vendor Relationship
      Policy, effective July 1, 2008, at www.umassmemorial.org.

289 *When integrity in:* DeAngelis CD. Fontanarosa PB. Impugning the integrity of medi-
      cal science: the adverse effects of industry influence. *JAMA* 2008;299:1833–34.

290 *More recently, a:* Association of American Medical Colleges. Report of the AAMC
      task force on industry funding of medical education to the AAMC Council, June
      18–19, 2008, at www.aamc.org. Rothman DJ, et al. Professional medical associations
      and their relationships with industry. *JAMA* 2009;301:1367–72.

290 *We take the liberty:* Khuly P. How do vets recommend pet foods? (Part 3: in practice).
      Vet P.O.V., June 17, 2007, at www.dolittler.com.

Chapter 25. Is Pet Food Research Ethical?

292 *Throughout this book:* Roberts RM, et al. Farm animal research in crisis. *Science* 2009;
      324:468–69.

293 *Beyond the lack:* People for the Ethical Treatment of Animals. Support brands that do
      not test on animals, at www.iamscruelty.com/notTested.asp.

293 *In 2007, PETA:* Procter & Gamble. Notice of annual meeting and proxy statement,
      annual meeting of shareholders, October 9, 2007:54–55.

294 *But we have:* PETA sues MSU for violations of public records act. PETA Media Center,
      January 16, 2006, at www.peta.org/mc. Norton I, Miss. Supreme Court Rules against

PETA in research-data case. News Blog, *The Chronicle of Higher Education*, August 5, 2008, at http://chronicle.com/news.

295 *One result of:* Waltham pet food symposia are published as supplements to the *J Nutrition* (see 1998;128:2363s–2815s, 2002;132:1579s–1800s, and 2006;136:1923s–2119s).

296 *But undefined diets:* Center SA, et al. *J Veterinary Internal Medicine* 2000;14:598–608. Ibraham WH, et al. G. Effects of carnitine and taurine on fatty acid metabolism and lipid accumulation in the liver of cats during weight gain and weight loss. *Am J Veterinary Research* 2003;64:1265–77.

296 *Another example:* Milgram NW, et al. Learning ability in dogs is preserved by behavioral enrichment and dietary fortification: a two-year longitudinal study. *Neurobiology of Aging* 2005;26:77–90.

297 *As a result of:* Hill's Science Diet. Our devotion to healthy, happy animals, 2008, at www.hillspet.com.

297 *Researchers are:* National Research Council. *Scientific and Humane Issues in the Use of Random Source Dogs and Cats in Research.* Washington, DC.: National Academies Press, 2009.

297 *Researchers must think:* Dahlberg CP. Clues to cat deaths found in UCD study. *Sacramento Bee*, November 14, 2007, at www.sacbee.com. Puschner B, et al. Assessment of melamine and cyanuric acid toxicity in cats. *J Veterinary and Diagnostic Investigation* 2007;19:616–24.

298 *We began with:* Singer P. *Animal Liberation.* New York: New York Review Books, 1990.

299 *Finally, we queried:* The Physicians Committee for Responsible Medicine is at www .pcrm.org.

Appendix 3. The History of Pet Food Regulation

322 *Wheat bran, for:* Federal Trade Commission. *Report of the Federal Trade Commission on Commercial Feeds.* Washington, DC.: Government Printing Office, March 29, 1921.

323 *A commercial feed:* Upton Sinclair's muckraking account of the meatpacking industry, *The Jungle*, has been in print continuously since 1906; eight editions were available on Amazon.com in July 2009. See Pure Food and Drug Act. *United States Statutes at Large*, 59th Cong., Sess. I, Chp. 3915, p. 768–72; cited as *34 U.S. Stats. 768*), 1906.

323 *The Chairman:* U.S. Senate and House of Representatives. *Adulteration of Mixed Feeds. Hearing Before the Committee on Conference of the Committees on Agriculture and Forestry on Food Production Act*, 1919, H.R. 11945, September 16 and 17, 1918. Dr. Haywood's testimony begins on page 23. The telegram is discussed on page 9. The New York State information is on p. 38.

324 *In 1938, Congress:* Federal Food, Drug, and Cosmetic Act, as amended, and Chronological history of CVM, at www.fda.gov.

324 *In 1958, an:* Gruber GS. The Pet Food Industry. AAFCO. *Official Publication 1958*: 97–100.

325 *In 1966, Congress:* Part 501-Animal Food Labeling. *Federal Register*, September 10, 1976:38619–27. The rules first appeared in the *Code of Federal Regulations* in 1977; in 2008 they were located in Title 21: Foods and Drugs, Part 501–Animal Food Labeling, with a reference to the 1976 *Federal Register* notice as the source, subject to amendments (these were few and did not make substantive changes).

Index

Page numbers in *italics* refer to figures and tables; those with *n* refer to notes.

About the Authors

Marion Nestle is Paulette Goddard Professor in the Department of Nutrition, Food Studies, and Public Health at New York University, which she chaired from 1988 to 2003. She also holds appointments as professor of sociology at NYU and visiting professor of nutritional sciences at Cornell. Her degrees include a Ph.D. in molecular biology and an MPH in public health nutrition, both from the University of California, Berkeley. She has held faculty positions at Brandeis University and the UCSF School of Medicine. From 1986 to 1988, she was senior nutrition policy advisor in the Department of Health and Human Services and managing editor of the 1988 *Surgeon General's Report on Nutrition and Health.* She has been a member of several federal advisory committees, including the 1995 Dietary Guidelines Advisory Committee (USDA and DHHS) and the FDA's Food Advisory Committee and Science Advisory Board. She is a fellow of the American Society of Nutrition and of the New York Academy of Medicine. Her research examines scientific, economic, and social influences on food choice. She is the author of three prize-winning books: *Food Politics, Safe Food,* and *What to Eat.* Her most recent book, *Pet Food Politics: The Chihuahua in the Coal Mine,* was published in 2008. She writes the Food Matters column for the *San Francisco Chronicle,* is co-contributing editor (with Malden Nesheim) for *The Bark* magazine, blogs daily (almost) at www.foodpolitics.com and the Atlantic Food Channel, and twitters@marionnestle.

Malden C. Nesheim is professor of nutrition emeritus and provost emeritus at Cornell University. He has a B.S. degree in agricultural science, an M.S. degree in animal nutrition from the University of Illinois, and a Ph.D. in nutrition from Cornell University. He joined the Cornell faculty in 1959, where his research and teaching interests have included diverse aspects of human and animal nutrition. In 1974 he was named professor of nutrition and director of the newly formed Division of Nutritional Sciences at Cornell, a post he held until the summer of 1987, when he was appointed vice president for planning and budgeting. From 1989 to 1995, he was provost of Cornell University. In that position, he was the chief academic officer of Cornell University, responsible for oversight of all programs on the Ithaca campus.

Nesheim received the American Society of Nutrition's (ASN) Conrad A. Elvehjem Award for public service and was elected fellow of the American Academy of Arts and Sciences and fellow of the ASN. He has served as president of the American Institute of Nutrition (now American Society of Nutrition) and on several review panels for the National Institutes of Health and the Department of Agriculture. He chaired the NIH Nutrition Study Section from 1983 to 1986, and was a member of the Food and Nutrition Board of the Institute of Medicine for nine years. He also chaired the 1990 joint USDA/HHS Dietary Guidelines Advisory Committee. In 1995 he was appointed chair of a Presidential Commission on Dietary Supplement Labels. He finished his term as chairman of the board of trustees of the Pan American Health and Education Foundation in 2008.